radiographic anatomy

The National Medical Series for Independent Study

radiographic anatomy

Frank Slaby, Ph.D.
Associate Professor
Department of Anatomy
George Washington University
Medical Center
Washington, D.C.

Eugene R. Jacobs, M.D.
Associate Professor
General Diagnostic Radiology Section
Musculoskeletal Radiology
George Washington University
Medical Center
Washington, D.C.

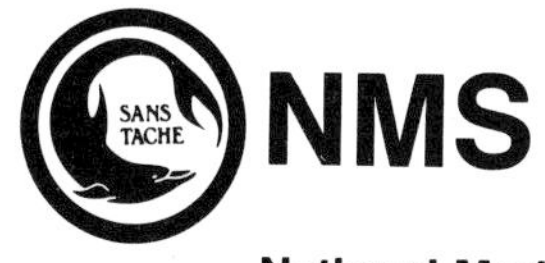

National Medical Series from Williams & Wilkins
Baltimore, Hong Kong, London, Sydney

Harwal Publishing Company, Media, Pennsylvania

Managing Editor: Debra Dreger
Project Editor: Gloria Hamilton
Art Direction and Illustrations: Wieslawa B. Langenfeld
Editorial Assistant: Judy Johnson
Compositors: June Sangiorgio Mash, Richard Doyle
Layout: Steffany Verna Trueman

Figures 1-1C, 1-7C, 1-9C, 1-10C, 1-11C, 1-20C, 2-1C, 2-5C, 2-6C, 2-7C, 2-21C, 2-24C, 2-25C, 5-7C, 5-8C, and 5-12C were modified from Bontrager KL, Anthony BT: *Textbook of Radiographic Positioning and Related Anatomy*, 2nd ed. St. Louis, CV Mosby, 1987.

Library of Congress Cataloging-in-Publication Data

Slaby, Frank.
Radiographic anatomy/Frank Slaby, Eugene R. Jacobs.
p. cm.—(The National medical series for independent study)
(A Wiley medical publication)
ISBN 0-471-51352-0
1. Diagnosis, Radioscopic—Outlines, syllabi, etc. 2. Diagnosis, Radioscopic—Examinations, questions, etc. 3. Human anatomy—Outlines, syllabi, etc. 4. Human anatomy—Examinations, questions, etc. I. Jacobs, Eugene R. II. Title. III. Series. IV. Series: A Wiley medical publication.
[DNLM: 1. Radiography—examination questions. 2. Radiography—outlines. WN 18 S631r]
RC78.15.S53 1990
616.07′572′076—dc20
DNLM/DLC
for Library of Congress 90-4321
CIP

10 9 8 7 6 5 4 3 2

Dedication

This book is dedicated to the memory of my dear grandmother, Anna Markewicz, and to the future of my son, Christopher.

Frank Slaby

Affectionately dedicated to my dear wife, Janet.

Eugene R. Jacobs

Contents

Preface

This radiographic anatomy text introduces the reader to the examination of the most common radiographs of the body. The discussion of the radiograph or set of radiographs of each body region begins with a review of the anatomy of the region. This is followed by a comprehensive description of the normal anatomy that is imaged in the radiographs. The presentation concludes with a discussion of frequently encountered abnormal findings. Thus, the intent of each presentation is not only to account for the normal anatomy apparent in the radiographs but also to show the anatomic basis of common abnormal findings.

Specifically, the material covered is as follows. Chapter 1 on the upper limb addresses the AP radiograph of the shoulder; the lateral, AP, internal oblique, and external oblique radiographs of the elbow; the PA radiograph of the hand; and the lateral radiograph of the wrist. Chapter 2 on the lower limb discusses the AP radiograph of the pelvis; the AP, tunnel, lateral, and axial radiographs of the knee; the mortise radiograph of the ankle; and the lateral, oblique, and AP radiographs of the foot; two additional sections describe T1-weighted magnetic resonance images (MRIs) of coronal and sagittal sections of the normal knee. Chapter 3 on the thorax outlines the examination of PA and lateral chest films; an additional section describes CT scans of the thorax, with the emphasis on the normal mediastinal relationships at six distinct levels within the superior mediastinum and the upper part of the inferior mediastinum. The abdominal plain film of the abdomen is discussed in Chapter 4; an additional section describes CT scans of the abdomen, with an emphasis on the abdominal viscera that are imaged at four broad abdominal levels. Chapter 5 on the head and neck introduces the Waters' view and lateral radiographs of the face and neck, with an additional section on CT scans of the cranium.

The text is designed for use by medical personnel and students interested in learning radiographic anatomy. In the first year of medical school, the reviews of gross anatomy in each chapter can be used as study aids; the sections that describe CT scans of the thorax and abdomen provide a clinically relevant, cross-sectional perspective to the organization of the trunk. Second-year medical students can quickly review appropriate chapters in preparation for learning pathologic processes. The radiologic sections of each chapter teach the reader to distinguish normal from abnormal findings on plain film radiographs. The questions at the end of each chapter assist in review for the Boards Part I exam and test the reader's mental images of radiographs and CT scans. Prior to each clerkship, third-year medical students can quickly review the relevant radiographs and CT scans presented here. The cases at the end of the book duplicate the format of radiologic presentation in the clinical setting, and they test the reader's ability to recognize major abnormal findings. Based on the material in this book, the reader should acquire a good understanding of the anatomic basis of radiographs and CT scans and an ability to recognize major common abnormalities. The reader will then be able to appreciate the more difficult diagnostic features presented in these radiographs.

Finally, we would like to emphasize that the ability to "read" a specific radiograph (especially chest and abdominal films) is almost directly proportional to the number of such radiographs that are examined. With each chest film or abdominal plain film that is examined, whether pathologic or not, there is an incremental increase in the ability to recognize the spectrum of normal features, especially as they relate to habitus, age, and sex. It is frustrating and yet exciting to discover that, for example, what is seen in the 100th PA chest film was not recognized in the first 99. The reader will find that experience and repetition are truly the best teachers of the distinction between normal variant and incipient abnormal findings.

Frank Slaby
Eugene R. Jacobs

Acknowledgments

The first author wishes to acknowledge the support and assistance of his wife, Susan K. McCune, M.D., without whose guidance and perspective this project could not have been initiated. The first author also would like to thank Dr. Frank D. Allan, Acting Chairman of the Anatomy Department at the George Washington University Medical Center, for his support and assistance during the writing of this text. Both authors want to thank James Kendrick and the personnel of the Biomedical Communications division at the George Washington University Medical Center for their professional and superb reproduction of all the radiologic images in this text. Lastly, we would like to thank Jim Harris, Matt Harris, Debra Dreger, and Wiesia Langenfeld of Harwal Publishing Company for their considerations and contributions; their cooperation and understanding made the writing of this text exceptionally enjoyable.

To the Reader

Since 1984, the *National Medical Series for Independent Study* has been helping medical students meet the challenge of education and clinical training. In this climate of burgeoning knowledge and complex clinical issues, a medical career is more demanding than ever. Increasingly, medical training must prepare physicians to seek and synthesize necessary information and to apply that information successfully.

The *National Medical Series* is designed to provide a logical framework for organizing, learning, reviewing, and applying the conceptual and factual information covered in basic and clinical studies. Each book includes a concise but comprehensive outline of the essential content of a discipline, with up to 500 study questions. The combination of distilled, outlined text and tools for self-evaluation allows easy retrieval and enhanced comprehension of salient information. Each question is accompanied by the correct answer, a paragraph-length explanation, and specific reference to the text where the topic is discussed. Study questions that follow each chapter use current National Board formats to reinforce the chapter content. Study questions appearing at the end of the text in the Challenge Exam vary in format depending on the book; the unifying goal of this exam, however, is to challenge the student to synthesize and expand on information presented throughout the book. Wherever possible, Challenge Exam questions are presented in the context of a clinical case or scenario intended to simulate real-life application of medical knowledge.

Each book in the *National Medical Series* is constantly being updated and revised to remain current with the discipline and with subtle changes in educational philosophy. The authors and editors devote considerable time and effort to ensuring that the information required by all medical school curricula is included and presented in the most logical, comprehensible manner. Strict editorial attention to accuracy, organization, and consistency also is maintained. Further shaping of the series occurs in response to biannual discussions held with a panel of medical student advisors drawn from schools throughout the United States. At these meetings, the editorial staff considers the complicated needs of medical students to learn how the *National Medical Series* can better serve them. In this regard, the staff at Harwal Publishing Company welcomes all comments and suggestions. Let us hear from you.

1
Upper Limb

I. SHOULDER

A. Anatomy of the shoulder and axillary regions

1. Bones

a. Clavicle

(1) The S-shaped clavicle is palpable along its entire length within the anterior part of the shoulder region.

(2) The clavicle is the first bone in the body to undergo ossification, which occurs via the intramembranous mode.

b. Scapula

(1) The acromion process of the scapula underlies the point of the shoulder.

(2) In its anatomic position, the inferior angle of the scapula lies at the level of the seventh intercostal space.

c. Proximal end of the humerus

(1) Longitudinal growth of the humeral shaft during childhood and adolescence occurs more actively at the proximal than at the distal end of the bone. The proximal end has two prominent secondary centers of ossification.

(a) The center for the head appears during the first 3 months after birth.

(b) The center for the greater tuberosity appears at 1 to 2 years of age.

(2) The surgical neck of the humerus is the most common fracture site in the proximal half of the bone.

2. Joints

a. Sternoclavicular joint. This joint provides for protraction and retraction of the pectoral girdle.

(1) The sternoclavicular joint articulates the medial end of the clavicle with the manubrium sterni.

(2) The costoclavicular ligament stabilizes the joint by serving as the strongest nonmuscular structure binding the clavicle to the rib cage.

b. Acromioclavicular joint. This joint provides for lateral and medial rotation of the scapula.

(1) The acromioclavicular joint articulates the acromion process of the scapula with the lateral end of the clavicle.

(2) The coracoclavicular ligament stabilizes the joint by serving as the strongest nonmuscular structure suspending the scapula from the clavicle.

c. Shoulder joint. This joint provides for flexion, extension, and medial and lateral rotation of the arm. It also provides for about 60° arm abduction and adduction.

(1) The shoulder joint articulates the head of the humerus with the glenoid fossa of the scapula.

(2) Two prominent **bursae** are associated with the joint.

(a) The **subacromion–subdeltoid bursa** separates the tendinous insertion of supraspinatus onto the joint capsule from the overlying deltoid.

(b) The **subscapular bursa** intervenes between the scapular fossa and the tendinous insertion of subscapularis onto the joint capsule; the bursa is an extracapsular extension of the joint's synovial lining.

3. Muscles

a. Muscles that suspend the pectoral girdle from the back

(1) **Trapezius** is the most powerful elevator and retractor of the pectoral girdle and one of

the two prime movers that raise the arm above the level of the shoulder.
(a) The spinal part of the accessory nerve provides motor fibers to the muscle, and C3 and C4 provide proprioceptive fibers.
(b) Loss of trapezius function produces a **drooped shoulder**.
(2) **Levator scapulae, rhomboid major, and rhomboid minor** assist the trapezius in elevation and retraction of the pectoral girdle. All three muscles are innervated by the dorsal scapular nerve; levator scapulae also receives innervation from C3 and C4.

b. **Muscles that pull upon the pectoral girdle from the anterior surface of the rib cage**
(1) **Serratus anterior** is the most powerful protractor of the pectoral girdle and the other prime mover used to raise the arm above the shoulder.
(a) Innervation is by the long thoracic nerve.
(b) Loss of function of serratus anterior produces a **winged scapula**.
(2) **Pectoralis minor** assists serratus anterior in protraction of the pectoral girdle; it is innervated by the medial and lateral pectoral nerves.
(3) **Subclavius** can depress the pectoral girdle; it is innervated by the nerve to subclavius.

c. **Muscles of the rotator cuff**
(1) **Supraspinatus** is one of the two prime movers that initiate arm abduction from the anatomic position (deltoid is the other prime mover); it is innervated by the suprascapular nerve.
(2) **Infraspinatus** is a lateral rotator of the arm; it is innervated by the suprascapular nerve.
(3) **Teres minor** is a lateral rotator of the arm; it is innervated by C5 and C6 fibers in the axillary nerve.
(4) **Subscapularis** is a medial rotator of the arm; it is innervated by the upper and lower subscapular nerves.

d. **Prime movers of arm abduction and adduction**
(1) **Deltoid** is the prime mover of arm abduction up to about the level of the shoulder; it is innervated by C5 and C6 fibers in the axillary nerve.
(2) **Latissimus dorsi** is a powerful extensor, adductor, and medial rotator of the arm; it is innervated by the thoracodorsal (middle subscapular) nerve. Latissimus dorsi accounts for most of the muscle mass of the posterior axillary fold.
(3) **Pectoralis major** is a powerful flexor, adductor, and medial rotator of the arm; it is innervated by the medial and lateral pectoral nerves. Pectoralis major accounts for most of the muscle mass of the anterior axillary fold.
(4) **Teres major** is a major adductor and medial rotator of the arm; it is innervated by the lower subscapular nerve.

4. Nerves

a. **Brachial plexus**
(1) **Roots.** The anterior rami of C5, C6, C7, C8, and T1 form the five roots of the brachial plexus. Only two nerves arise from the roots.
(a) The **dorsal scapular nerve** arises from the C5 root.
(b) The **long thoracic nerve** arises from the C5, C6, and C7 roots.
(2) **Trunks**
(a) The unions and extension of the roots form the three trunks of the brachial plexus.
(i) The **upper trunk** is formed from the union of the C5 and C6 roots.
(ii) The **middle trunk** is an extension of the C7 root.
(iii) The **lower trunk** is formed from the union of the C8 and T1 roots.
(b) Only two nerves arise from the trunks—the **suprascapular nerve** and the **nerve to subclavius**—both of which arise from the upper trunk.
(3) **Divisions.** The divisions of the trunks form the six divisions of the brachial plexus; each trunk divides to form an anterior and a posterior division. No nerves arise from the divisions.
(4) **Cords**
(a) The unions and extension of the divisions form the cords of the brachial plexus; each cord is named for its relationship relative to the second part of the axillary artery.
(i) The **lateral cord** is formed from the union of the anterior divisions of the upper and middle trunks.
(ii) The **posterior cord** is formed from the union of all three posterior divisions.
(iii) The **medial cord** is a continuation of the anterior division of the lower trunk.
(b) Several nerves arise from each cord.
(i) The lateral cord gives rise to the **lateral pectoral nerve**, the **musculocutaneous nerve**, and the **lateral root of the median nerve**.

(ii) The posterior cord gives rise to the **upper**, **middle** (thoracodorsal), and **lower subscapular nerves**; the **axillary nerve**; and the **radial nerve**.

(iii) The medial cord gives rise to the **medial pectoral nerve**, the **medial cutaneous nerves** of the arm and forearm, the **ulnar nerve**, and the **medial root of the median nerve**.

b. Brachial plexus injuries

(1) Erb-Duchenne paralysis (waiter's tip palsy) is caused by irreversible damage to the C5 and C6 roots or to the upper trunk. In this condition, the upper limb hangs by the side of the body (due to loss of deltoid function) and the forearm is noticeably pronated (due to loss of biceps brachii function).

(2) Klumpke's paralysis is caused by irreversible damage to the C8 and T1 roots or to the lower trunk.

(a) This condition is characterized by absence of oppositional movement of the thumb (due to loss of function of opponens pollicis) and inability to abduct or adduct the fingers (due to loss of function of the palmar and dorsal interossei and abductor digiti minimi).

(b) Affected persons have disfigurement of the hand resulting from hyperextension of the fingers at the metacarpophalangeal joints (due to loss of function of the lumbricals).

5. Blood vessels and lymph nodes

a. Axillary artery

(1) The axillary artery begins at the lateral border of the first rib as a continuation of the subclavian artery and ends at the lower border of the insertion of teres major onto the humerus. At its end, the axillary artery is continuous with the **brachial artery**.

(2) The axillary artery is divided into three parts.

(a) The first part has only one branch—the **superior thoracic artery**.

(b) The second part lies behind pectoralis minor and has two branches—the **thoracoacromial trunk** and the **lateral thoracic artery**. The lateral thoracic artery is the chief artery supplying the lateral half of the mammary gland.

(c) The third part has three branches—the **subscapular artery** and the **anterior and posterior humeral circumflex arteries**.

(i) Branches of the subscapular artery anastomose with branches of the suprascapular and transverse cervical arteries to form an arterial network around the scapula.

(ii) This network provides a route across the shoulder joint collateral to the axillary artery.

b. Axillary vein

(1) The axillary vein begins at the union of the basilic vein with the venae comitantes of the brachial artery and ends at the lateral border of the first rib. At its end, the axillary vein is continuous with the **subclavian vein**.

(2) The **cephalic vein**, the largest tributary of the axillary vein, passes deeply through the deltopectoral triangle before joining the axillary vein.

c. Axillary lymph nodes are divided into six groups.

(1) The **anterior** (pectoral) **group** drains the superficial tissues of the anterolateral region of the trunk, down to the level of the umbilicus; these nodes also drain the lateral half of the mammary gland. The anterior group of axillary lymph nodes can be palpated posterior to the lateral border of pectoralis major.

(2) The **posterior** (subscapular) **group** drains the superficial tissues of the posterior region of the trunk, down to the level of the iliac crest. These nodes can be palpated anterior to the lateral border of latissimus dorsi.

(3) The **lateral group** drains all the tissues of the hand, forearm, and arm with the exception of the superficial tissues on the lateral side of the upper limb. These nodes can be palpated along the axillary vein.

(4) The **central group** drains efferent lymphatic vessels from the pectoral, subscapular, and lateral groups. These nodes can be palpated against the chest wall in the center of the axilla.

(5) The **deltopectoral group** drains the superficial tissues on the lateral side of the hand, forearm, and arm. These nodes can be palpated in the deltopectoral triangle beneath the clavicle.

(6) The **apical group**, which lies immediately lateral to the lateral border of the first rib, drains efferent lymphatic vessels from all of the other five groups of axillary lymph nodes.

B. Major features of the AP radiograph of the shoulder (Figure 1-1)

1. The radiograph shows all or parts of the following **most proximal bones of the upper limb**:
   a. Most or all of the **clavicle**
   b. The coracoid process, acromion process, and glenoid fossa of the **scapula**
   c. The head, anatomic neck, and surgical neck of the **humerus**
      (1) The radiograph shows the **greater tuberosity in profile** (see Figures 1-1A and 1-1B) if the humerus is **externally rotated** to the extent that the line between the epicondyles of the humerus lies in a **coronal plane**.
      (2) The radiograph shows the **lesser tuberosity in profile** if the humerus is **internally rotated** to the extent that the line between the epicondyles of the humerus lies in a **parasagittal plane**.

2. The radiograph shows the following **most proximal joints of the upper limb**:
   a. The **sternoclavicular joint**, which in some instances (as in Figure 1-1A) lies medial to the medial extent of the radiograph
   b. The **acromioclavicular joint**
   c. The **shoulder joint**

3. The radiograph shows a radiolucent space called the **coracoclavicular space** between the coracoid process and the clavicle; the coracoclavicular space marks the location of the coracoclavicular ligament.

4. The radiograph shows a radiolucent space called the **acromioclavicular space** between the acromion process and the lateral end of the clavicle; the acromioclavicular space represents the apposed articular cartilages in the acromioclavicular joint.

5. The perspective of the radiograph superimposes the head of the humerus over an obliquely oriented glenoid fossa; the region of superimposition approximates an ellipse in shape.

C. Clinical and radiographic features of common traumatic injuries

1. **Subluxation or dislocation of the acromioclavicular joint.** Simple sprains, subluxations (i.e., partial dislocations), and dislocations of the acromioclavicular joint are different grades of injuries known as **shoulder separations**. These injuries generally occur as a result of a downward blow on the point of the shoulder. Shoulder separations are graded I to III.
   a. A **grade I shoulder separation** is a simple sprain of the fibrous capsule of the acromioclavicular joint. Neither the fibrous capsule nor the coracoclavicular ligament is significantly damaged; the radiograph therefore shows acromioclavicular and coracoclavicular spaces of normal width.
   b. A **grade II shoulder separation** is a subluxation of the acromioclavicular joint. Subluxation occurs when significant damage to the joint's ligamentous supports is limited to its fibrous capsule; the radiograph shows a coracoclavicular space of normal width but an acromioclavicular space that is at least 50% wider than that measured in an AP radiograph of the contralateral, uninjured shoulder (Figure 1-2).
   c. A **grade III shoulder separation** is a dislocation of the acromioclavicular joint. Dislocation occurs when both the joint's fibrous capsule and the coracoclavicular ligament are significantly disrupted; the radiograph shows the acromioclavicular and coracoclavicular spaces both to be at least 50% wider than the corresponding spaces in the AP radiograph of the contralateral, uninjured shoulder (Figure 1-3).

2. **Dislocation of the shoulder joint.** The shoulder joint is the joint most commonly dislocated in adults.
   a. **Anterior dislocation of the humeral head** is the most common type of shoulder joint dislocation.
      (1) **Description of injury.** Anterior dislocation is produced by trauma that drives the humeral head anteroinferiorly from its articulation with the glenoid fossa. In many cases, the injury is accompanied by a cleave-shaped indentation (called a **hatchet**, or **Hill-Sachs, defect**) in the posterolateral aspect of the humeral head, which is produced by abutment of the displaced head onto the inferior rim of the glenoid fossa.
      (2) **Clinical features**
         (a) The patient presents with a shoulder that has lost its normal rounded contour and acquired the contour of the acromion process.
         (b) Damage to the axillary nerve (which extends posteriorly through the quadrangular space beneath the fibrous capsule of the shoulder joint) should be tested via assessment of pinprick sensation on the lateral aspect of the upper arm.

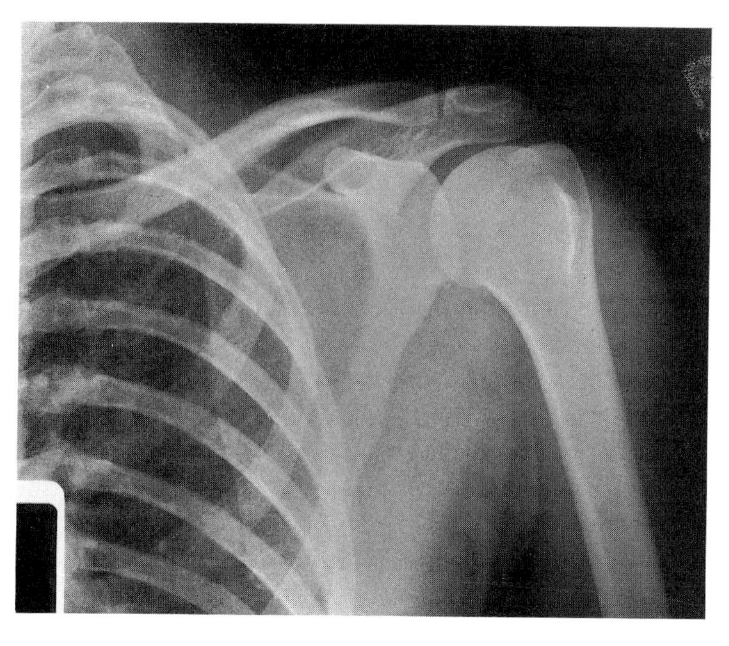

Figure 1-1. (*A*) An AP radiograph of the shoulder and (*B*) its schematic representation. (C) The orientation of a patient's shoulder relative to the x-ray beam and film cassette for an AP radiograph of the shoulder (the film cassette is located beneath the tabletop). In this instance, the arm is externally rotated to the extent that the line between the humeral epicondyles lies in a coronal plane. Such external rotation projects the greater tuberosity in profile, as seen in Figure 1-1A. (See section I B.)

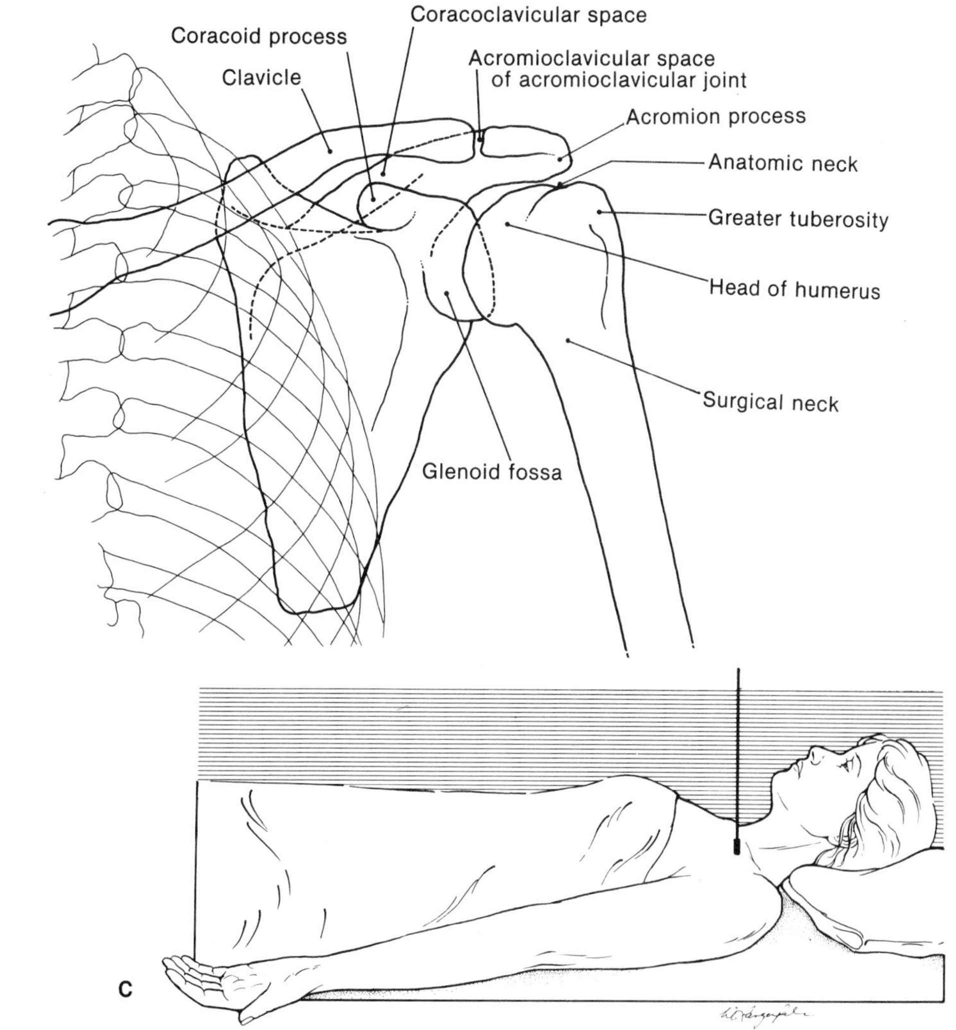

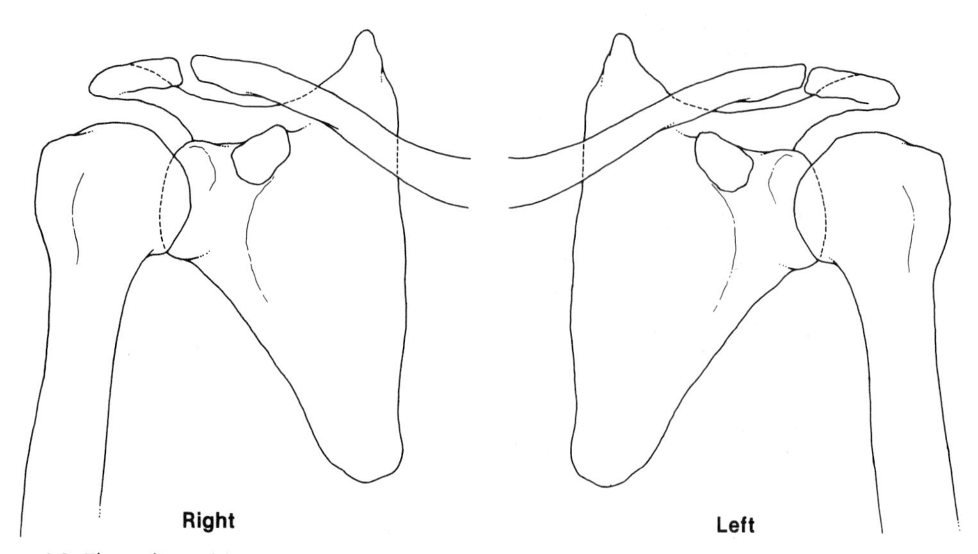

Figure 1-2. The outlines of the AP radiographs of the normal (*left*) and injured (*right*) shoulders of a person who has suffered a grade II shoulder separation on the right side. (See section I C 1 b.)

(3) Radiographic features

(a) The radiograph shows the humeral head in a subglenoid (Figure 1-4), subcoracoid, or subclavicular position.

(b) Following reduction of the dislocation, an AP radiograph of the shoulder taken with the arm internally rotated provides the best view for detection of a hatchet defect.

b. Posterior dislocation of the humeral head

(1) Description of injury. Posterior dislocation is produced by trauma that drives the humeral head posteriorly from its articulation with the glenoid fossa.

(2) Clinical features. The patient presents with a shoulder that is flattened anteriorly and bulging posteriorly; abduction and external rotation of the arm are markedly limited.

(3) Radiographic features. Posterior dislocations are difficult to ascertain in AP radiographs of the shoulder, because the humeral head almost always assumes a subacromial position and thus lies at approximately its normal "level" within the shoulder region. However, most posterior dislocations are associated with the following abnormal findings:

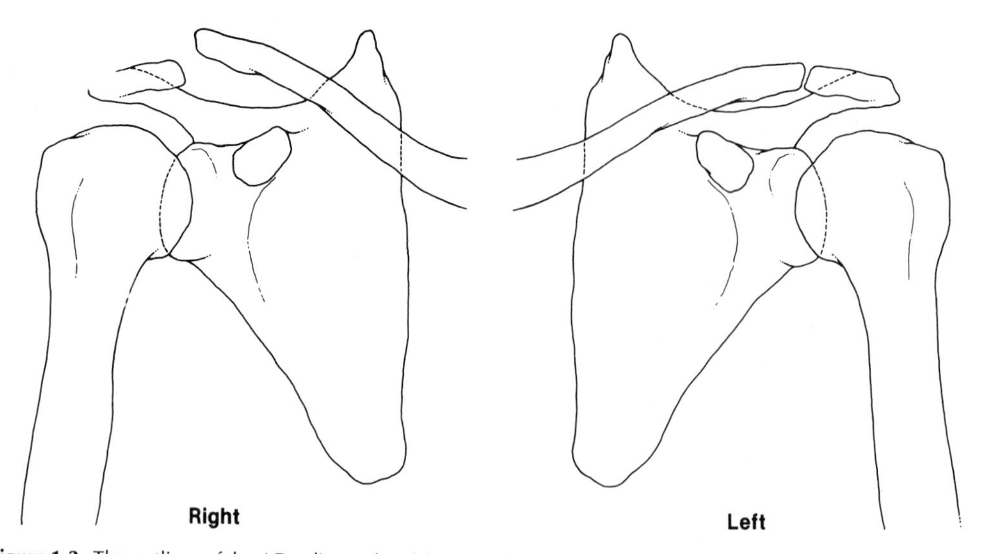

Figure 1-3. The outlines of the AP radiographs of the normal (*left*) and injured (*right*) shoulders of a person who has suffered a grade III shoulder separation on the right side. (See section I C 1 c.)

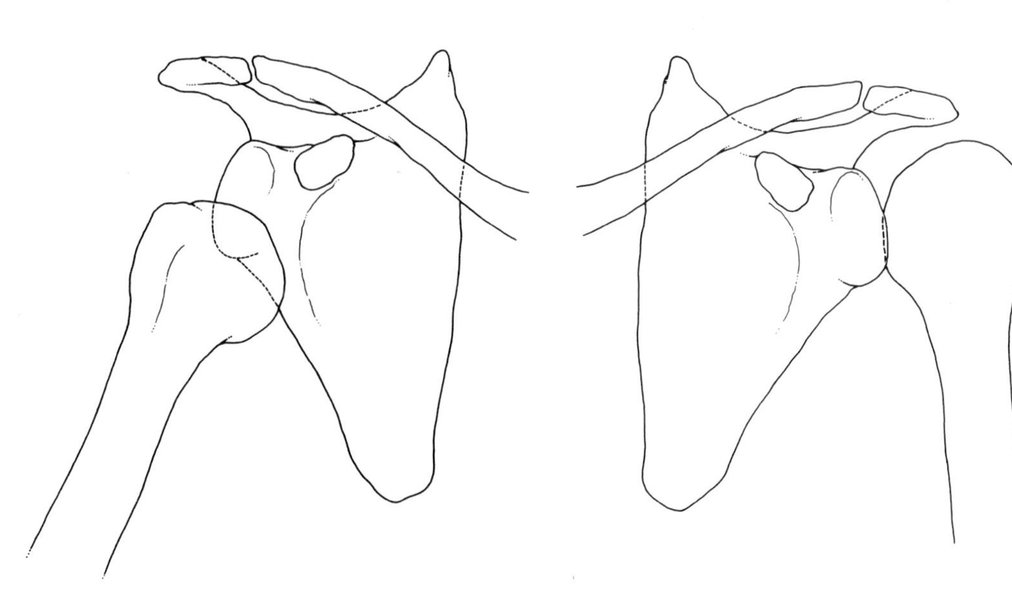

Figure 1-4. An outline of an AP radiograph of an anterior shoulder dislocation, in which the humeral head rests in a subglenoid position. [See section I C 2 a (3) (a).]

Figure 1-5. An outline of an AP radiograph of a posterior shoulder dislocation, in which the humeral head only marginally overlaps the glenoid fossa. [See section I C 2 b (3) (a).]

(a) The partially overlapped images of the humeral head and glenoid fossa do not present a normal elliptic outline (Figure 1-5).

(b) An angled AP radiograph of the shoulder, in which the patient's body is turned 35° to 40° toward the x-ray film cassette, shows the glenoid fossa in profile. In a normal shoulder, such a projection shows a radiolucent space between the humeral head and the profiled glenoid fossa; a shoulder bearing a posteriorly dislocated humeral head always shows a partially overlapped humeral head and glenoid fossa (Figure 1-6).

3. Fractured clavicle. The clavicle participates in the transmission of all forces between the arm and the trunk of the body; it is the most commonly fractured bone of the body.

a. Clinical features. Normally, the clavicle props the shoulder posterosuperiorly on the trunk of the body. A person with a fractured clavicle thus presents with a shoulder that is anteroinferiorly displaced.

b. Radiographic features. The most common fracture site is the border region between the middle and lateral thirds of the bone. The fracture site generally is evident because of angulation of the fragments.

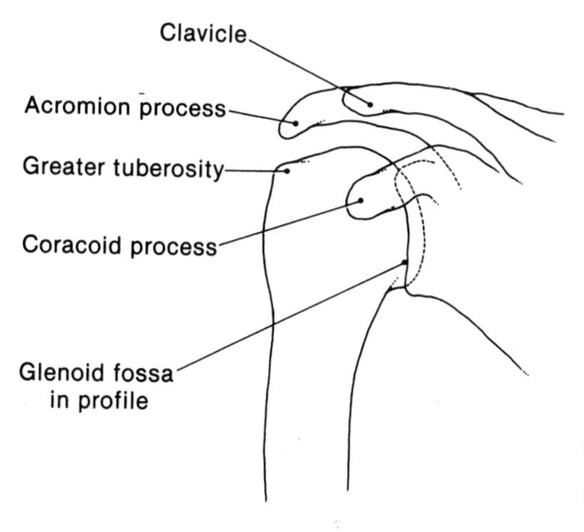

Figure 1-6. An outline of an angled AP radiograph of a posterior shoulder dislocation, in which the patient's body was rotated 35° to 40° toward the dislocated shoulder before the radiograph was taken. The body was rotated to project the glenoid fossa in profile. [See section I C 2 b (3) (b).]

II. ELBOW

A. Anatomy of the elbow region

1. Bones

a. Distal end of the humerus

(1) The **medial and lateral epicondyles** of the humerus are palpable on the sides of the elbow.

(2) The distal end of the humerus bears four secondary **centers of ossification** during childhood and adolescence.

(a) The center for the capitulum appears during the first 6 months after birth.

(b) The center for the medial epicondyle appears at 4 to 6 years of age.

(c) The center for the trochlea appears at 8 to 9 years of age.

(d) The center for the lateral epicondyle appears at 11 to 12 years of age.

b. Proximal ends of the ulna and radius

(1) The **olecranon process of the ulna** is palpable in the posterior elbow region.

(a) When the forearm is flexed 90° at the elbow, the olecranon process and the humeral epicondyles lie at the vertices of an equilateral triangle.

(b) When the forearm is fully extended at the elbow, the three bony prominences are colinear.

(2) The **head of the radius** is palpable on the lateral side of the elbow, immediately distal to the lateral epicondyle of the humerus.

2. Joints

a. Elbow joint. This joint provides for flexion and extension of the forearm, and consists of two **articulations**.

(1) In the **humeroulnar articulation**, the trochlear notch of the ulna articulates with the trochlea of the humerus. When forces are transmitted from the forearm to the arm under normal conditions, the humeroulnar articulation bears most of the force transmitted.

(2) In the **humeroradial articulation**, the head of the radius articulates with the capitulum of the humerus.

b. Proximal radioulnar joint. The proximal and distal radioulnar joints provide for pronation and supination of the forearm. (The distal radioulnar joint is discussed in section III A 2 a).

(1) The proximal radioulnar joint articulates the radial head with the radial notch of the ulna and the annular ligament.

(2) The synovial cavity of the proximal radioulnar joint is continuous with that of the elbow joint.

3. Muscles

a. Biceps brachii is a major **flexor** and the chief **supinator of the forearm**; it is innervated by the musculocutaneous nerve. The **biceps brachii tendon reflex test** is a phasic stretch reflex test of the integrity of neuronal pathways at the C5 and C6 spinal cord segment levels.

b. Brachialis is a major **flexor of the forearm**; it is innervated by the musculocutaneous nerve.

c. Triceps brachii is the chief **extensor of the forearm**; it is innervated by the radial nerve. The **triceps brachii tendon reflex test** is a phasic stretch reflex test of the integrity of neuronal pathways at the C7 and C8 spinal cord segment levels.

d. Pronator teres is a **flexor and pronator of the forearm**; it is innervated by the median nerve.

e. Pronator quadratus assists pronator teres in **pronation of the forearm**; it is innervated by the anterior interosseous branch of the median nerve.

f. Brachioradialis stabilizes the forearm in the midprone position; it is innervated by the radial nerve. The **brachioradialis tendon reflex test** is a phasic stretch reflex test of the integrity of neuronal pathways at the C5 and C6 spinal cord segment levels.

g. Supinator assists biceps brachii in **supination of the forearm**; it is innervated by the deep branch of the radial nerve.

4. Nerves

a. The **ulnar nerve** exits the arm by passing directly behind the medial epicondyle of the humerus; fracture of the medial epicondyle thus places the ulnar nerve at risk. A **cubitus val-**

gus deformity [i.e., an elbow with an abnormally small carrying angle (see Figure 1-9B)] frequently places increased pressure on the ulnar nerve in the elbow region.

b. The **median nerve** crosses the elbow region by extending obliquely through the cubital fossa alongside the brachial artery.

c. The **radial nerve** crosses the elbow region by extending through the cubital fossa under the cover of brachioradialis.

d. The **lateral cutaneous nerve of the forearm**, which is the terminal extent of the musculocutaneous nerve, extends across the elbow region in the lateral aspect of the superficial fascia overlying the cubital fossa.

e. The **medial cutaneous nerve of the forearm** extends across the elbow region in the medial aspect of the superficial fascia overlying the cubital fossa.

5. Blood vessels and lymph nodes

a. The **brachial artery** is the chief artery that extends across the elbow region; it courses through the cubital fossa deep to the bicipital aponeurosis. At the level of the radial neck, the brachial artery bifurcates into the **ulnar and radial arteries.**

b. The major superficial veins of the upper limb, namely, the **basilic and cephalic veins**, extend across the elbow region in the medial and lateral aspects, respectively, of the superficial fascia overlying the cubital fossa. The two veins commonly are connected by a median cubital vein, which courses superomedially from the cephalic to the basilic vein.

c. The **supratrochlear nodes** of the cubital fossa receive lymph drained from the medial half of the hand and the middle, ring, and little fingers. The efferent lymphatics from the supratrochlear nodes drain into the lateral group of axillary nodes.

B. Major features of radiographs of the elbow

1. Lateral radiograph. A lateral radiograph of the elbow has the following distinguishing features (Figure 1-7).

a. The radiograph shows the **placement of the bones and fat pads in the elbow region** when the forearm is flexed 90° at the elbow joint and placed in the midprone position (i.e., positioned midway between the fully supine and fully prone positions—see Figure 1-7C).

(1) The **trochlea** casts a highly radiopaque, circular profile at the distal end of the humerus; the coronoid and olecranon fossae are seen separated by a thin plate of bone proximal to the trochlea.

(2) The round, anterior border of the **capitulum** is visible anterior to the trochlear profile.

(3) The wrench-shaped proximal end of the **ulna**, with its olecranon process, trochlear notch, and coronoid process, encircles the lower outline of the trochlea.

(4) The radiograph provides an unobstructed view of the radial tuberosity and most of the neck of the **radius**; most of the head of the radius, however, lies partially overlapped by the coronoid process of the ulna.

(5) The coronoid fossa and olecranon fossa of the **humerus** each bear a fat pad called, respectively, the **anterior and posterior fat pads** of the elbow region. A lateral radiograph of a normal elbow shows the presence of the anterior but not the posterior fat pad.

(a) When the forearm is flexed 90° at the elbow joint, the superficial part of the **anterior fat pad** lies anterior to the bony rim of the coronoid fossa. Fat is more radiolucent than muscle; therefore, in a normal lateral radiograph, the superficial part of the anterior fat pad appears as a small radiolucent area sandwiched between the highly radiopaque, bony rim of the coronoid fossa and the moderately radiopaque shadows of brachialis and biceps brachii.

(b) By contrast, the **posterior fat pad** lies deep to the bony rim of the olecranon fossa, and, thus, only the moderately radiopaque shadow of triceps brachii is seen posterior to the bony rim of the olecranon fossa.

b. In a lateral radiograph of a child's elbow (Figure 1-8), the ossified core of the **capitulum** exhibits the following relationships:

(1) The center of the capitulum is colinear with the central axis of the radial shaft. The line defining this colinear relationship is called the **radiocapitellar line**.

(2) The **anterior humeral line**, which is the line coincident with the anterior margin of the humeral shaft, projects through the middle one-third of the capitulum.

(3) The **midhumeral line**, which is the line coincident with the central axis of the humeral shaft, projects just posterior to the posterior margin of the capitulum.

Figure 1-7. (*A*) A lateral radiograph of the elbow and (*B*) its schematic representation. (*C*) The orientation of a patient's elbow relative to the x-ray beam and film cassette for a lateral radiograph of the elbow. (See section II B 1.)

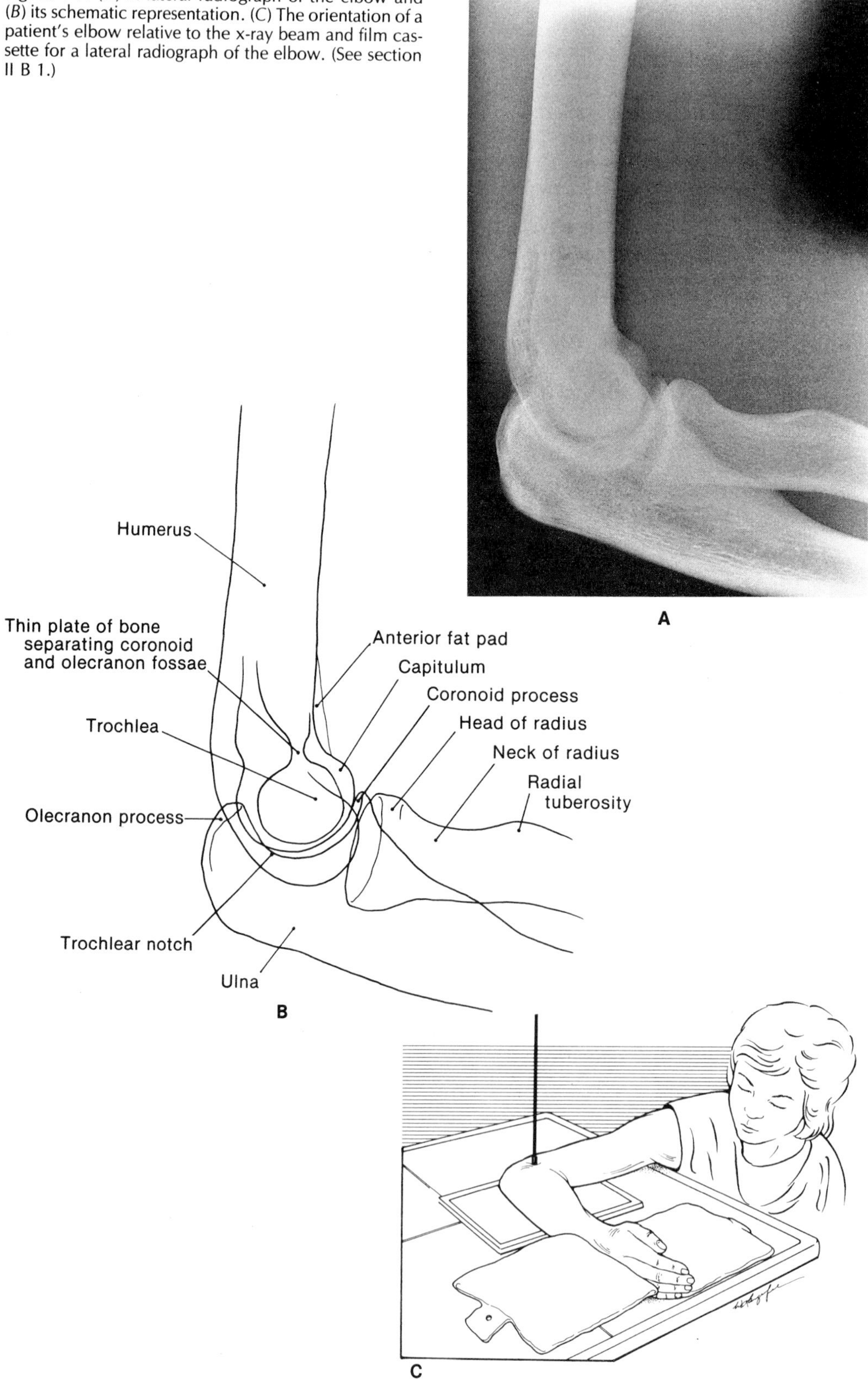

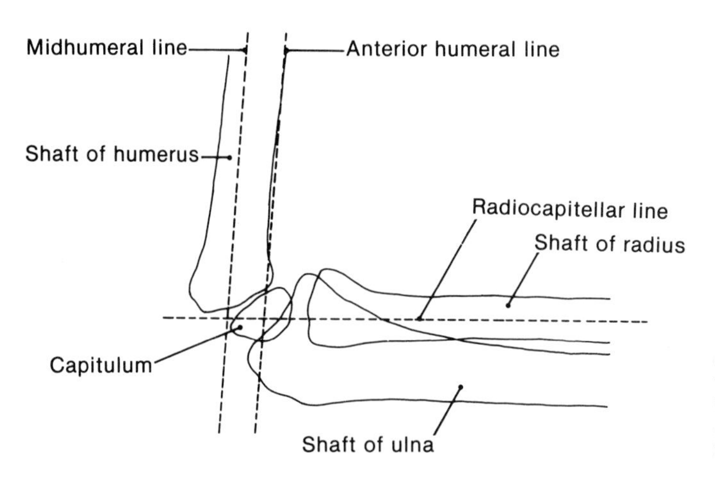

Figure 1-8. An outline of a lateral radiograph of a child's elbow. Note the relationships of the capitulum to the radiocapitellar, anterior humeral, and midhumeral lines. (See section II B 1 b.)

2. **AP radiograph.** An AP radiograph of the elbow has the following distinguishing features (Figure 1-9).
   a. The radiograph presents an unobstructed view of the **medial and lateral epicondyles** of the humerus.
   b. The trochlea and olecranon fossa overlap the olecranon process; the sinuous radiolucent space distal to the trochlear surface represents the apposed articular cartilages in the **humeroulnar articulation** of the elbow joint.
   c. The radiolucent space distal to the capitulum represents the apposed articular cartilages in the **humeroradial articulation** of the elbow joint.
   d. The **proximal ulna** overlaps the radial tuberosity and the medial margin of the head of the radius.
   e. The angle on the radial side of the elbow between the lines that project along the central axes of the humeral and ulnar shafts is called the **carrying angle** of the elbow (see Figure 1-9B). The carrying angle averages 169° for males and 167° for females.
3. **Internal oblique radiograph.** An internal oblique radiograph of the elbow has the following distinguishing features (Figure 1-10).
   a. The radiograph shows the **trochlear notch of the ulna** encircling the posterior aspect of the pulley-shaped trochlea.
   b. The radiograph shows the tip of the **olecranon process of the ulna** pressed into the **olecranon fossa of the humerus**.
   c. The radiograph provides an unobstructed view of the **medial epicondyle of the humerus** and most of the **coronoid process of the ulna**.
4. **External oblique radiograph.** An external oblique radiograph of the elbow has the following distinguishing features (Figure 1-11).
   a. The radiograph provides an unobstructed view of the **capitulum of the humerus** and the **head and neck of the radius**.
   b. The radiolucent space between the head of the radius and the radial notch of the ulna represents the apposed articular cartilages in the **proximal radioulnar joint**.

C. Clinical and radiographic features of common traumatic injuries

1. **Dislocation at the elbow**
   a. **Posterior dislocation of the ulna and radius** is the most common dislocation at the elbow in adults.
      (1) **Clinical features.** The patient generally presents with a flexed forearm bearing a posteriorly protruding olecranon process.
      (2) **Radiographic features.** A lateral radiograph of the elbow best displays the dislocation.
   b. **Subluxation of the head of the radius** from its encirclement by the annular ligament is a common elbow injury among young children; the injury is called a **nursemaid's elbow**.
      (1) **Description of injury.** The subluxation of the radial head generally results from a sudden pull on the upper limb, such as that exerted by an adult to prevent a child from falling.
      (2) **Clinical features and diagnosis.** The child presents with a flexed and pronated forearm

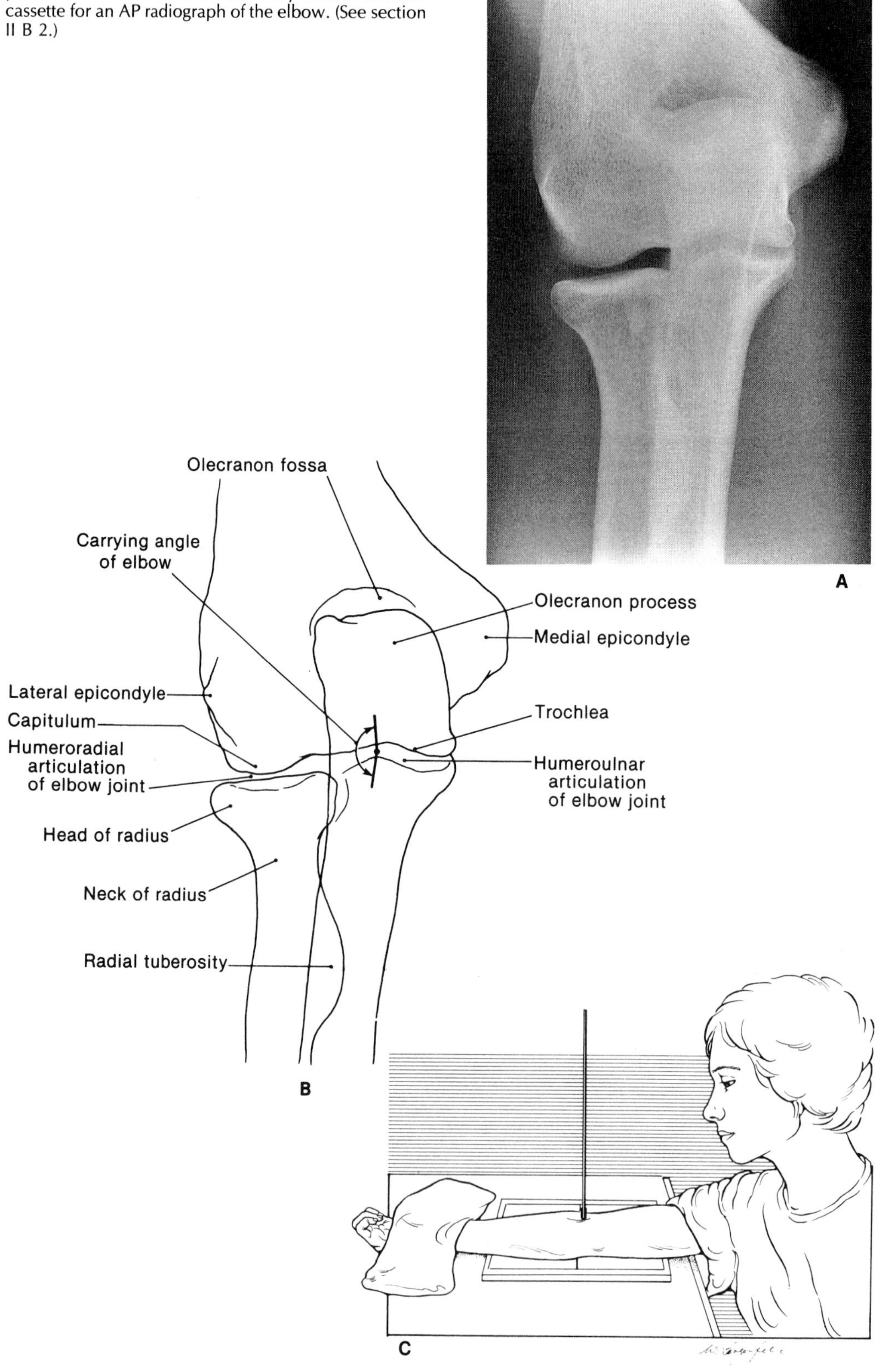

Figure 1-9. (*A*) An AP radiograph of the elbow and (*B*) its schematic representation. (C) The orientation of a patient's elbow relative to the x-ray beam and film cassette for an AP radiograph of the elbow. (See section II B 2.)

Figure 1-10. (*A*) An internal oblique radiograph of the elbow and (*B*) its schematic representation. (*C*) The orientation of a patient's elbow relative to the x-ray beam and film cassette for an internal oblique radiograph of the elbow. (See section II B 3.)

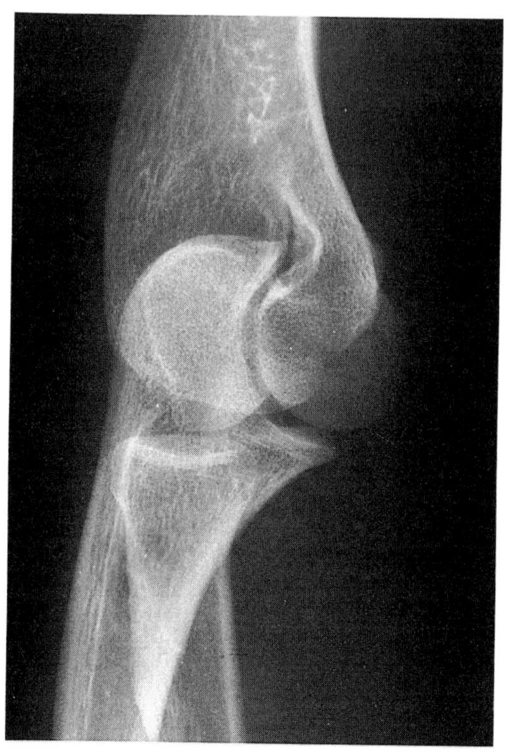

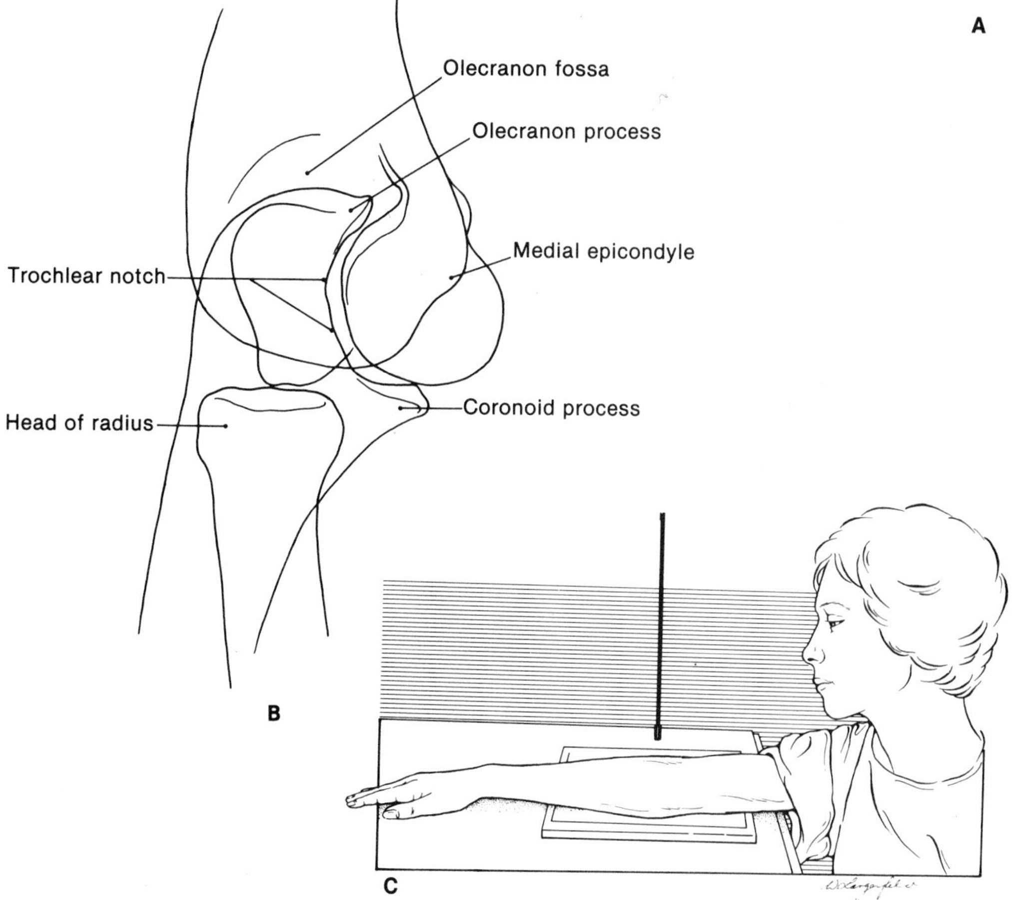

Figure 1-11. (*A*) An external oblique radiograph of the elbow and (*B*) its schematic representation. (*C*) The orientation of a patient's elbow relative to the x-ray beam and film cassette for an external oblique radiograph of the elbow. (See section II B 4.)

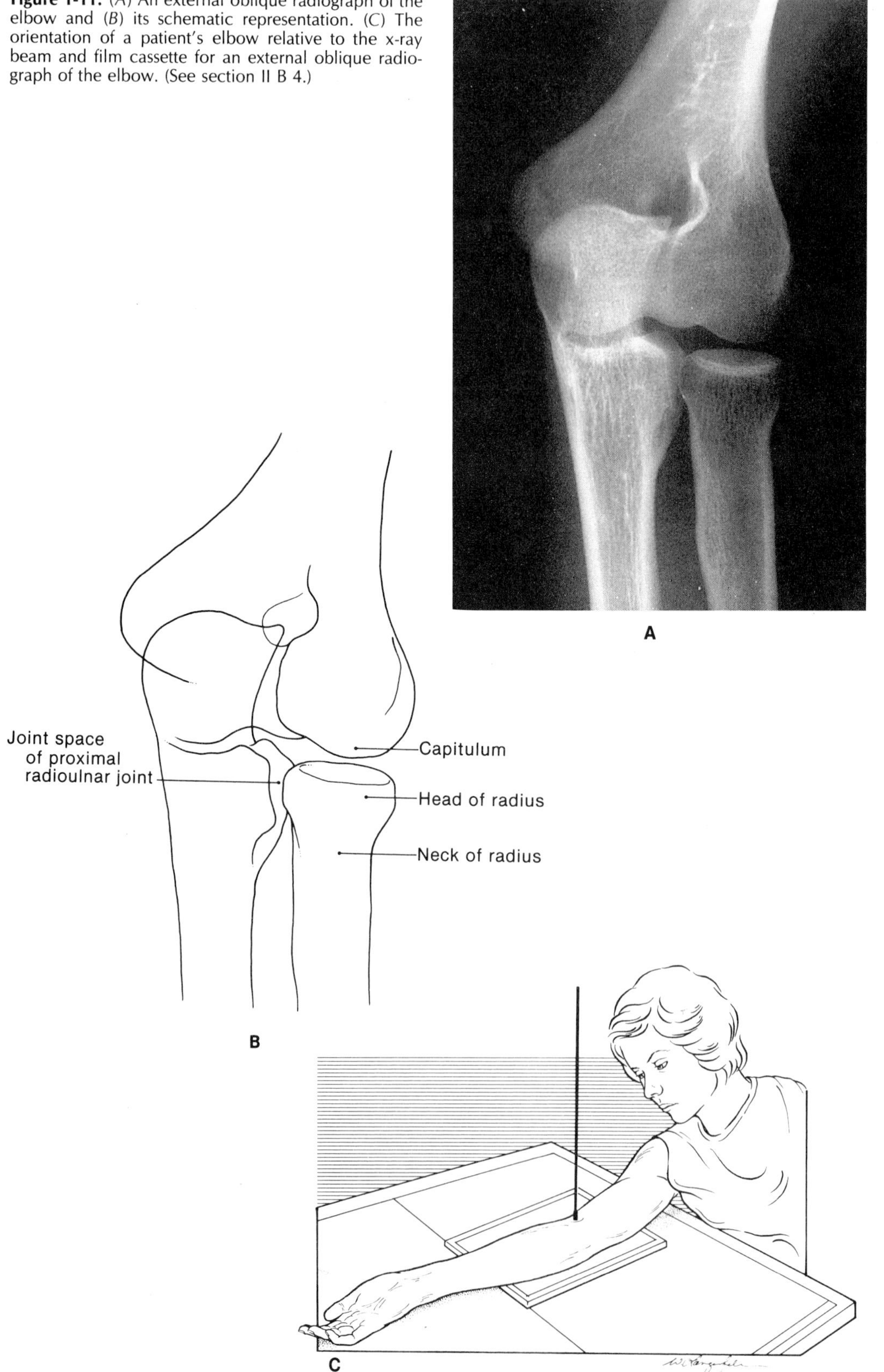

supported closely to the trunk of the body. The patient complains of pain around the radial head. Diagnosis can be made on the basis of the history and physical examination; however, radiographs should be examined to determine that there are no fractures or dislocations.

(3) Radiographic features. It is important to note that it is the annular ligament (not the head of the radius) that is displaced in a nursemaid's elbow at the time of presentation (the proximal part of the annular ligament lies entrapped between the capitulum and the radial head). Consequently, a lateral radiograph of a nursemaid's elbow does not show a break in the colinear relationship between the capitulum and the central axis of the radius.

(4) Reduction of a nursemaid's elbow can be achieved in the office setting by applying posteriorly directed pressure on the head of the radius while slowly, but firmly, supinating and extending the forearm; these manipulations screw the radial head into the annular ligament.

c. Fracture of the proximal third of the ulnar shaft commonly is accompanied by a dislocation of the head of the radius, with the radial head most often displaced anteriorly. This injury combination is called a **Monteggia fracture-dislocation** (Figure 1-12). Almost all radial head dislocations involve a complete tear of the annular ligament.

2. Fracture of the distal humerus

a. Description of injury

(1) Distal humeral fractures are most common in children, adolescents, and adults over 50 years of age; generally, the fracture is caused by a fall on an outstretched hand.

(2) In older children and adolescents, the growth plates at the ends of the long bones of the extremities are the regions of these bones most susceptible to fracture. Consequently, most distal humeral fractures in older children and adolescents involve the growth plate.

(3) Distal humeral fracture sometimes occurs in association with a fracture of the surgical neck of the humerus.

b. Clinical features. Distal humeral fracture causes edema in the region of the elbow, which can significantly compromise blood supply to the muscles of the forearm. **Volkmann's contracture** (ischemic muscular atrophy) always is a potential complication of these fractures.

c. Radiographic features of growth plate fractures. Growth plate fractures are classified as one of five types on the basis of the **Salter-Harris classification scheme**.

(1) A **Salter-Harris Type I fracture** extends through only the growth plate (Figure 1-13). Radiographic evidence of such a fracture in the distal humerus often is difficult to detect. The following four criteria should be examined.

(a) Fractures and dislocations at the elbow commonly produce an effusion within the synovial cavity of the joint, which anteriorly displaces the anterior fat pad and posteriorly displaces the posterior fat pad (Figure 1-14).

(i) The displacement of the anterior fat pad increases the size of the fat-density area anterior to the coronoid fossa in the lateral elbow radiograph (this feature is called the **sail sign** since the fat-density area is shaped like a triangular sail).

(ii) The displacement of the posterior fat pad generates a fat-density area posterior to the olecranon fossa in the lateral elbow radiograph (this feature is called the **positive posterior fat pad sign**).

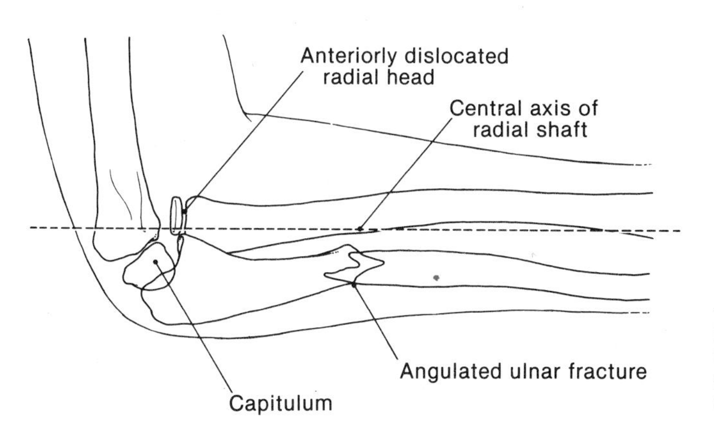

Figure 1-12. An outline of a lateral radiograph of a Monteggia fracture-dislocation in a pediatric patient. (See section II C 1 c.)

(b) The alignment of the capitulum with respect to the anterior humeral and midhumeral lines in the lateral radiograph provides for recognition of subtle anterior or posterior displacements of the distal humeral epiphysis.

(c) An increase or decrease of the carrying angle, as determined by comparison of the angles in the AP radiographs of the traumatized and contralateral elbows, provides for recognition of medial or lateral angular displacement of the distal humeral epiphysis.

(d) The widths of the growth plates in the traumatized and contralateral elbows should be carefully measured; such comparison usually is required to reveal a subtle increase in the width of a fractured growth plate.

(2) A **Salter-Harris Type II fracture** extends through most of the growth plate and a small part of the metaphysis; the growth plate may be widened on the side contralateral to the metaphyseal fragment (Figure 1-15). Type II fractures account for more than 50% of all growth plate fractures.

(3) A **Salter-Harris Type III fracture** extends through part of the growth plate and part of the epiphysis (Figure 1-16).

(4) A **Salter-Harris Type IV fracture** extends through the metaphysis, the growth plate, and the epiphysis (Figure 1-17).

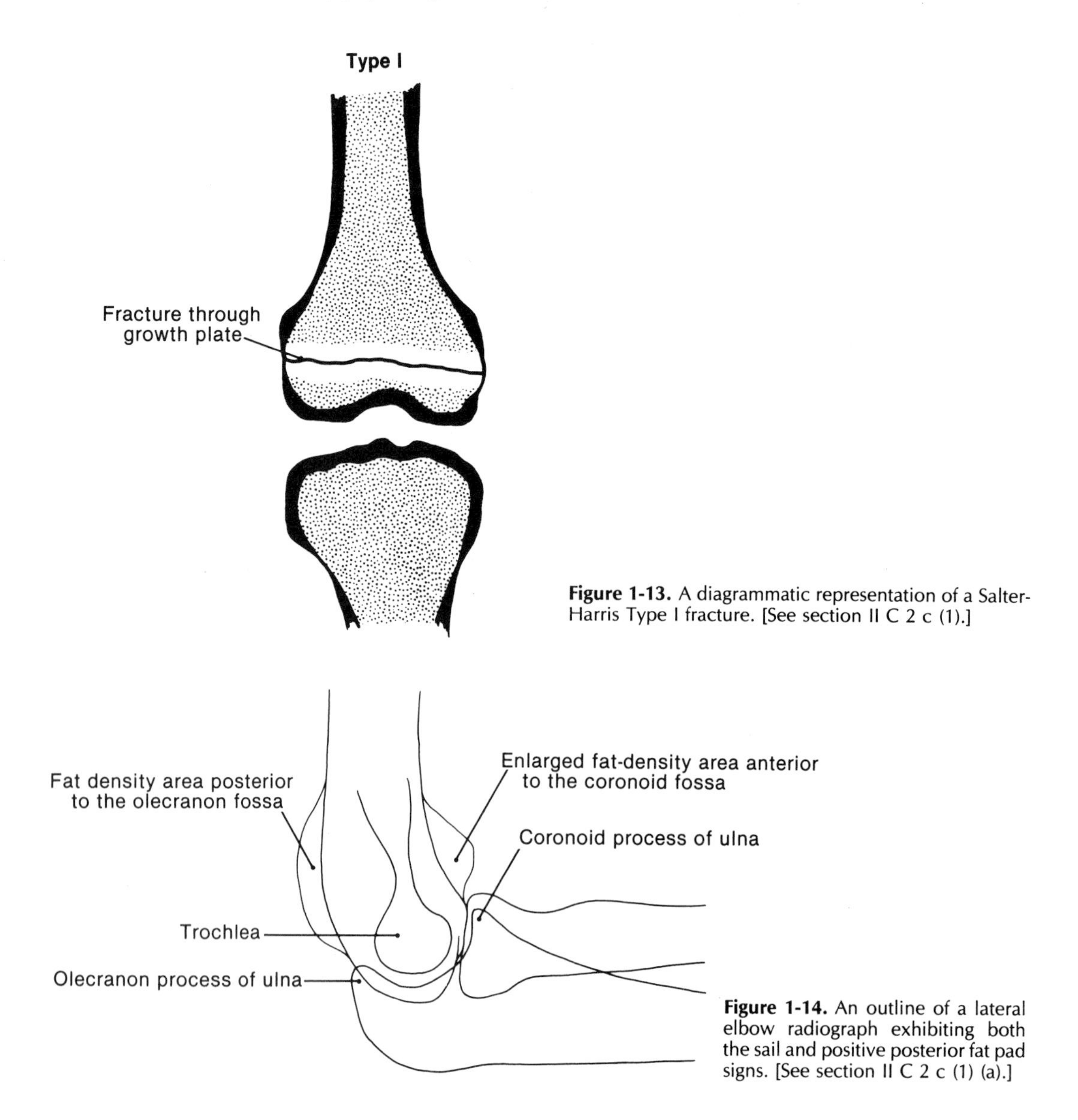

Figure 1-13. A diagrammatic representation of a Salter-Harris Type I fracture. [See section II C 2 c (1).]

Figure 1-14. An outline of a lateral elbow radiograph exhibiting both the sail and positive posterior fat pad signs. [See section II C 2 c (1) (a).]

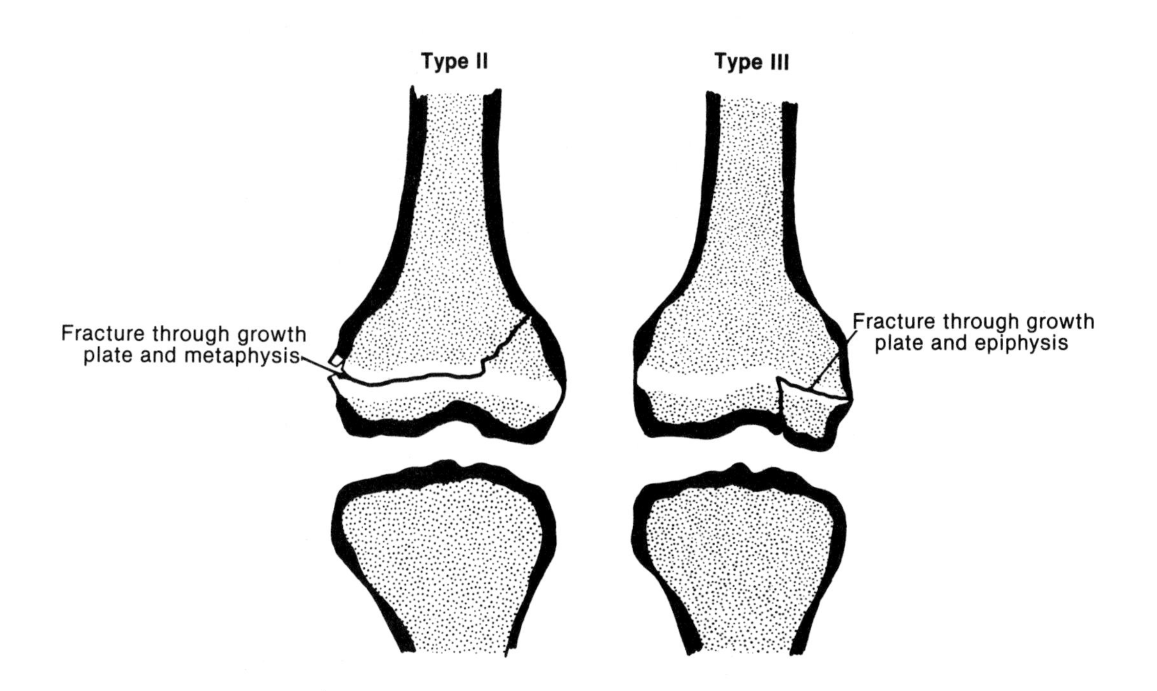

Figure 1-15. A diagrammatic representation of a Salter-Harris Type II fracture. [See section II C 2 c (2).]

Figure 1-16. A diagrammatic representation of a Salter-Harris Type III fracture. [See section II C 2 c (3).]

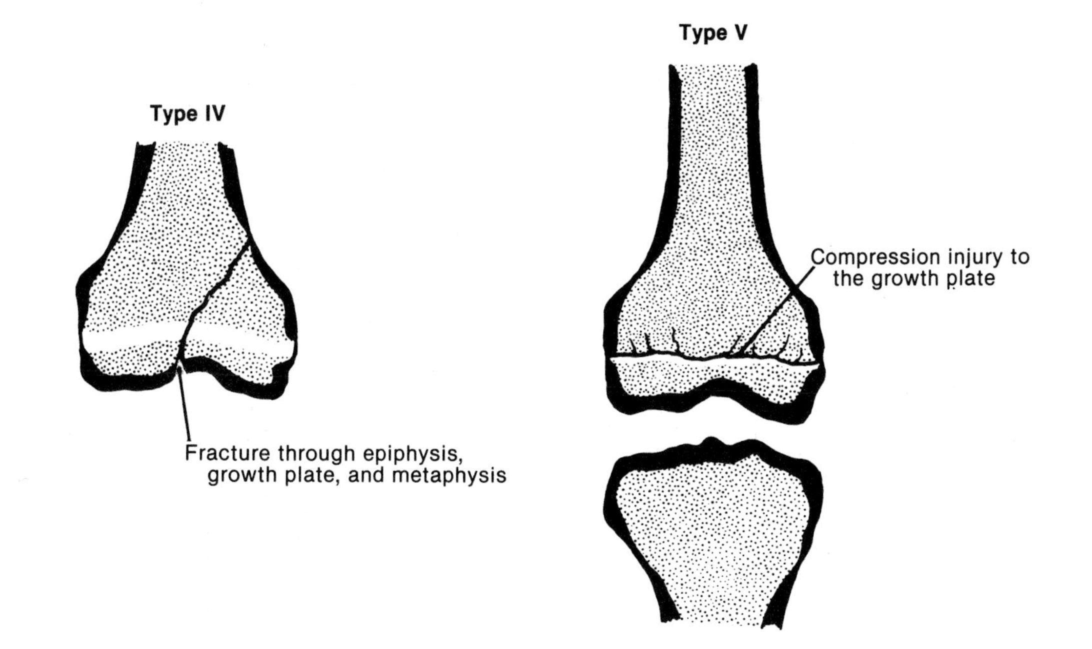

Figure 1-17. A diagrammatic representation of a Salter-Harris Type IV fracture. [See section II C 2 c (4).]

Figure 1-18. A diagrammatic representation of a Salter-Harris Type V fracture. [See section II C 2 c (5).]

(5) A **Salter-Harris Type V fracture** is a compression injury to the growth plate (Figure 1-18). Radiographs of such a fracture generally do not show any changes of growth plate width or evidence of epiphyseal displacement; however, the fracture does produce elbow joint effusion, with its attendant displacements of the anterior and posterior fat pads.

d. Prognosis. Type I and Type II fractures have a more favorable prognosis than do Type III, Type IV, and Type V fractures. The latter group of fractures extend through the epiphyseal side of the growth plate and thus injure the proliferating chondrocytes of the growth plate. Injury to these cells increases the likelihood of retarded longitudinal growth at the end of the bone and of premature fusion of the epiphysis with the diaphysis.

3. Fracture of the head and neck of the radius

a. Description of injury

(1) A fracture of the head or neck of the radius generally results from a hard fall on an outstretched hand. The impact of the fall drives the head of the radius axially onto the capitulum of the humerus.

(2) A radial head or neck fracture sometimes occurs in association with a fracture of the capitulum, a fracture of the distal radius, or a dislocation of the distal radioulnar joint.

b. Radiographic features

(1) Radial head fracture is the most common type of elbow fracture in adults; the fracture generally extends vertically through the radial head to include its superior articular surface.

(2) A Salter-Harris Type II fracture is the most common type of radial head and neck fractures in children. These fractures often are characterized by the presence of one or both of the following radiographic findings:

(a) The sail and positive posterior fat pad signs

(b) Subtle anterior or posterior displacement of the radial head or shaft, as determined by use of the radiocapitellar line

III. HAND AND WRIST

A. Anatomy of the wrist and hand

1. Bones

a. Distal ends of the ulna and radius

(1) The **styloid processes** of the ulna and radius are respectively palpable on the medial and lateral sides of the wrist.

(2) The **dorsal tubercle** of the radius is palpable on the posterior aspect of the distal end of the radius.

(3) The **epiphyses** at the distal end of the ulna and at the distal end of the radius are the last epiphyses to fuse with the metaphyses of these bones during late adolescence.

b. Carpals

(1) The **scaphoid (navicular)** and **trapezium (greater multangular)** are palpable in the floor of the anatomic snuffbox.

(2) The order of appearance of the carpal ossification centers is quite variable. The ossification centers for the capitate and hamate are generally present at birth; the ossification center for the pisiform is commonly the last to appear.

c. Metacarpals

(1) The **knuckles** represent the heads of the second to fifth metacarpals.

(2) Each metacarpal bears only a single epiphysis during childhood and adolescence. Whereas the epiphysis of the first metacarpal resides at the base of the bone, the epiphyses of the second to fifth metacarpals reside at the heads of the bones.

d. Phalanges

(1) There are two methods for **assessing rotational malalignment of phalangeal fractures** in the index, middle, ring, and little fingers.

(a) Normally, when the fingers are flexed so as to form a fist, the index, middle, ring, and little fingers each point to roughly the same spot at the wrist (this spot overlies the proximal pole of the scaphoid). Rotational malalignment of a phalangeal fracture in any of these digits invariably makes that finger point toward a different spot.

(b) Normally, when the index, middle, ring, and little fingers of each hand are flexed so as to form a fist, and the medial edges of the two fists are then brought into contact with each other, the orientation of each fingernail in the left hand is a mirror image of the orientation of its counterpart in the right hand. Rotational malalignment of a phalangeal fracture in any of these digits invariably alters the orientation of the finger's nail.

(2) Each phalanx, during childhood and adolescence, bears only a single epiphysis, residing at the bone's base.

2. Joints

a. Distal radioulnar joint

(1) The distal radioulnar joint articulates the head of the ulna with the ulnar notch of the radius.

(2) The triangular disk of fibrous cartilage that lies immediately distal to the head of the ulna separates the synovial cavity of the distal radioulnar joint from that of the wrist joint.

b. Wrist (radiocarpal) joint

(1) The wrist joint articulates the scaphoid, lunate, and triquetrum with the distal end of the radius and the above-mentioned disk of fibrous cartilage.

(2) The wrist joint provides for abduction, adduction, flexion, and extension of the hand.

c. Metacarpophalangeal and interphalangeal joints

(1) The head of the metacarpal articulates with the base of the proximal phalanx within each metacarpophalangeal joint. Each of the metacarpophalangeal joints provides for abduction, adduction, flexion, and extension of the proximal phalanx of the digit.

(2) Each of the interphalangeal joints provides for only flexion and extension of the more distal phalanx.

3. Muscles

a. Extrinsic muscles of the wrist and hand

(1) Six muscles commonly function as **fixators of the hand** at the wrist joint whenever the digits are moved.

(a) **Flexor carpi ulnaris** flexes and adducts the hand at the wrist joint; it is innervated by the ulnar nerve.

(b) **Palmaris longus** flexes the hand at the wrist joint; it is innervated by the median nerve.

(c) **Flexor carpi radialis** flexes and abducts the hand at the wrist joint; it is innervated by the median nerve.

(d) **Extensor carpi ulnaris** extends and adducts the hand at the wrist joint; it is innervated by the deep branch of the radial nerve.

(e) **Extensors carpi radialis longus and brevis** extend and abduct the hand at the wrist joint; extensor carpi radialis longus is innervated by the radial nerve, and extensor carpi radialis brevis is innervated by the deep branch of the radial nerve.

(2) Four muscles commonly serve as powerful **flexors or extensors of the thumb**.

(a) **Flexor pollicis longus** chiefly acts to flex the distal phalanx of the thumb; it is innervated by the anterior interosseous branch of the median nerve.

(b) **Extensors pollicis brevis and longus** chiefly act to extend the proximal and distal phalanges of the thumb, respectively. Both muscles are innervated by the deep branch of the radial nerve.

(c) **Abductor pollicis longus** extends and abducts the thumb at its carpometacarpal joint; it is innervated by the deep branch of the radial nerve.

(3) Five muscles commonly serve as powerful **flexors or extensors of the fingers**.

(a) **Flexors digitorum superficialis and profundus** chiefly act to flex the middle and distal phalanges of the fingers, respectively. The ulnar nerve innervates the medial half of flexor digitorum profundus, and the anterior interosseous branch of the median nerve innervates the lateral half of profundus. Flexor digitorum superficialis is innervated by the median nerve.

(b) **Extensor digitorum** extends the fingers at their metacarpophalangeal and interphalangeal joints; it is innervated by the deep branch of the radial nerve.

(c) **Extensors indicis and digiti minimi** respectively extend the index and little fingers at their metacarpophalangeal and interphalangeal joints. Both muscles are innervated by the deep branch of the radial nerve.

b. Intrinsic muscles of the hand

(1) The hand bears four short **muscles of the thumb**.

(a) **Abductor pollicis brevis** abducts the thumb at its carpometacarpal and metacarpophalangeal joints.

(b) **Flexor pollicis brevis** flexes the proximal phalanx of the thumb.
(c) **Opponens pollicis** is the muscle chiefly responsible for the thumb's capacity to form a pincer with any of the fingers.
(d) **Adductor pollicis** adducts the thumb at its carpometacarpal and metacarpophalangeal joints.

(2) The **lumbricals** serve in large measure to counteract the extensive forces exerted across the metacarpophalangeal joints of the fingers by the extensors digitorum, indicis, and digiti minimi.

(3) The **palmar and dorsal interossei** are prime **abductors and adductors of the fingers**.
(a) The first palmar interosseous adducts the thumb.
(b) The first dorsal interosseous abducts the index finger.
(c) The second palmar interosseous adducts the index finger.
(d) The second dorsal interosseous abducts the middle finger.
(e) The third dorsal interosseous abducts the middle finger.
(f) The third palmar interosseous adducts the ring finger.
(g) The fourth dorsal interosseous abducts the ring finger.
(h) The fourth palmar interosseous adducts the little finger.

(4) The hand bears three short **muscles of the little finger**.
(a) **Abductor digiti minimi** abducts the little finger.
(b) **Flexor digiti minimi** flexes the proximal phalanx of the little finger.
(c) **Opponens digiti minimi** flexes and rotates the fifth metacarpal; in so doing, it deepens the hollow of the palmar surface.

(5) **Palmaris brevis** wrinkles the skin covering the hypothenar eminence, and thus enhances the grip of this region of the palmar surface.

4. Nerves

a. Median nerve

(1) **Route.** The median nerve extends across the wrist region by passing through the carpal tunnel along with the tendons of flexor digitorum profundus, flexor digitorum superficialis, and flexor pollicis longus.

(2) **Motor and sensory supply**
(a) The median nerve innervates five intrinsic muscles of the hand.
(i) The three muscles of the thenar eminence; namely, abductor pollicis brevis, flexor pollicis brevis, and opponens pollicis
(ii) The first and second lumbricals, which serve the index and middle fingers
(b) The median nerve provides cutaneous innervation for the lateral two-thirds of the palm and the palmar surfaces of the lateral three and one-half digits.

(3) **Tests of motor and sensory supply**
(a) A quick test of the median nerve's **motor supply** within the hand is to request the patient to make an O with the thumb and index finger and to keep the O intact as you try to separate the two digits by passing a probe between them. This procedure tests the action of opponens pollicis.
(b) A quick test of the median nerve's **sensory supply** in the hand is to ascertain whether the patient can sense a probe lightly applied to the palmar tip of the index finger.

b. Ulnar nerve and its branches

(1) **Route.** The ulnar nerve extends across the wrist region by passing over (i.e., superficial to) the flexor retinaculum; here the ulnar nerve lies immediately medial to the ulnar artery. Upon entering the hand, the ulnar nerve divides into **deep and superficial branches**.

(2) **Motor and sensory supply**
(a) The **superficial branch** innervates palmaris brevis.
(b) The **deep branch** innervates all the intrinsic muscles of the hand except for palmaris brevis and the five intrinsic muscles innervated by the median nerve. Thus, the deep branch of the ulnar nerve innervates:
(i) Adductor pollicis
(ii) All the palmar and all the dorsal interossei
(iii) The third and fourth lumbricals
(iv) The muscles of the hypothenar eminence, namely, abductor digiti minimi, flexor digiti minimi, and opponens digiti minimi
(c) The ulnar nerve provides cutaneous innervation for the medial third of the palm,

the palmar surfaces of the medial one and one-half digits, and roughly the medial half of the dorsum of the hand.

(3) Tests of motor and sensory supply

(a) A quick test of the ulnar nerve's **motor supply** within the hand is to request the patient to clench a piece of paper tightly between the middle and ring fingers as you attempt to dislodge the paper. This procedure tests the actions of the third palmar and the third dorsal interossei.

(b) A quick test of the ulnar nerve's **sensory supply** in the hand is to ascertain whether the patient can sense a probe lightly applied to the palmar tip of the little finger.

c. Superficial branch of the radial nerve

(1) Route. The superficial branch of the radial nerve extends from the forearm into the hand within the superficial fascia of the dorsolateral aspect of the wrist.

(2) Sensory supply. The superficial branch of the radial nerve provides cutaneous innervation for roughly the lateral half of the dorsum of the hand.

(3) Test of sensory supply. A quick test of the nerve's sensory supply in the hand is to ascertain whether the patient can sense a probe lightly applied to the dorsal aspect of the skin web between the thumb and index finger.

5. Blood vessels and lymph nodes

a. Arterial supply

(1) Palpable pulsations

(a) The pulsations of the **ulnar artery** can be palpated on the anteromedial surface of the forearm about 1 cm proximal to the distal crease of the wrist.

(b) The pulsations of the **radial artery** can be palpated on the anterolateral surface of the forearm about 2 to 3 cm proximal to the distal crease of the wrist.

(2) The palmar arterial arches and their derivations

(a) The **superficial palmar arch** is a direct continuation of the ulnar artery in the hand.

(b) The **deep palmar arch** is a direct continuation of the radial artery in the hand.

(3) The **Allen test** can determine whether the ulnar and radial arteries both contribute blood supply to a patient's hand. Each artery is tested separately as follows:

(a) The patient is asked to make a tight fist. The capillary beds within the skin of the palm are thereby emptied of much of their blood content.

(b) The physician then applies pressure to both the ulnar and radial arteries at their palpation sites in the anterior forearm. This significantly blocks the blood flow into the palmar arches.

(c) The patient is asked to unclench the fist, exposing the blanched pallor of the palmar surface.

(d) The physician releases the pressure on one artery and ascertains whether color is restored to the palmar surface within 2 to 4 seconds. The return of color indicates that the artery is a chief source of blood supply to the hand.

(e) The entire test is then repeated with the other artery to ascertain that both arteries are supplying the palmar arches.

b. Venous and lymphatic drainage of the hand

(1) On the **medial side of the hand**, the superficial tissues are primarily drained of blood and lymph by the **basilic vein** and its accompanying lymphatics.

(2) On the **lateral side of the hand**, the superficial tissues are primarily drained of blood and lymph by the **cephalic vein** and its accompanying lymphatics.

(3) Much of the venous and lymph flow within the hand is transferred from the palmar to the dorsal side. Consequently, injury and infection of the palmar surface commonly produces edema of the dorsum of the hand.

B. Major features of radiographs of the hand and wrist

1. PA radiograph of the hand. A PA radiograph of the hand has the following distinguishing features (Figure 1-19).

a. The radius and ulna

(1) The radiograph provides an unobstructed view of the **styloid process of the radius** and the **styloid process of the ulna**.

(2) The radiograph shows the **medial (ulnar) angulation** of the articular surface at the distal end of the radius [this surface articulates with the scaphoid and lunate bones in the radiocarpal (wrist) joint]. The medial angulation is quantitated by measuring the acute angle between two imaginary lines: one drawn from the tip of the radial styloid process

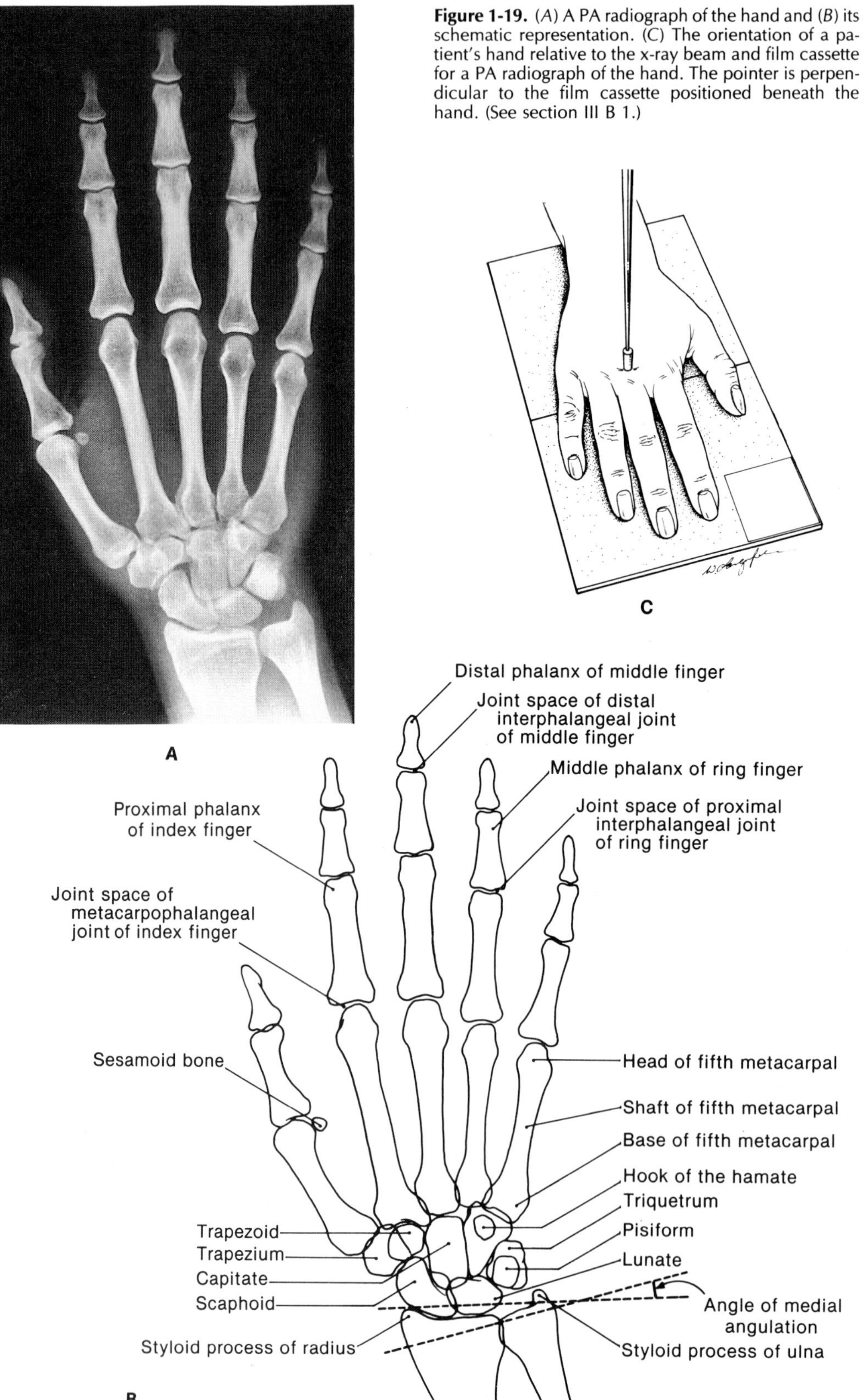

Figure 1-19. (*A*) A PA radiograph of the hand and (*B*) its schematic representation. (*C*) The orientation of a patient's hand relative to the x-ray beam and film cassette for a PA radiograph of the hand. The pointer is perpendicular to the film cassette positioned beneath the hand. (See section III B 1.)

to the base of the ulnar styloid process, and the other drawn perpendicular to the central axis of the radius (see Figure 1-19B). The normal range of the angle is 7° to 18°.

(3) The apposed **articular cartilages** in the distal radioulnar joint appear as a radiolucent space between the head of the ulna and the ulnar notch of the radius.

b. The carpals

(1) The four most **proximal carpals**—the **scaphoid (navicular), lunate, triquetrum, and pisiform**—form a semilunar array of radiopaque shadows immediately distal to the distal end of the radius and the head of the ulna.

(a) The roughly circular outline of the pisiform overlies the triquetrum.

(b) The lunate casts a quadrangular (four-sided) shadow.

(2) The **fibrocartilaginous disk** of the wrist joint lies within the gaping, radiolucent space between the head of the ulna and the proximal edges of the lunate and triquetrum.

(3) The **capitate** and **hamate** occupy the concavity in the semilunar array of the four most proximal carpals. The ovoid radiopacity overlying the distal part of the hamate represents the **hook of the hamate**.

(4) The radiopaque shadows of the **trapezium (greater multangular)** and **trapezoid (lesser multangular)** largely overlap each other, and lie interposed between the distal pole of the scaphoid and the bases of the first and second metacarpals.

c. The metacarpals, phalanges, and sesamoid bones

(1) The **central axis of the third metacarpal** lies along the major axis by which forces are transmitted from the hand across the wrist to the forearm. From the third metacarpal, this axis extends proximally as follows:

(a) Along the central axis of the capitate

(b) Between the scaphoid and lunate

(c) Along the central axis of the radius

(2) The **bases of the metacarpals** partially overlap each other or one of the distal carpals.

(3) The radiograph provides an unobstructed view of the **metacarpophalangeal and interphalangeal joints** of all five digits.

(4) The radiograph shows one or both of the **sesamoid bones** on the anterior side of the first metacarpophalangeal joint.

(a) The more medial sesamoid bone lies embedded in the common tendon of insertion of adductor pollicis and the first palmar interosseous.

(b) The more lateral sesamoid bone lies embedded in the common tendon of insertion of flexor pollicis brevis and abductor pollicis brevis.

2. Lateral radiograph of the wrist. A lateral radiograph of the wrist has the following distinguishing features (Figure 1-20).

a. The radiograph shows the **anterior (volar) angulation** of the articular surface at the distal end of the radius. The anterior angulation is quantitated by measuring the acute angle between a line drawn through the anterior and posterior margins of the radial articular surface and a line drawn perpendicular to the central axis of the radius (see Figure 1-20B). The angle normally measures 15° to 23°.

b. Two convex bony outlines overlap the distal end of the **radius**.

(1) The more proximal outline represents the proximal surface of the **lunate**.

(2) The more distal outline represents the proximal surface of the **scaphoid**.

c. The rounded **head of the capitate** lies immediately distal to the concave bony outline cast by the distal surface of the lunate.

d. The **tuberosity of the scaphoid** projects anterior to the head of the capitate.

e. The **central axis of the third metacarpal** extends proximally as follows:

(1) Along the central axis of the capitate

(2) Through the center of the lunate

(3) Along the central axis of the radius

C. Clinical and radiographic features of common traumatic injuries and arthritides

1. Dislocation of one or more of the carpals

a. Dislocations of the lunate

(1) Whenever the lunate is dislocated either anteriorly or posteriorly, it undergoes an anterior rotation on its convex, proximal surface. This rotation transforms its PA outline from a quadrangular to a triangular shadow (Figure 1-21).

(2) Dislocations of the lunate displace the center of the bone from the line in the lateral wrist radiograph that extends from the central axes of the third metacarpal and capitate to the central axis of the radius (Figure 1-22).

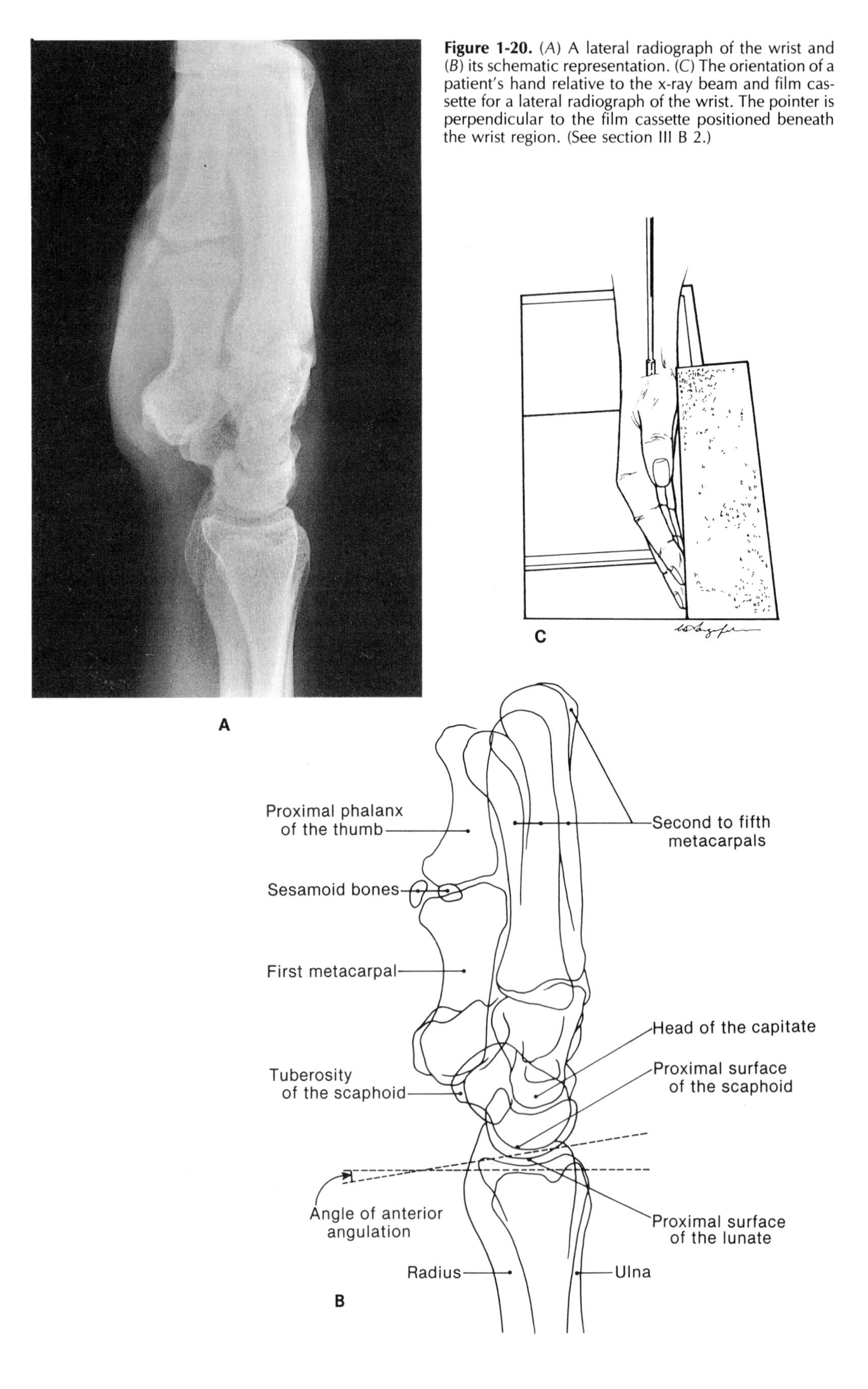

Figure 1-20. (*A*) A lateral radiograph of the wrist and (*B*) its schematic representation. (*C*) The orientation of a patient's hand relative to the x-ray beam and film cassette for a lateral radiograph of the wrist. The pointer is perpendicular to the film cassette positioned beneath the wrist region. (See section III B 2.)

(3) **Anterior dislocation of the lunate** is one of the most common carpal dislocations. Anterior dislocation of the lunate thrusts the bone into the carpal tunnel and thus may result in injury to the median nerve.

b. **Posterior dislocation of all the carpals relative to the lunate (posterior perilunate dislocation)** is another common carpal dislocation. A lateral radiograph of such a dislocation characteristically shows that the central axis of the capitate extends proximally posterior to the central axis of the radius (Figure 1-23).

c. A tear of the scapholunate ligament can lead to a **rotational dislocation of the scaphoid** in which the proximal pole of the bone is directed posteriorly and the distal pole is directed anteriorly. Such a dislocation increases the width of the radiolucent space between the scaphoid and lunate in a PA radiograph of the hand (Figure 1-24).

2. **Fracture of the distal radius**

a. Fractures of the distal third of the radial shaft commonly occur in association with a dislocation of the distal radioulnar joint (a **Galeazzi fracture-dislocation**; Figure 1-25).

b. Fractures in a **young child** commonly reflect the fact that the bones of a young child are relatively supple and easily deformed.

(1) **Compression failure of the cortical bone** in the distal third of a young child's radial shaft can cause the cortical bone to buckle outward. Such a fracture is called a **torus fracture** because the radiographic outline of the fracture site resembles the outline of an architectural column bearing a torus molding at its base (Figure 1-26).

(2) Fractures of the distal radius in a young child are frequently incomplete. Radiographs show a discontinuity of the cortical bone on one side of the shaft and a bent cortical bone on the opposite side (Figure 1-27). These fractures are called **greenstick fractures** because of their similarity to a break in a supple branch of a tree or bush.

c. A **Colles' fracture** is a fracture of the distal radius in which there is **posterior displacement and rotation** of the distal fragment (Figure 1-28). A Colles' fracture is generally produced by a fall on an outstretched hand. More than 50% of Colles' fractures are accompanied by a fracture of the ulnar styloid process.

d. A **Smith's (reversed Colles') fracture** is a fracture of the distal radius in which there is **anterior displacement and rotation** of the distal fragment (Figure 1-29). Smith's fractures are encountered much less frequently than Colles' fractures.

e. **Reduction of fractures** at the distal end of the radius require that:

(1) The anterior angulation of the articular surface be restored in order to ensure adequate grip function

(2) The medial angulation of the articular surface be restored in order to ensure sufficient adduction of the hand at the wrist joint

3. **Fracture of the scaphoid.** The scaphoid is the most frequently fractured carpal bone. Fully 80% of scaphoid fractures occur in its waist (the narrowed midregion that joins the proximal and distal poles of the carpal).

a. **Clinical features and diagnosis.** A fractured scaphoid is indicated if pain in the anatomic snuffbox occurs with two or all three of the following procedures:

(1) Deep palpation of the anatomic snuffbox

(2) Axial compression of the thumb toward the anatomic snuffbox

(3) An attempt by the patient to supinate the forearm against resistance (with the examiner holding the patient's hand in a neutral position)

b. **Radiographic features**

(1) A fracture of the scaphoid is commonly difficult to detect radiographically during the first 1 to 2 days after the injury. The subsequent bone resorption which occurs at the fracture site renders the site more radiolucent and thus more apparent in radiographs taken 7 to 10 days after the injury. It is advisable to order a PA radiograph of the wrist with the hand ulnar-deviated, or adducted, at the wrist joint, because adduction diminishes the extent to which the surrounding carpals overlap the image of the scaphoid.

(2) It is not uncommon for bony union of the fragments to be delayed or not occur at all. Failure of bony union frequently results in avascular necrosis of the proximal fragment; this is because most or all of the scaphoid's nutrient foramina are located on the surface of the distal half of the bone.

4. **Primary osteoarthritis**

a. **Affected joints.** Within the hand, primary osteoarthritis most commonly affects the distal and proximal interphalangeal joints of the fingers and the carpometacarpal joint of the thumb.

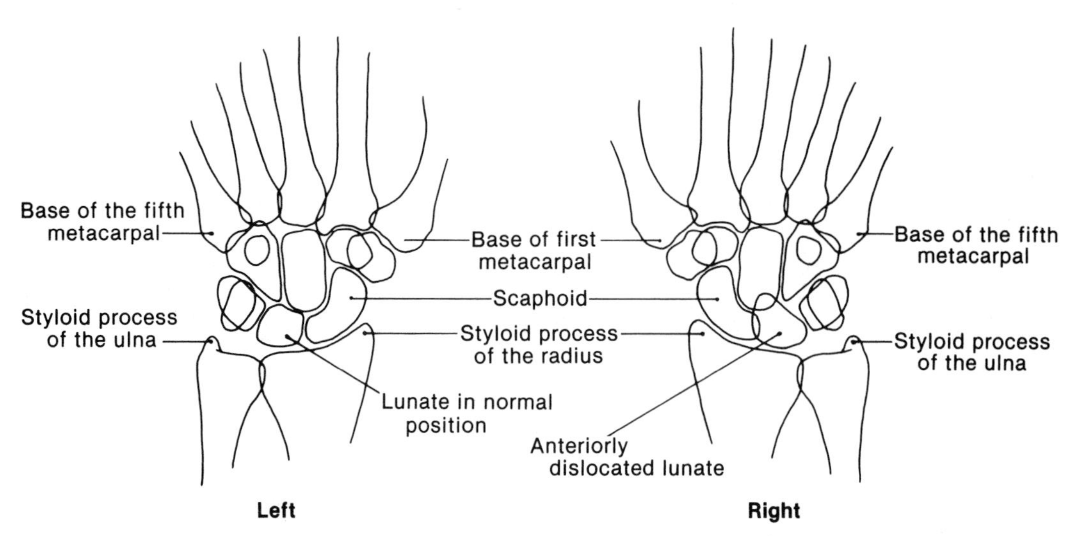

Figure 1-21. The outlines of the PA radiographs of the normal (*left*) and injured (*right*) wrists of a person who has suffered an anteriorly dislocated lunate in the right wrist. [See section III C 1 a (1).]

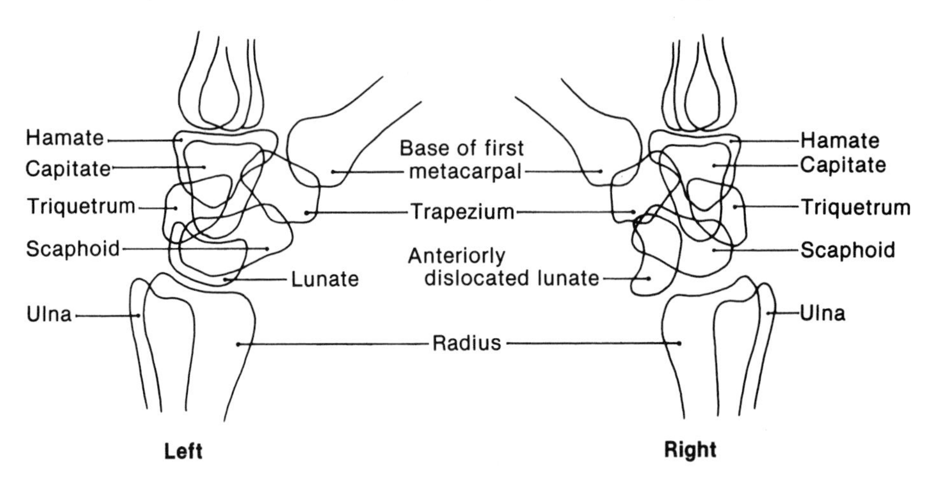

Figure 1-22. The outlines of the lateral radiographs of the normal (*left*) and injured (*right*) wrists of a person who has suffered an anteriorly dislocated lunate in the right wrist. The outlines of the trapezoid and pisiform bones are not shown, for the purpose of clarity. [See section III C 1 a (2).]

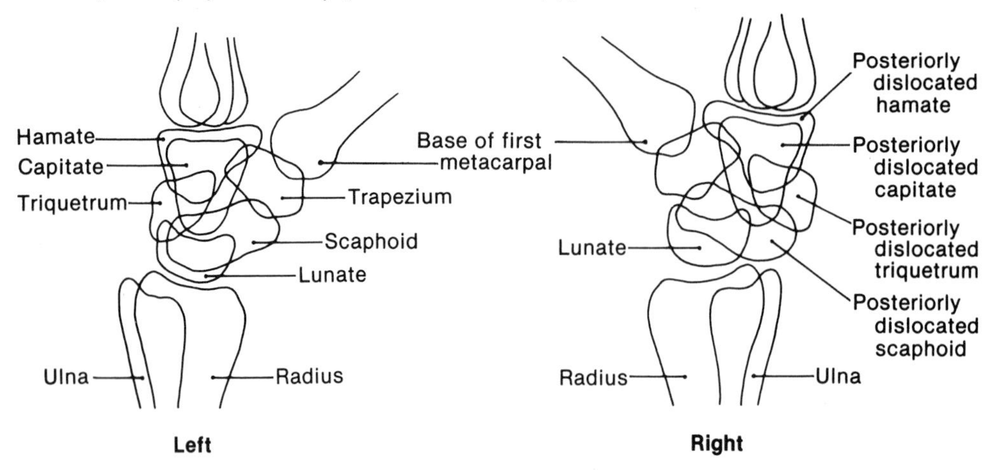

Figure 1-23. The outlines of the lateral radiographs of the normal (*left*) and injured (*right*) wrists of a person who has suffered a posterior perilunate dislocation in the right wrist. The outlines of the trapezoid and pisiform bones are not shown, for the purpose of clarity. (See section III C 1 b.)

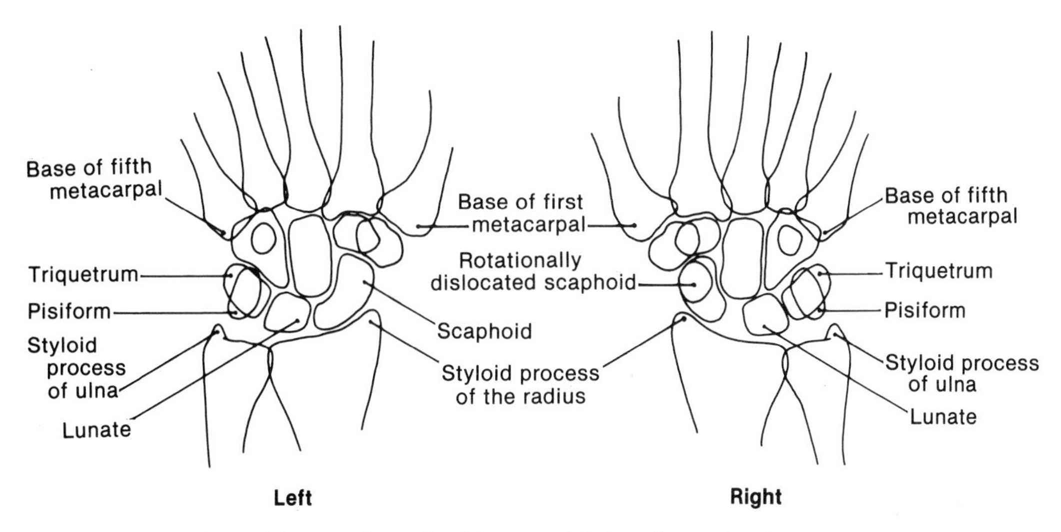

Figure 1-24. The outlines of the PA radiographs of the normal (*left*) and injured (*right*) wrists of a person who has suffered a rotationally dislocated scaphoid in the right wrist. (See section III C 1 c.)

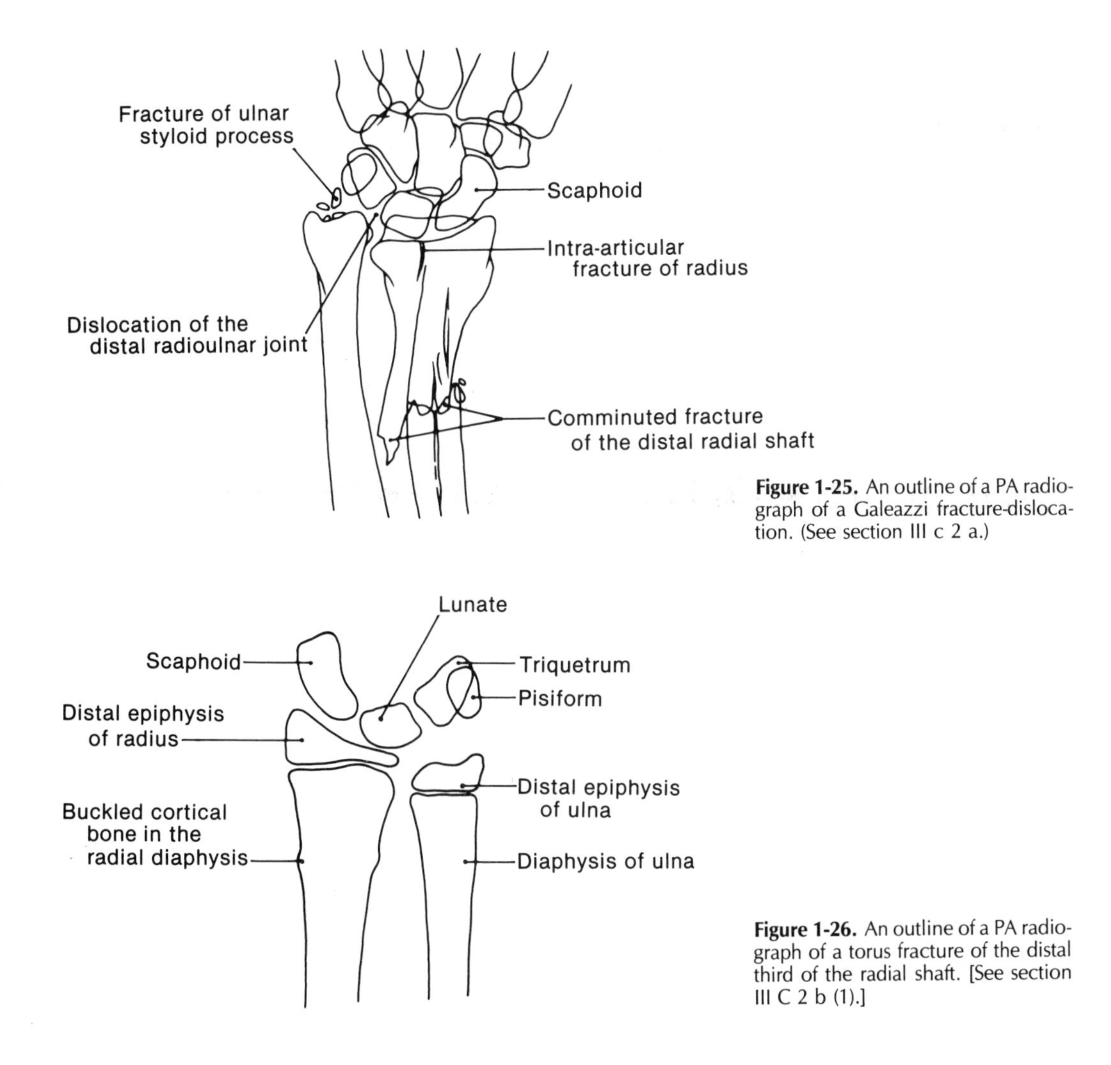

Figure 1-25. An outline of a PA radiograph of a Galeazzi fracture-dislocation. (See section III c 2 a.)

Figure 1-26. An outline of a PA radiograph of a torus fracture of the distal third of the radial shaft. [See section III C 2 b (1).]

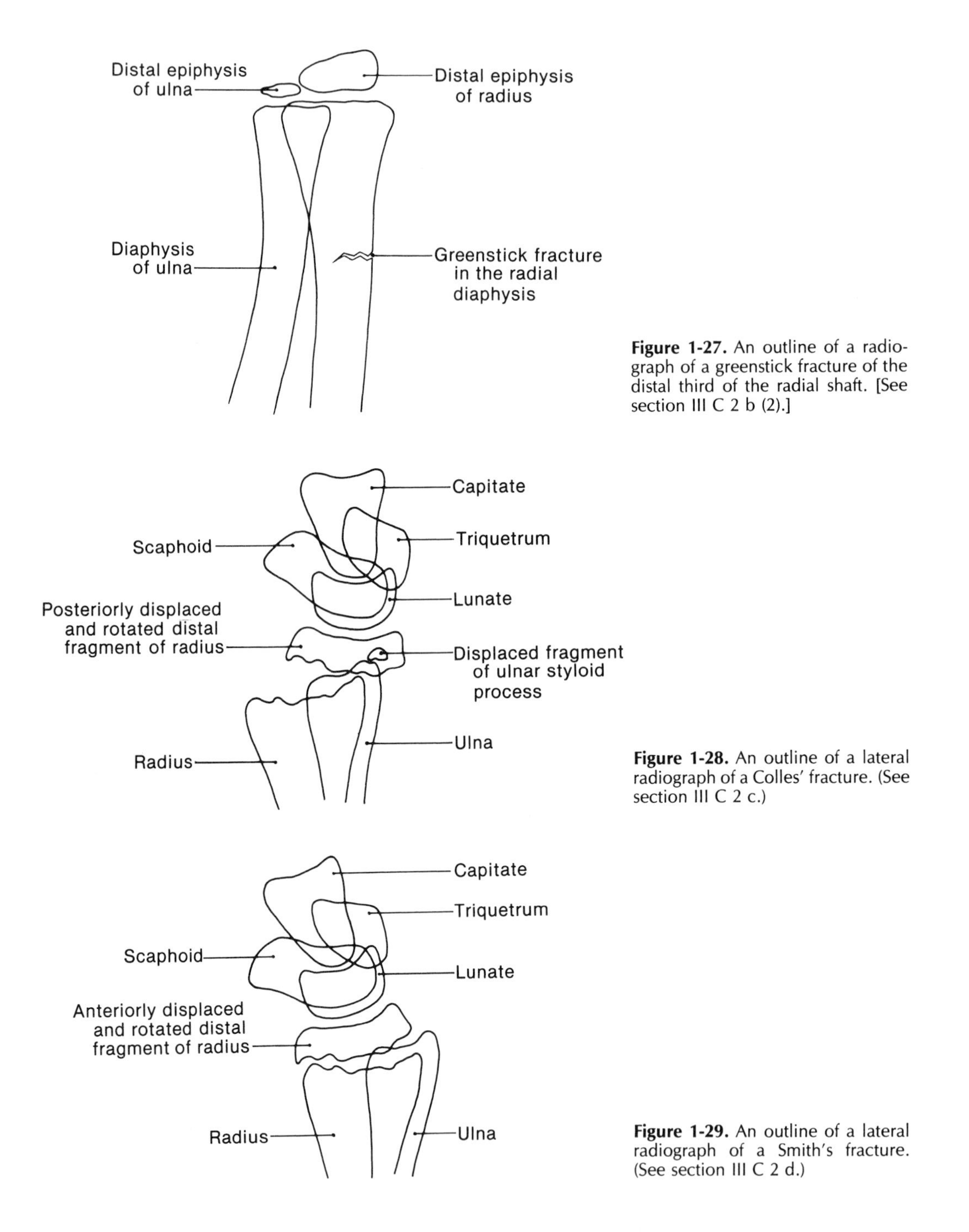

Figure 1-27. An outline of a radiograph of a greenstick fracture of the distal third of the radial shaft. [See section III C 2 b (2).]

Figure 1-28. An outline of a lateral radiograph of a Colles' fracture. (See section III C 2 c.)

Figure 1-29. An outline of a lateral radiograph of a Smith's fracture. (See section III C 2 d.)

b. Radiographic features

(1) The radiolucent **joint space** narrows in width as a result of degeneration and thinning of the articular cartilage surfaces.

(2) The subchondral bone areas exhibit **osteosclerosis**; in other words, the bone areas underlying the articular cartilage surfaces become **more radiopaque**.

(3) Hypertrophy of the subchondral bone areas generates **osteophytes** (amorphous outgrowths).

(a) Heberden's nodes are osteophytes of the distal interphalangeal joints.

(b) Bouchard's nodes are osteophytes of the proximal interphalangeal joints.

5. **Rheumatoid arthritis**
   a. **Affected joints.** Within the hand, rheumatoid arthritis most commonly affects the proximal interphalangeal and metacarpophalangeal joints of the fingers and joints of the wrist region.
   b. **Radiographic features**
      (1) The radiolucent **joint space** narrows in width as a result of degeneration and thinning of the articular cartilage surfaces.
      (2) The periarticular bone areas exhibit **osteopenia**; in other words, the bone areas around the articular cartilage surfaces become **more radiolucent**. The osteopenia is a result of **osteoporosis** (i.e., diminished bone mass).
      (3) The peripheral regions of subchondral bone exhibit **erosions** (seen as notch-shaped deficiencies).
      (4) In **advanced rheumatoid arthritis**, the fingers become deformed or malaligned.
         (a) Permanent flexion of the distal interphalangeal joint and hyperextension of the proximal interphalangeal joint produces a **swan-neck deformity**, so called because the outline of such fingers resembles that of a swan's neck.
         (b) Permanent hyperextension of the distal interphalangeal joint and flexion of the proximal interphalangeal joint produces a **boutonniere deformity**, so called because the fingers assume this configuration when tucking a boutonniere in the buttonhole of a lapel.
         (c) The fingers may also exhibit ulnar deviation at the metacarpophalangeal joints.

6. **Determining the degree of bone mineralization**
   a. The mineral content of a patient's bones can be determined by measuring the **thickness of cortical bone in the second metacarpal** as displayed in a PA radiograph of the hand.
   b. The thickness of the cortex is measured on both the medial and the lateral sides at the midpoint of the diaphysis. **Bone loss** (as in **osteoporosis**) is indicated if the sum of these two cortical thicknesses is less than 4 mm.

STUDY QUESTIONS

Directions: Each question below contains five suggested answers. Choose the **one best** response to each question.

1. Radiographically, a grade III shoulder separation shows the acromioclavicular and coracoclavicular spaces of the injured shoulder to be wider than the corresponding spaces of the uninjured shoulder. For diagnosis of a grade III separation, the spaces must be wider by at least

(A) 25%
(B) 33%
(C) 50%
(D) 75%
(E) 100%

2. Which nerve is most likely to be damaged by trauma that produces an anterior shoulder dislocation?

(A) Musculocutaneous nerve
(B) Radial nerve
(C) Ulnar nerve
(D) Axillary nerve
(E) Upper subscapular nerve

3. A muscle that can extend, adduct, and internally rotate the arm is

(A) pectoralis major
(B) latissimus dorsi
(C) deltoid
(D) teres major
(E) subscapularis

4. A winged scapula is produced by loss of function of which of the following muscles?

(A) Serratus anterior
(B) Infraspinatus
(C) Teres minor
(D) Trapezius
(E) Subclavius

5. All of the following are muscles of the rotator cuff EXCEPT

(A) subscapularis
(B) supraspinatus
(C) infraspinatus
(D) teres major
(E) teres minor

6. The posterior cord of the brachial plexus gives rise to all of the following nerves EXCEPT

(A) upper subscapular nerve
(B) suprascapular nerve
(C) thoracodorsal nerve
(D) axillary nerve
(E) radial nerve

7. Correct statements regarding Erb-Duchenne paralysis include all of the following EXCEPT

(A) the condition is produced by a tear of the lower trunk of the brachial plexus
(B) the affected person walks with the arm hanging by the side of the body
(C) the affected forearm is noticeably pronated
(D) there is diminished power of flexion of the affected forearm at the elbow joint
(E) opposition of the thumb in the affected limb is normal

8. Which of the following axillary lymph node groups can be palpated against the chest wall in the center of the axilla?

(A) Anterior group
(B) Posterior group
(C) Lateral group
(D) Central group
(E) Deltopectoral group

9. Which of the following axillary lymph node groups is palpable posterior to the lateral border of pectoralis major?

(A) Anterior group
(B) Posterior group
(C) Lateral group
(D) Central group
(E) Deltopectoral group

10. Which secondary center of ossification is the last to appear in the humerus?

(A) The center for the medial epicondyle
(B) The center for the lateral epicondyle
(C) The center for the capitulum
(D) The center for the trochlea
(E) The center for the greater tuberosity

11. Growth plate fractures are divided into five types according to the Salter-Harris classification scheme. Which type accounts for more than 50% of all growth plate fractures?

(A) Type I
(B) Type II
(C) Type III
(D) Type IV
(E) Type V

12. Which type of Salter-Harris fracture extends through the growth plate and part of the epiphysis but not through part of the metaphysis?

(A) Type I
(B) Type II
(C) Type III
(D) Type IV
(E) Type V

13. Which muscle is innervated by both the ulnar nerve and the anterior interosseous branch of the median nerve?

(A) Flexor carpi ulnaris
(B) Flexor pollicis longus
(C) Flexor pollicis brevis
(D) Flexor digitorum superficialis
(E) Flexor digitorum profundus

14. Which nerve commonly is subject to increased pressure by a marked cubitus valgus deformity?

(A) Median nerve
(B) Radial nerve
(C) Lateral cutaneous nerve of the forearm
(D) Medial cutaneous nerve of the forearm
(E) Ulnar nerve

15. The dorsal aspect of the skin web between the thumb and index finger is innervated by which of the following nerves?

(A) Median nerve
(B) Ulnar nerve
(C) Superficial branch of the radial nerve
(D) Lateral cutaneous nerve of the forearm
(E) None of the above

16. Which of the following muscles is innervated by the deep branch of the ulnar nerve?

(A) Opponens pollicis
(B) Adductor pollicis
(C) Abductor pollicis brevis
(D) Abductor pollicis longus
(E) Extensor pollicis brevis

Directions: Each question below contains four suggested answers. Choose the **one best** response to each question.

17. An AP radiograph is taken after injection of a radiopaque solution into the synovial cavity of a normal shoulder joint. The solution should appear in

(A) the subacromion–subdeltoid bursa
(B) the subscapularis bursa
(C) both bursae
(D) neither bursa

18. The lunate casts a quadrangular outline in a PA radiograph of the hand if the lunate is

(A) anteriorly dislocated
(B) posteriorly dislocated
(C) both
(D) neither

19. A patient has a lateral radiograph of the wrist taken, which shows the center of the lunate colinear with the central axis of the radius and the head of the capitate lying posterior to the central axis of the radius. This patient's injury includes

(A) an anteriorly dislocated lunate
(B) a posterior perilunate dislocation
(C) both
(D) neither

20. A young boy accidentally smashes his hand through a glass window. He is cut across the entire length of the distal transverse crease on the anterior surface of the wrist; the cut extends down to the superficial surface of the flexor retinaculum, but not into it. Structures that are partially or completely severed include

(A) the ulnar nerve
(B) the median nerve
(C) both
(D) neither

Directions: Each question below contains four suggested answers of which **one or more** is correct. Choose the answer

A if **1, 2, and 3** are correct
B if **1 and 3** are correct
C if **2 and 4** are correct
D if **4** is correct
E if **1, 2, 3, and 4** are correct

21. An AP radiograph of a normal shoulder typically shows

(1) an oblique view of the glenoid fossa
(2) partially superimposed images of the humeral head and glenoid fossa
(3) a radiolucent space between the acromion process and the lateral end of the clavicle
(4) a greater tuberosity in profile if the arm is internally rotated to the extent that the line between the humeral epicondyles lies in a parasagittal plane

22. A significant drop, or inferior displacement, of the point of the shoulder occurs with which of the following injuries?

(1) A grade I shoulder separation
(2) A fractured clavicle
(3) An anterior shoulder dislocation
(4) Denervation of the trapezius

23. True statements regarding a grade III shoulder separation include which of the following?

(1) The acromion process and clavicle are dislocated at the acromioclavicular joint
(2) The fibrous capsule of the shoulder joint is often intact
(3) A downward blow on the point of the shoulder usually is the cause
(4) The sternoclavicular ligament is torn significantly

24. True statements regarding posterior shoulder dislocations include which of the following?

(1) Abduction and external rotation of the patient's arm are markedly limited
(2) The patient's shoulder is flattened anteriorly and bulging posteriorly
(3) An AP radiograph of the shoulder generally shows the humeral head in a subacromial position
(4) The humeral head is partially superimposed upon the glenoid fossa when the AP radiograph is taken with the patient's body turned 35° to 40° toward the x-ray film cassette

25. A normal lateral radiograph of a child's elbow characteristically shows which of the following features?

(1) A fat-density region representing the anterior fat pad is visible
(2) A fat-density region representing the posterior fat pad is visible
(3) The midhumeral line projects just posterior to the posterior margin of the capitulum
(4) The anterior humeral line projects just anterior to the anterior margin of the capitulum

26. Radiographs that provide an unobstructed view of the articulation of the radial head with the radial notch of the ulna include

(1) an AP radiograph of the elbow
(2) a lateral radiograph of the elbow
(3) an internal oblique radiograph of the elbow
(4) an external oblique radiograph of the elbow

27. The deep branch of the radial nerve innervates which of the following muscles?

(1) Extensor carpi radialis brevis
(2) Extensor carpi radialis longus
(3) Supinator
(4) Brachioradialis

28. True statements regarding Salter-Harris Type I and Type V fractures at the distal end of the humerus include which of the following?

(1) Type I fractures are associated with a better prognosis than are Type V fractures
(2) Both types usually show evidence of displacement of the distal humeral epiphysis
(3) Both types are likely to show evidence of fat pad displacement
(4) Both types typically show evidence of change in growth plate width

29. Statements that accurately describe nursemaid's elbow include which of the following?

(1) The injury commonly occurs as a result of a child's hard fall on an outstretched hand
(2) The child presents with an extended and supinated forearm
(3) A lateral radiograph shows a break in the colinear relationship between the capitulum and the central axis of the radius
(4) Posterior pressure is directed against the head of the radius during reduction of the subluxation

30. A PA radiograph of the hand shows which of the following features?

(1) The long axis of the capitate is colinear with the long axis of the third metacarpal
(2) The lunate has a semilunar outline
(3) The image of the pisiform is superimposed upon that of the triquetrum
(4) The radiolucent space between the scaphoid and the distal end of the radius is wider than that between the lunate and the head of the ulna

31. A lateral radiograph of the wrist shows which of the following features?

(1) The proximal surface of the lunate casts the more proximal of the two convex bony outlines that overlap the distal end of the radius
(2) The central axis of the capitate projects proximally through the center of the lunate
(3) The tuberosity of the scaphoid projects directly anterior to the head of the capitate
(4) The central axes of the third metacarpal and radius are colinear

32. The PA radiograph of the hand shows the ulnar angulation of the articular surface at the distal end of the radius. Angles that fall within the normal range of the ulnar angulation include

(1) 12°
(2) 9°
(3) 18°
(4) 4°

33. The lateral radiograph of the wrist shows the volar angulation of the articular surface at the distal end of the radius. Angles that fall within the normal range of the volar angulation include

(1) 15°
(2) 10°
(3) 20°
(4) 30°

34. Statements that accurately describe primary osteoarthritis of the hand include which of the following?

(1) The distal interphalangeal joints are affected more often than the metacarpophalangeal joints
(2) An affected joint has a narrowed joint space
(3) Subchondral bone areas of an affected joint exhibit osteosclerosis
(4) The periphery of subchondral bone areas of an affected joint exhibit erosions

35. Characteristic features of rheumatoid arthritis of the hand include

(1) more common involvement of the metacarpophalangeal joints than the distal interphalangeal joints
(2) narrowed joint space of affected joints
(3) osteopenia of periarticular bone areas of affected joints
(4) osteophytes of subchondral bone areas of affected joints

SUMMARY OF DIRECTIONS

A	B	C	D	E
1, 2, 3 only	1, 3 only	2, 4 only	4 only	All are correct

36. Statements that accurately describe a fractured scaphoid include which of the following?

(1) Most fractures occur in the proximal one-third of the scaphoid
(2) Pain in the anatomic snuffbox upon deep palpation is an indication of a fracture
(3) The fracture site is most apparent in radiographs taken 1 to 2 days after the injury
(4) Bony union of the fragments commonly is delayed or does not occur

37. Muscles that receive most or all of their innervation from the C5 and C6 spinal cord segment levels include

(1) brachioradialis
(2) teres minor
(3) biceps brachii
(4) triceps brachii

38. Lymph drained from the ring finger is filtered through which of the following nodes?

(1) Supratrochlear nodes of the elbow region
(2) Apical group of axillary nodes
(3) Lateral group of axillary nodes
(4) Central group of axillary nodes

Directions: The group of questions below consists of lettered choices followed by several numbered items. For each numbered item, select the one lettered choice with which it is most closely associated. Each lettered choice may be used once, more than once, or not at all. Choose the answer

A if the item is associated with **(A) only**
B if the item is associated with **(B) only**
C if the item is associated with **both (A) and (B)**
D if the item is associated with **neither (A) nor (B)**

Questions 39 and 40

For each of the following movements, select the muscle or muscles of the shoulder acting as prime movers of the movement.

(A) Serratus anterior
(B) Trapezius
(C) Both
(D) Neither

39. Elevating the arm to comb the hair

40. Shrugging the shoulder

ANSWERS AND EXPLANATIONS

1. The answer is C. [*I C 1 c*] An AP radiograph of a grade III shoulder separation shows the acromioclavicular and coracoclavicular spaces of the injured shoulder to be at least 50% wider than the corresponding spaces of the uninjured shoulder. A 50% or greater increase in the width of the acromioclavicular space confirms dislocation of the acromioclavicular joint. A 50% or greater increase in the width of the coracoclavicular space confirms significant disruption of the coracoclavicular ligament.

2. The answer is D. [*I C 2 a (2) (b)*] As the axillary nerve extends posteriorly through the quadrangular space, it lies directly beneath the fibrous capsule of the shoulder joint. Accordingly, the axillary nerve is likely to be damaged by trauma that produces an anterior shoulder dislocation, as such trauma would drive the humeral head anteroinferiorly from its articulation with the glenoid fossa.

3. The answer is B. [*I A 3 d (2)*] Latissimus dorsi is a powerful extensor, adductor, and medial rotator of the arm; it comprises most of the muscle mass of the posterior axillary fold. Pectoralis major and teres major cannot extend the arm, deltoid cannot adduct the arm, and subscapularis can neither extend nor adduct the arm.

4. The answer is A. [*I A 3 b (1) (b)*] The muscle tone of serratus anterior is the force that holds the lower platelike part of the scapula flat against the upper posterolateral aspect of the chest wall. If a person with a paralyzed serratus anterior muscle pushes forward against an unyielding object (such as a wall of a room) with the affected upper limb, the lower part of the scapula protrudes posteriorly from the chest wall. The protruding scapula is called a winged scapula because it resembles a rudimentary wing.

5. The answer is D. [*I A 3 c*] The muscles of the rotator cuff include supraspinatus, infraspinatus, teres minor, and subscapularis. All of these muscles insert onto the fibrous capsule of the shoulder joint, forming a musculotendinous cuff about the capsule. This cuff dynamically stabilizes the joint when prime movers of the arm exert their actions across the joint.

6. The answer is B. [*I A 4 a (4) (b) (ii)*] The suprascapular nerve arises from the upper trunk of the brachial plexus. The upper subscapular, middle subscapular (thoracodorsal), lower subscapular, axillary, and radial nerves are the five nerves that arise from the posterior cord of the brachial plexus.

7. The answer is A. [*I A 4 b (1)*] Erb-Duchenne paralysis is caused by irreversible damage to the C5 and C6 roots or to the upper trunk of the brachial plexus. The damage completely denervates deltoid and severely denervates biceps brachii. The loss of deltoid action abolishes the normal swinging arm movement that accompanies walking; the loss of biceps brachii action diminishes the power of forearm flexion and the extent to which the forearm is supinated. Thumb opposition is normal because the prime mover for this movement, opponens pollicis, is innervated by C8 and T1 fibers.

8. The answer is D. [*I A 5 c (4)*] The central group of axillary lymph nodes drains efferent lymphatics from the anterior (pectoral), posterior (subscapular), and lateral groups. The central group is therefore the second group of axillary nodes to be infiltrated when bacteria or malignant cells disseminate via lymphatics from superficial tissues of the upper trunk of the body or from the deep or medial superficial tissues of the upper limb.

9. The answer is A. [*I A 5 c (1)*] The anterior (pectoral) group of axillary lymph nodes drains the superficial tissues of the anterolateral region of the trunk down to the level of the umbilicus; these tissues include the lateral half of the mammary gland. The anterior group is therefore the first group of axillary nodes to receive malignant cells which metastasize via lymphatics from sites in the lateral half of the mammary gland.

10. The answer is B. [*I A 1 c (1); II A 1 a (2)*] The centers for the humeral head and the capitulum are the first to appear; they appear during the first 6 months after birth. The center for the greater tuberosity appears at 1 to 2 years of age, that for the medial epicondyle at 4 to 6 years, that for the trochlea at 8 to 9 years, and, finally, that for the lateral epicondyle at 11 to 12 years.

11. The answer is B. [*II C 2 c (2)*] The growth plate at the end of a developing long bone is the region most susceptible to fracture. An undue burden of stress forces extending across the end of the bone is the mechanism which generates Salter-Harris Type I to IV fractures; Type V fractures are the product of excessive axial compression forces.

12. The answer is C. [*II C 2 c (3); Figure 1-16*] A Type I Salter-Harris fracture extends through only the growth plate. A Type II fracture extends through the growth plate and part of the metaphysis. As indicated in the question, a Type III fracture extends through the growth plate and part of the epiphysis. A Type IV fracture extends through the metaphysis, growth plate, and epiphysis. A Type V fracture is a compression injury to the growth plate.

13. The answer is E. [*III A 3 a (3) (a)*] Flexor digitorum profundus flexes the distal phalanges of the fingers. The ulnar nerve innervates the medial half of flexor digitorum profundus; the anterior interosseous branch of the median nerve innervates the lateral half of the muscle. Flexor carpi ulnaris is innervated by the ulnar nerve. Flexor pollicis longus is innervated by the anterior interosseous branch of the median nerve. Flexor pollicis brevis and flexor digitorum superficialis are both innervated by the median nerve.

14. The answer is E. [*II A 4 a*] A cubitus valgus deformity diminishes the carrying angle of the elbow (i.e., the angle on the radial side of the elbow). This deformity increases pressure on the ulnar nerve along its course behind the medial epicondyle of the humerus; such pressure may affect the nerve's motor and sensory supply. The median and radial nerves cross the elbow region by extending through the cubital fossa, and the medial and lateral cutaneous nerves of the forearm cross the elbow region in the superficial fascia overlying the cubital fossa.

15. The answer is C. [*III A 4 c (3)*] The superficial branch of the radial nerve provides cutaneous innervation for roughly the lateral half of the dorsum of the hand. The median nerve provides cutaneous innervation for the lateral two-thirds of the palm and the palmar surfaces of the lateral three and one-half digits; the ulnar nerve provides cutaneous innervation for the medial one-third of the palm, the palmar surfaces of the medial one and one-half digits, and roughly the medial half of the dorsum of the hand. The lateral cutaneous nerve of the forearm is the terminal branch of the musculocutaneous nerve; it provides cutaneous innervation for the lateral aspect of the forearm.

16. The answer is B. [*III A 4 b (2) (b) (i)*] The deep branch of the ulnar nerve innervates two thumb muscles: adductor pollicis and the first palmar interosseous. The median nerve innervates three thumb muscles: opponens pollicis, abductor pollicis brevis, and flexor pollicis brevis. The anterior interosseous branch of the median nerve innervates one thumb muscle: flexor pollicis longus. The deep branch of the radial nerve innervates three thumb muscles: abductor pollicis longus, extensor pollicis brevis, and extensor pollicis longus.

17. The answer is B. [*I A 2 c (2)*] The subscapular bursa is an extracapsular extension of the synovial lining of the shoulder joint; the subacromion–subdeltoid bursa is not. Radiopaque solution commonly is injected into the shoulder joint to confirm or exclude a suspected tear of the supraspinatus portion of the rotator cuff. Such a tear establishes direct communication between the synovial cavity of the shoulder joint and the subdeltoid bursa.

18. The answer is D. [*III B 1 b (1) (b), C 1 a (1); Figures 1-19 and 1-22*] Anterior and posterior dislocations of the lunate cause an anterior rotation of this carpal bone on its convex, proximal surface. This rotation transforms its PA outline from a quadrangular to a triangular shadow.

19. The answer is B. [*III C 1 a (2), b; Figures 1-22 and 1-23*] In a lateral radiograph of the normal wrist, the central axis of the third metacarpal extends proximally as follows: (1) along the central axis of the capitate, (2) through the center of the lunate, and (3) along the central axis of the radius. When a patient's injury causes a posterior dislocation of all the carpals relative to the lunate (a posterior perilunate dislocation), a lateral radiograph of the hand will show the head of the capitate to lie posterior to the central axis of the radius.

20. The answer is A. [*III A 4 a (1), b (1)*] The ulnar nerve and ulnar artery extend across the wrist region by passing over the flexor retinaculum; here both the nerve and artery are susceptible to transection by fairly superficial cuts. Since the median nerve extends across the wrist region by passing through the carpal tunnel, it is not susceptible to transection by superficial cuts in the anterior wrist suface. Complete loss of the ulnar nerve's motor supply to the intrinsic muscles of the hand results in an inability to abduct or adduct the fingers (due to loss of function of the palmar and dorsal interossei and abductor digiti minimi) and hyperextension of the ring and little fingers at the metacarpophalangeal joints (due to loss of function of the third and fourth lumbricals).

21. The answer is A (1, 2, 3). [*I B 1 c, 4, 5; Figures 1-1A and 1-1B*] An AP radiograph of a normal shoulder shows the humeral head partially superimposed over the obliquely oriented glenoid fossa. The radiolucent space between the acromion process and the lateral end of the clavicle represents the apposed articular cartilages in the acromioclavicular joint. The radiograph shows the lesser, not the greater, tuberosity in profile if the arm is rotated internally to the extent that the line between the humeral epicondyles lies in a parasagittal plane. The greater tuberosity is seen in profile if the humerus is rotated externally, putting the line between the humeral epicondyles into a coronal plane.

22. The answer is C (2, 4). [*I A 1 b (1), 3 a (1) (b), C 1 a, 2 a (2) (a), 3 a*] The acromion process of the scapula underlies the point of the shoulder. The scapula is suspended in the shoulder region from both the vertebral column (chiefly by the action of trapezius) and the clavicle (chiefly by the coracoclavicular ligament). Consequently, the point of the shoulder drops if trapezius is denervated or if the clavicle is fractured. A grade I shoulder separation is merely a simple sprain of the acromioclavicular joint capsule, and, therefore, does not affect the scapula's suspension from the clavicle. Shoulder dislocations are injuries involving displacement of the humeral head within the shoulder region. With an anterior dislocation, the normally rounded contour is replaced by the contour of the acromion process.

23. The answer is A (1, 2, 3). [*I C 1*] A grade III shoulder separation is a dislocation of the acromioclavicular joint. A downward blow to the point of the shoulder can produce such an injury because it strains the suspension of the scapula from the clavicle via the coracoclavicular ligament and the acromioclavicular joint's fibrous capsule. The trauma which produces a grade III shoulder separation generally does not damage the sternoclavicular ligament or the fibrous capsule of the shoulder joint.

24. The answer is E (all). [*I C 2 b*] With a posterior shoulder dislocation, abduction and external rotation of the arm are markedly limited. Posterior displacement of the humeral head flattens the shoulder anteriorly and causes it to bulge posteriorly. The humeral head occupies a subacromial position in the AP radiograph because the head is generally not superiorly or inferiorly displaced. The angled AP radiograph of the shoulder offers the best projection for confirming a posterior shoulder dislocation because the radiograph unambiguously demonstrates the medial displacement of the humeral head posterior to the glenoid fossa.

25. The answer is B (1, 3). [*II B 1 a (5), b (2), (3); Figure 1-8*] A fat-density region representative of the anterior fat pad is observed in a normal lateral radiograph of a child's (or adult's) elbow. However, a comparable fat-density region representing the posterior fat pad is not observed because triceps brachii is pressing the posterior fat pad deep into the olecranon fossa. The midhumeral line does project just posterior to the margin of the capitulum, as stated in the question, but the anterior humeral line projects through the middle one-third of the capitulum.

26. The answer is D (4). [*II B 4 b; Figures 1-11A and 1-11B*] Of the radiographs listed in the question, only an external oblique radiograph of the elbow provides an unobstructed view of the proximal radioulnar joint. The AP projection superimposes the proximal end of the ulna on the articulation of the radial head with the radial notch of the ulna. The lateral and internal oblique projections do not provide a view of the joint space in the proximal radioulnar joint.

27. The answer is B (1, 3). [*II A 3 f, g; III A 3 a (1) (e)*] Supinator and extensor carpi radialis brevis (but not longus) are innervated by the deep branch of the radial nerve. Brachioradialis and extensor carpi radialis longus are both innervated by the radial nerve. Extensors carpi radialis longus and brevis extend and abduct the hand at the wrist joint. Supinator assists biceps brachii in supination of the forearm. Brachioradialis stabilizes the forearm in the midprone position; its tendon reflex tests the integrity of neuronal pathways at the C5 and C6 spinal cord segment levels.

28. The answer is B (1, 3). [*II C 2 c (1), (5), d*] Salter-Harris Type V fractures generally do not show any evidence of epiphyseal displacement or changes in growth plate width. The prognosis associated with Type I fractures is more favorable than that associated with Type V fractures because the former do not injure the proliferating chondrocytes of the growth plate. Elbow joint effusion with its attendant fat pad displacement is a consequence of all types of fractures about the elbow joint; effusion and fat pad displacement commonly occur with elbow dislocations as well.

29. The answer is D (4). [*II C 1 b*] The injury known as "nursemaid's elbow" generally results from a sudden pull on a child's upper limb. The child presents with a flexed and pronated forearm supported close to the trunk of the body. A lateral radiograph shows a normal colinear relationship between the capitulum and the central axis of the radius. A nursemaid's elbow can often be reduced by applying posterior pressure on the head of the radius while supinating and extending the forearm slowly and firmly.

30. The answer is B (1, 3). [*III B 1 b (1), (2), c (1); Figures 1-19A and 1-19B*] The long axis of the third metacarpal is colinear with the long axis of the capitate; this line represents the major axis for forces transmitted from the hand across the wrist to the forearm. The lunate itself casts a quadrangular shadow, but all four proximal carpals together (scaphoid, lunate, triquetrum, and pisiform) form a semilunar array of radiopaque shadows. The radiolucent space between the lunate and the head of the ulna (which bears the fibrocartilaginous disk of the wrist joint) is wider than the space between the scaphoid and the distal end of the radius.

31. The answer is E (all). [*III B 2 b, d, e; Figures 1-20A and 1-20B*] The lunate is the carpal with the most proximal surface in the wrist joint. The tuberosity of the scaphoid projects anterior to the head of the capitate. The central axis of the third metacarpal is colinear with the central axis of the capitate, the center of the lunate, and the central axis of the radius.

32. The answer is A (1, 2, 3). [*III B 1 a (2)*] The normal range of the angle of ulnar angulation of the articular surface at the distal end of the radius is 7° to 18°. A patient will suffer diminished adduction of the hand at the wrist joint if this angle is significantly diminished by improper reduction of a fracture at the distal end of the radius.

33. The answer is B (1, 3). [*III B 2 a*] The normal range of the angle of volar angulation of the articular surface at the distal end of the radius is 15° to 23°. A patient will suffer diminished grip function if this angle is significantly diminished by improper reduction of a fracture at the distal end of the radius.

34. The answer is A (1, 2, 3). [*III C 4*] The distal and proximal interphalangeal joints of the fingers and the carpometacarpal joint of the thumb are the joints of the hand most commonly affected by primary osteoarthritis. The affected joints exhibit narrowed joint spaces, subchondral osteosclerosis, and subchondral osteophytes. Subchondral erosions are seen in rheumatoid arthritis, not osteoarthritis.

35. The answer is A (1, 2, 3). [*III C 5*] The proximal interphalangeal and metacarpophalangeal joints of the fingers and joints of the wrist region are the joints of the hand most commonly affected by rheumatoid arthritis. The affected joints exhibit narrowed joint spaces, periarticular osteopenia, and subchondral erosions. Osteophytes are characteristic of primary osteoarthritis, not rheumatoid arthritis.

36. The answer is C (2, 4). [*III C 3*] Most scaphoid fractures occur in the narrowed midregion of the scaphoid. The fracture site is most apparent in radiographs taken 7 to 10 days after the injury, because bone absorption occurs at the site during the 7- to 10-day period, rendering the site more radiolucent. Deep palpation of the anatomic snuffbox is painful when the scaphoid is fractured. Axial compression of the thumb toward the anatomic snuffbox or an attempt by the patient to supinate the forearm against resistance are two other procedures which also generally elicit pain in the anatomic snuffbox if the scaphoid is fractured.

37. The answer is A (1, 2, 3). [*I A 3 c (3), 4 a (2)–(4); II A 3 a, c, f*] Brachioradialis and biceps brachii both receive most of their innervation from the C5 and C6 levels; the tendon reflex test of each muscle tests the integrity of neuronal pathways at these spinal cord segment levels. Deltoid and teres minor, which are innervated by the axillary nerve, are the two muscles of the upper limb that receive all, or almost all, of their innervation from the C5 and C6 levels. Triceps brachii receives most of its innervation from C7 and C8 levels.

38. The answer is E (all). [*I A 5 c (3), (4), (6); II A 5 c*] Much of the lymph drained from the medial half of the hand and the middle, ring, and little fingers is filtered through the supratrochlear nodes of the elbow region. The efferent lymphatics from the supratrochlear nodes drain into the lateral group of axillary nodes. The efferent lymphatics from the lateral group drain into the central group of axillary nodes, and the efferent lymphatics from the central group drain into the apical group of axillary nodes.

39 and 40. The answers are: 39-C, 40-B. [*I A 3 a (1), b (1)*] Elevation of the arm above the level of the shoulder requires lateral rotation of the pectoral girdle, a movement whose prime movers are serratus anterior and trapezius. Lateral rotation of the pectoral girdle occurs at the sternoclavicular and acromioclavicular joints.

Elevation of the pectoral girdle is the principal movement that occurs during shrugging of the shoulder, and trapezius is the sole prime mover of the movement. The spinal part of the accessory nerve innervates trapezius; the nerve is most vulnerable to injury along its superficial course through the posterior triangle of the neck.

2
Lower Limb

I. GLUTEAL REGION AND THIGH

A. Anatomy of the gluteal region and thigh

1. Bones

a. Innominate bone

(1) At birth, the innominate bone consists of three bones—the **ilium**, **ischium**, and **pubis**—united by cartilage. The iliac crest, acetabulum, ischiopubic ramus, and ischial tuberosity are all cartilaginous at birth.

(2) The **anterior superior iliac spine** and most of the **iliac crest** are palpable on the lateral aspect of the hip region.

(a) The most superior point of the iliac crest lies at the level of the spinous process of the fourth lumbar vertebra. This relationship is used to identify the L3–L4 and L4–L5 interspinous process spaces for the site of needle entry when performing procedures such as lumbar puncture or lumbar epidural anesthesia.

(b) Contusions of the muscles attached to the iliac crest and its anterior end, the anterior superior iliac spine, are colloquially called **hip pointers**.

(3) The **ischial tuberosity** is palpable in the gluteal region. The paired ischial tuberosities are the parts of the bony pelvis upon which a person rests when seated. Tenderness upon palpation of the ischial tuberosity is a cardinal sign of **ischial bursitis** (i.e., inflammation of the ischial bursa).

(4) The **pubic tubercle** is palpable near the medial end of the inguinal, or groin, region. The neck of a direct **inguinal hernia** lies superolateral to the pubic tubercle; the neck of a **femoral hernia** lies inferolateral to the pubic tubercle.

b. Proximal end of the femur

(1) The proximal femur (i.e., that part of the femur extending from the head of the femur to the immediate subtrochanteric region) in clinical practice is commonly called the **hip**.

(2) The proximal end of the femur has three secondary **centers of ossification** during childhood and adolescence:

(a) The **center for the head** appears during the first 6 months after birth.

(b) The **center for the greater trochanter** appears at 4 years of age.

(c) The **center for the lesser trochanter** appears at 12 to 14 years of age.

(3) The soft tissues overlying the greater trochanters are susceptible to ulceration in bedridden individuals.

2. Joints

a. Symphysis pubis

(1) The symphysis pubis is a secondary cartilaginous joint that unites the pubic bodies of the paired innominate bones.

(2) The symphysis pubis, the pubic bodies, and the superior pubic rami of the innominate bones together form an **osseocartilaginous arch** in the anteroinferior part of the pelvic girdle. This arch serves as:

(a) A tie beam that resists the tendency of the upper body's weight to thrust the innominate bones apart laterally

(b) A compression strut that resists the tendency of the lower limbs to thrust the innominate bones medially against one another

b. Sacroiliac joint

(1) The sacroiliac joint articulates the ileal wing of the innominate bone with the sacrum.

(2) The sacroiliac, sacrotuberous, and sacrospinous ligaments stabilize the sacroiliac joints by resisting the tendency of the upper body's weight to rotate the sacrum anteriorly at the joints.

(3) The sacroiliac joints and ligaments, the sacrum, and the ileal bodies of the innominate bones together form an **osseoligamentous arch** in the posterosuperior part of the pelvic girdle. This arch transmits the upper body weight onto the lower limbs.

c. Hip joint

(1) The hip joint articulates the head of the femur with the lunate surface of the acetabulum and the acetabular labrum.

(2) The hip joint provides for flexion, extension, abduction, adduction, medial rotation, and lateral rotation of the thigh.

3. Muscles that move the thigh

a. Extensors of the thigh

(1) Gluteus maximus is the chief extensor of the body trunk relative to the thigh when someone rises from a seated position. The muscle is also active in extending the thigh when climbing stairs or running. Gluteus maximus is innervated by the inferior gluteal nerve.

(2) Semitendinosus, **semimembranosus**, and the long head of **biceps femoris** are commonly called the **hamstring muscles**. They are the chief extensors of the thigh when walking. All three muscles are innervated by the tibial portion of the sciatic nerve.

(3) The hamstring portion of **adductor magnus** is an extensor of the thigh; it is innervated by the tibial portion of the sciatic nerve.

b. Flexors of the thigh

(1) Iliacus and **psoas major** share a common tendon of insertion onto the lesser trochanter of the femur and commonly act together, and hence are frequently named in tandem as **iliopsoas**. Iliopsoas is the most powerful flexor of the thigh; it is also the chief flexor of the body trunk relative to the thigh when someone rises from a recumbent to a seated position. Iliacus is innervated by the femoral nerve; psoas major is innervated by branches of the anterior rami of L1–L3.

(2) Sartorius is an active flexor of the thigh when walking. It is innervated by the femoral nerve.

(3) Pectineus is an active flexor of the thigh when walking. It is commonly innervated by both the femoral and obturator nerves.

(4) Rectus femoris, one of the muscles of the **quadriceps femoris**, is a flexor of the thigh; it is innervated by the femoral nerve.

c. Abductors and medial rotators of the thigh

(1) Gluteus medius and **gluteus minimus** are the chief abductors and medial rotators of the thigh. Their principal contribution to the walking gait, however, is exerted by acting from their insertions onto their origins when one lower limb is the sole weight-bearing limb; their contraction supports and steadies the upper body over the contralateral, non–weight-bearing limb.

(2) Gluteus medius and minimus are innervated by the superior gluteal nerve.

d. Adductors of the thigh

(1) Adductor longus, **adductor brevis**, and the adductor portion of **adductor magnus** are the chief adductors of the thigh; they contribute to the walking gait by serving as:

(a) Antagonists of the abductor actions of gluteus medius and minimus when one lower limb is the sole weight-bearing limb

(b) Synergists of the actions of the flexors and extensors of both the thigh and leg

(2) All three muscles are innervated by the obturator nerve.

(3) The **reflex test** of the adductor portion of adductor magnus is a phasic stretch reflex test of the integrity of neuronal pathways at the L2, L3, and L4 spinal cord segment levels.

e. Lateral rotators of the thigh

(1) Pyriformis, **obturator externus**, **obturator internus**, **superior gemellus**, **inferior gemellus**, and **quadratus femoris** are the chief lateral rotators of the thigh.

(2) Pyriformis is innervated by nerve fibers derived from S1 and S2; obturator externus is innervated by the obturator nerve. Obturator internus and superior gemellus are innervated by the nerve to obturator internus; inferior gemellus and quadratus femoris are innervated by the nerve to quadratus femoris.

4. Sciatic nerve

a. The sciatic nerve is derived from the anterior rami of L4, L5, S1, S2, and S3.

b. The sciatic nerve follows a curved inferolateral course through the lower medial quadrant of the gluteal region; this course extends from the greater sciatic foramen to the midpoint between the ischial tuberosity and the greater trochanter of the femur.

c. Intramuscular injections in the buttock should be placed in the upper lateral quadrant of the buttock because this is the quadrant furthest removed from the course of the sciatic nerve through the gluteal region.

5. Anatomy of the femoral triangle

a. Boundaries

(1) The femoral triangle is the triangular-shaped region in the anterior compartment of the thigh bordered **superiorly** by the inguinal ligament, **medially** by the medial border of adductor longus, and **laterally** by the medial border of sartorius.

(2) **Four muscles** form the **floor of the femoral triangle**; they are, from the most medial to the most lateral, adductor longus, pectineus, psoas, and iliacus.

b. Nerves, blood vessels, and lymphatics

(1) The **femoral nerve** and **femoral artery** enter the femoral triangle by passing deep to the inguinal ligament; the **femoral vein** and **efferent lymphatics** from the deep group of inguinal lymph nodes exit the femoral triangle by passing deep to the inguinal ligament.

(a) The **femoral nerve**, which is derived from the anterior rami of L2, L3, and L4, extends onto the floor of the femoral triangle at a point midway between the anterior superior iliac spine and the pubic tubercle (the entrance site lies immediately deep to the midpoint of the inguinal ligament).

(b) The **femoral artery** extends deep to the inguinal ligament and onto the floor of the femoral triangle at a point midway between the anterior superior iliac spine and the symphysis pubis. **Palpation of the femoral pulse** and **obstructive compression of the artery** are best performed along the proximal 2- to 3-cm segment of the artery in the femoral triangle.

(c) As the **femoral vein** extends over the floor of the femoral triangle to exit the thigh, it lies directly medial to the femoral artery.

(d) The group of **deep inguinal lymph nodes** lies aligned along the medial side of the terminal segment of the femoral vein in the femoral triangle.

(i) The deep inguinal nodes receive lymph from the popliteal nodes, the deep tissues of the thigh, and some of the superficial inguinal nodes.

(ii) The efferent lymphatics from the deep inguinal nodes drain into the external iliac nodes.

(2) The **femoral sheath** envelops the proximal segment of the femoral artery, the terminal segment of the femoral vein, and the deep inguinal nodes in the femoral triangle. In an adult, the femoral sheath extends for a distance of 3 to 4 cm distal to the inguinal ligament.

(a) The **femoral canal** is a potential space within the femoral sheath; it bears the deep inguinal nodes and transmits their afferent and efferent lymphatics.

(b) The superior end of the femoral canal is called the **femoral ring**, and the loose connective tissue which occupies the femoral ring is called the **femoral septum**. A **femoral hernia** is a weakness or opening in the femoral septum through which a tissue or organ may protrude.

(3) The terminal segment of the **great saphenous vein** and the vertical and horizontal groups of **superficial inguinal lymph nodes** lie within the superficial fascia overlying the femoral triangle.

(a) The **great saphenous vein** ends by passing through the saphenous opening in the fascia lata overlying the femoral triangle and then uniting with the femoral vein.

(b) **The vertical group of superficial inguinal lymph nodes** lies aligned along the terminal segment of the great saphenous vein.

(i) This group of nodes receives lymph from all the lower limb's superficial tissues except those of the posterolateral aspect of the leg and the lateral side of the foot.

(ii) The efferent lymphatics from the vertical group of superficial inguinal nodes drain primarily into the external iliac nodes.

(c) **The horizontal group of superficial inguinal lymph nodes** lies aligned parallel and inferior to the inguinal ligament.

(i) This group of nodes receives lymph from the urethra, the lower half of the anal canal, the external genitalia (which includes the vagina below the hymen in the female but not the testes in the male), the anterolateral abdominal wall up to the level of the umbilicus, and the superficial tissues of the buttock.

(ii) The efferent lymphatics from the horizontal group of superficial inguinal nodes drain primarily into the external iliac nodes.

B. Major features of the AP radiograph of the pelvis (Figure 2-1)

1. **Innominate bone and femur.** The radiograph shows major parts of each innominate bone and the proximal end of each femur.
   a. **Innominate bone**
      (1) **Iliac crest** and **anterior superior iliac spine** of the iliac wing
      (2) **Ischial tuberosity** and **ischial spine**
      (3) Superior ramus, body, and inferior ramus of the **pubis**
      (4) **Obturator foramen**
      (5) Roof, anterior and posterior rims, and medial wall of the **acetabulum** (The teardrop-shaped radiopaque outline immediately superolateral to the obturator foramen is called **Kohler's teardrop**; it represents the AP image of the acetabulum's medial wall.)
   b. **Proximal end of the femur**
      (1) **Head** (with fovea capitis)
      (2) **Neck**, **greater trochanter**, and **intertrochanteric crest**
         (a) The radiograph shows the **lesser trochanter** in profile and the **neck** foreshortened if the lower limb is neutrally or laterally rotated at the hip joint. The neck is foreshortened because the neck is anteriorly angulated (anteverted) at its union with the shaft of the femur. The **angle of anteversion** decreases during childhood and adolescence from the 30° to 50° range seen at birth to the 10° to 15° range of adulthood.
         (b) The radiograph does not show the **lesser trochanter** in profile if the femur is internally rotated by 10° to 15°. Such internal rotation also compensates for most of the anteversion of the femoral neck, and thus provides for almost maximum projection of the length of the neck.
         (c) The medial angle between the axes of the neck and shaft of the femur decreases during childhood and adolescence from an average 146° at birth to an average 127° by adulthood.
   c. In a normal AP radiograph of the pelvis, a smoothly curved line called **Shenton's line** can be drawn from the superior margin of the obturator foramen onto the inferior margin of the neck of the femur (see Figure 2-1B).

2. **Vertebrae.** The radiograph shows the bodies and the spinous and transverse processes of the **fourth and fifth lumbar vertebrae**, the upper lateral parts of the **sacrum**, and the **coccyx**.

3. **Joints**
   a. The AP radiograph shows the major joints of the bony pelvis.
      (1) The paired **sacroiliac joints**
      (2) The **symphysis pubis**
      (3) The paired **hip joints**
   b. The radiograph permits assessment of the width of the **radiolucent joint spaces** in the hip joint at three distinct locations.
      (1) The **superior joint space** lies between the superior margin of the femoral head and the roof of the acetabulum. The superior joint space bears the apposed articular cartilages of the femoral head and the lunate surface of the acetabulum.
      (2) The **axial joint space** lies between the femoral head and acetabulum, and extends along the axis of the femoral neck. The axial joint space bears the apposed articular cartilages of the femoral head and the lunate surface of the acetabulum.
      (3) The **medial joint space** lies between the medial margin of the femoral head and Kohler's teardrop. The medial joint space bears the articular cartilage of the femoral head and the fat and ligamentum teres of the acetabular fossa. The medial joint space is approximately twice as wide as the superior and axial joint spaces.
   c. The radiograph shows three **curved radiolucent lines** around the hip joint.
      (1) The radiolucent line medial to the femoral neck is called the **psoas line** because it represents a fat layer between the hip joint's fibrous capsule and iliopsoas's tendon of insertion onto the lesser trochanter of the femur.
      (2) The radiolucent line medial to the acetabulum is called the **obturator line** because it represents a fat layer medial to obturator internus.
      (3) The radiolucent line lateral to the femoral neck is called the **gluteal line** because it represents a fat layer between the hip joint's fibrous capsule and gluteus minimus's tendon of insertion onto the greater trochanter of the femur.

4. The **absence of pelvic rotation** is best assessed by the following criteria:
   a. The symphysis pubis is aligned with the midline of the sacrum.

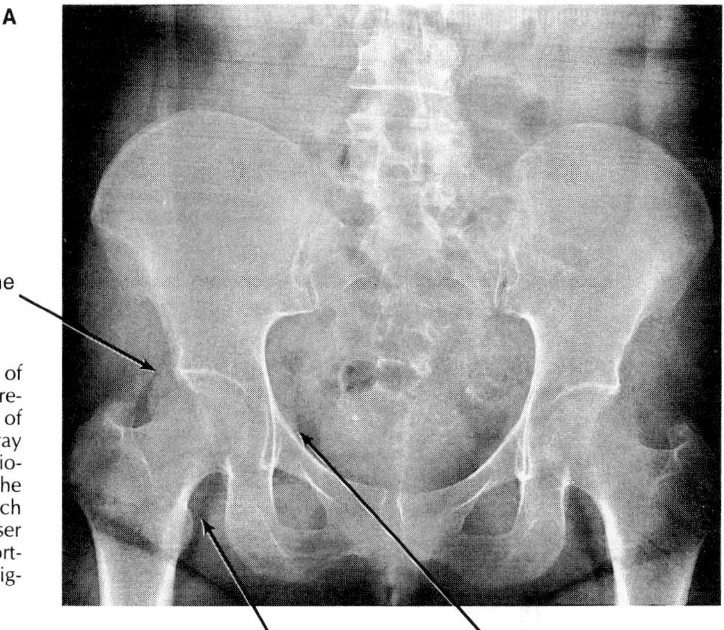

Figure 2-1. (*A*) An AP radiograph of the pelvis, (*B*) its schematic representation, and (*C*) the orientation of a patient's pelvis relative to the x-ray beam and film cassette for the radiograph. Note that in this instance the lower limb is neutrally rotated; such neutral rotation projects the lesser trochanter in profile and foreshortens the femoral neck, as seen in Figure 2-1A. (See section I B.)

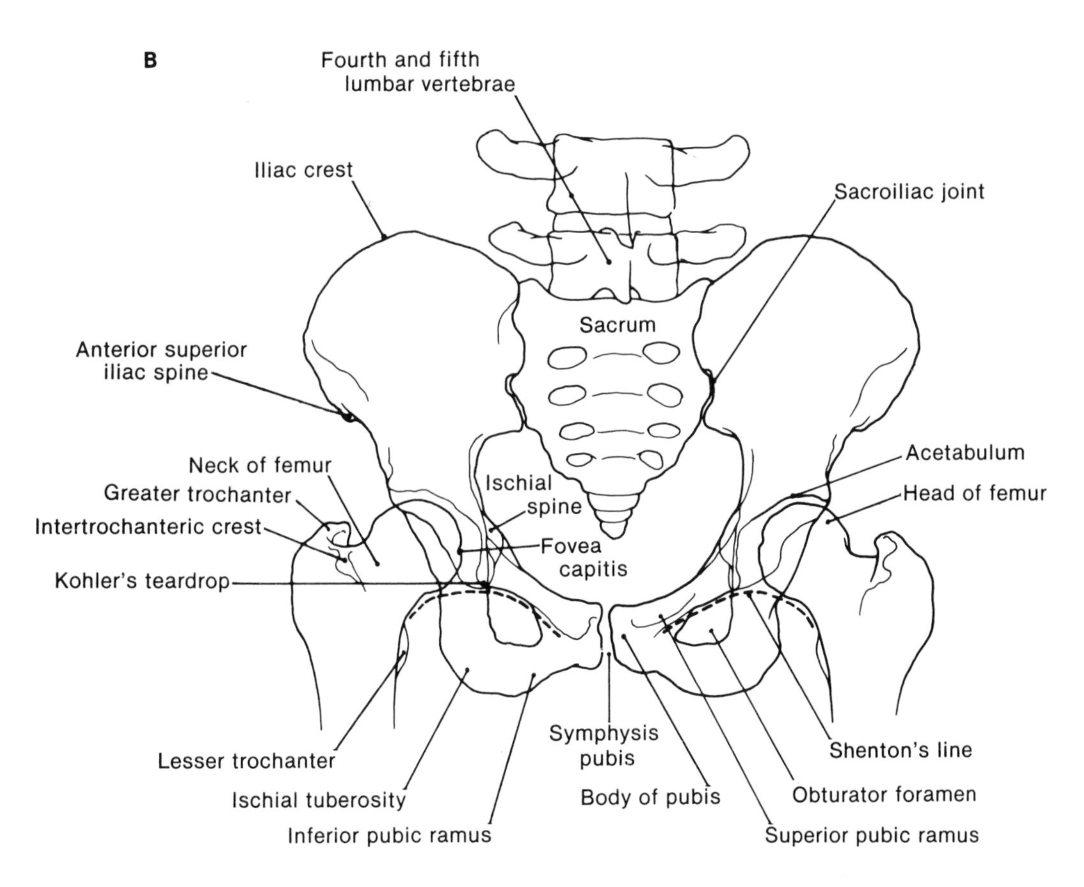

continued on next page

Figure 2-1. *continued*

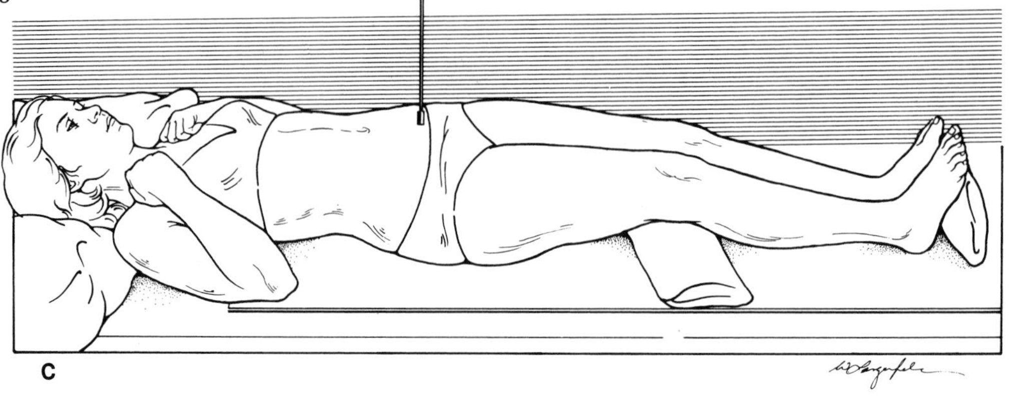

C

b. The paired obturator foramina are nearly identical in outline.
c. Kohler's teardrops are nearly identical in outline.

C. Clinical and radiographic features of common traumatic injuries, growth abnormalities, and diseases

1. Hip joint dislocations

a. Posterior dislocations of the femoral head from its articulation in the hip joint account for the majority of hip joint dislocations.

(1) Clinical features. A person with a posterior hip dislocation presents with a shortened, adducted, and internally rotated limb. The sciatic nerve commonly is compressed by the dislocated femoral head.

(2) Radiographic features. An AP radiograph of a posterior hip dislocation shows the head of the femur displaced superiorly from its normal alignment with the acetabular cavity.

b. Anterior dislocations of the femoral head account for most of the remainder of hip joint dislocations.

(1) Clinical features. A person with an anterior hip dislocation presents with an abducted and externally rotated limb. The limb may be cyanotic because of compression of the femoral vein by the dislocated femoral head.

(2) Radiographic features. An AP radiograph of an anterior hip dislocation shows the head of the femur displaced inferiorly from its normal alignment with the acetabular cavity.

c. Both posterior and anterior hip dislocations produce a discontinuity in Shenton's line.

d. Central dislocations of the femoral head are often associated with major acetabular fractures.

2. Fractures of the bony pelvis

a. Description of injury

(1) Since the bony pelvis is structurally a united ring of bones, breaks within the ring generally occur in pairs. The pair of breaks commonly are either a pair of fractures or a fracture accompanied by a joint dislocation.

(2) The superior and inferior pubic rami are the most commonly fractured parts of the bony pelvis; dislocation of the symphysis pubis is more common than dislocation of the sacroiliac joints.

b. Clinical features. There is a high morbidity and mortality associated with bony pelvis fractures because of attendant hemorrhagic shock and pelvic organ damage. In particular, it must always be assumed with bony pelvis fractures, until examination proves otherwise, that the bladder and urethra are also damaged.

c. Radiographic features. Bony pelvis fractures about or near the acetabulum may produce discontinuities in Shenton's line or changes in its curvature.

3. Femoral neck fractures

a. Clinical features

(1) Fractures of the femoral neck are especially common among the elderly; the contribution of osteoporosis to the genesis of such fractures accounts for the greater incidence of hip fractures among elderly women than among elderly men. Femoral neck fractures in young individuals occur as a consequence of severe physical trauma or pathologic bone disorders.

(2) Most femoral neck fractures in elderly individuals occur immediately distal to the femoral head (**subcapital fractures**). The attendant rupture of the circumflex femoral arterial branches to the head of the femur accounts for the common posttraumatic complication of avascular necrosis of the femoral head.

(3) External rotation of the foot is limited to 45° following **intracapsular fractures** of the femoral neck; this is because the fibrous capsule of the hip joint limits external rotation of the thigh (and foot) to 45°. External foot rotation can be as great as 90° following displacement of **extracapsular fractures** of the femoral neck.

b. Radiographic features

(1) Radiographs of acute, nondisplaced stress and impacted fractures of the femoral neck may show only an alteration of the trabecular pattern or a zone of increased radiopacity due to impaction.

(2) The integrity of the cortical bone in the femoral neck should be examined in all instances of suspected hip fractures.

4. Slipped capital femoral epiphysis

a. Pathogenesis

(1) The epiphyseal growth plate for the femoral head changes its orientation during the early years of adolescence, placing the plane of the growth plate in greater alignment with the direction of weight-bearing forces through the hip joint. This change in orientation subjects the growth plate to greater disruptive shear forces during the course of daily activities.

(2) The increased mechanical stress on the growth plate in combination with certain hormonal imbalances renders young adolescents vulnerable to a slipped capital femoral epiphysis; that is, vulnerable to a displaced, Salter-Harris Type I fracture of the epiphyseal plate for the head of the femur.

b. Clinical features. The patient presents with pain in the groin, thigh, or knee and with an **antalgic gait** (i.e., a gait in which the patient minimizes weight-bearing on the affected limb).

c. Radiographic features. An AP radiograph of a slipped capital femoral epiphysis exhibits one or more of the following radiographic signs (Figure 2-2):

(1) The medial edge of the growth plate abuts the lower rim of the acetabular cavity at an abnormally low point.

(2) The radiolucent space representing the growth plate is abnormally widened.

(3) A line drawn along the superior margin of the neck of the femur projects proximally above the level of the capital epiphysis.

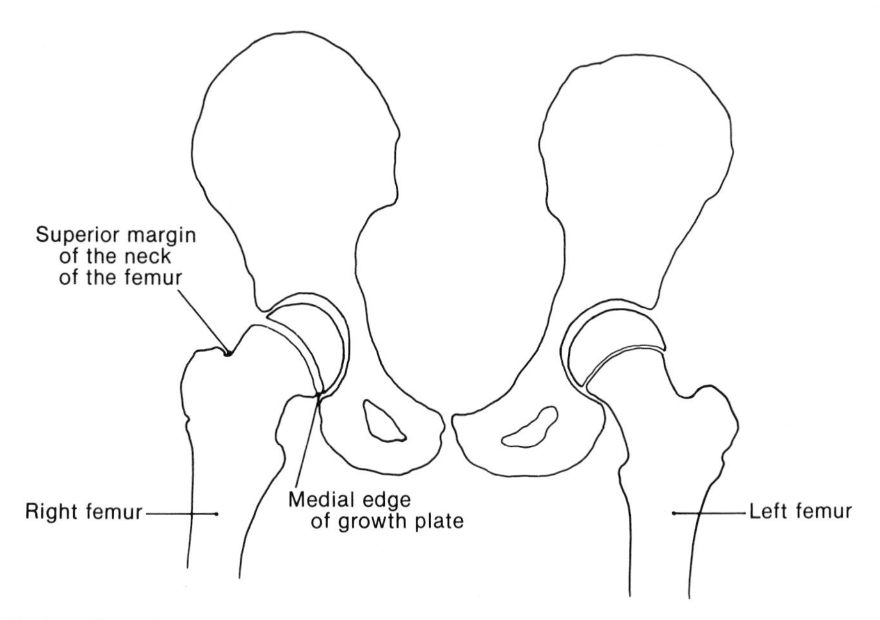

Figure 2-2. An outline of an AP radiograph of a pelvis with a normal capital femoral epiphysis (*left*) and a slipped capital femoral epiphysis (*right*). (See section I C 4 c.)

5. Legg-Perthes disease

a. Description and pathogenesis

(1) Legg-Perthes disease is idiopathic avascular necrosis of the head of the femur.

(2) During childhood, branches of the medial and lateral circumflex femoral arteries increasingly replace the artery of the ligament to the head of the femur as the principal source of blood supply to the head of the femur. This change in blood supply apparently increases the vulnerability of the femoral head to avascular necrosis as a result of mechanical or infectious insults.

b. Clinical features

(1) Legg-Perthes disease occurs almost exclusively in young Caucasian children, and is more common among boys than among girls.

(2) The onset of the disease is typically insidious. The child may complain of mild hip or knee pain and present with a slightly externally rotated thigh.

(3) The disease is unilateral in most patients; when present bilaterally, the disease is almost never in the same stage on both sides.

(4) The course of Legg-Perthes disease shows three major phases—initial, degenerative, and regenerative—and generally spans a 5- to 6-year period.

c. Radiographic features. AP radiographs of the pelvis in each phase appear as follows:

(1) **Early in the initial phase** of the disease, radiographs are generally normal. **Late in the initial phase**, radiographs may show one or both of the following signs:

(a) The widths of the superior, axial, and medial joint spaces of the hip joint may be increased.

(b) There may be a subchondral radiolucency in the femoral head; this finding represents a subchondral fracture.

(2) In the **degenerative phase**, radiographs show evidence of sclerosis and fragmentation of the epiphyseal ossification center for the femoral head (Figure 2-3A). Impaction of the fragments subsequently produces a flattened femoral head called a **coxa plana**.

(3) In the **regenerative phase**, during which the femoral head reossifies, radiographs show two characteristic changes:

(a) A femoral head that is ill-fitted to the acetabular cavity

(b) A truncated and widened femoral neck (Figures 2-3B and 2-3C)

(4) The time frames of the degenerative and regenerative phases generally overlap to a considerable extent.

6. Hip joint effusions

a. The **etiology** of hip joint effusions is extensive; some common causes are:

(1) Intracapsular fractures

(2) Transient synovitis

(3) Septic arthritis

(4) Osteomyelitis

(5) Legg-Perthes disease in children

b. Clinical features. A person suffering from a painful hip joint effusion is most comfortable when seated with the painful thigh slightly abducted and externally rotated at the hip joint. This orientation reduces the tension in the synovial membrane to a minimum because it maximizes the encapsulation of the femoral head by the acetabular cavity and labrum.

c. Radiographic features

(1) The most sensitive indicator of hip joint effusion in an AP radiograph is inferolateral displacement of the femoral head from the acetabular cavity.

(2) **In a child**, a reliable and sensitive indicator of hip joint effusion is medial displacement of the psoas line or the obturator line. However, lateral displacement of the gluteal line is not a reliable indicator because such displacement is artifactually generated if the pelvis is slightly rotated in the AP radiograph or if the thigh is slightly abducted or externally rotated.

(3) Displacements of the fat lines about the hip joint are unreliable indicators of hip joint effusion in adults.

7. Primary osteoarthritis of the hip joint

a. Clinical features

(1) Certain arthritides of the hip joint, such as osteoarthritis or acute suppurative arthritis, commonly elicit referred pain to the knee.

(2) The extent of the radiographic changes in an osteoarthritic hip does not always correspond with the severity of the pain and loss of function in the joint.

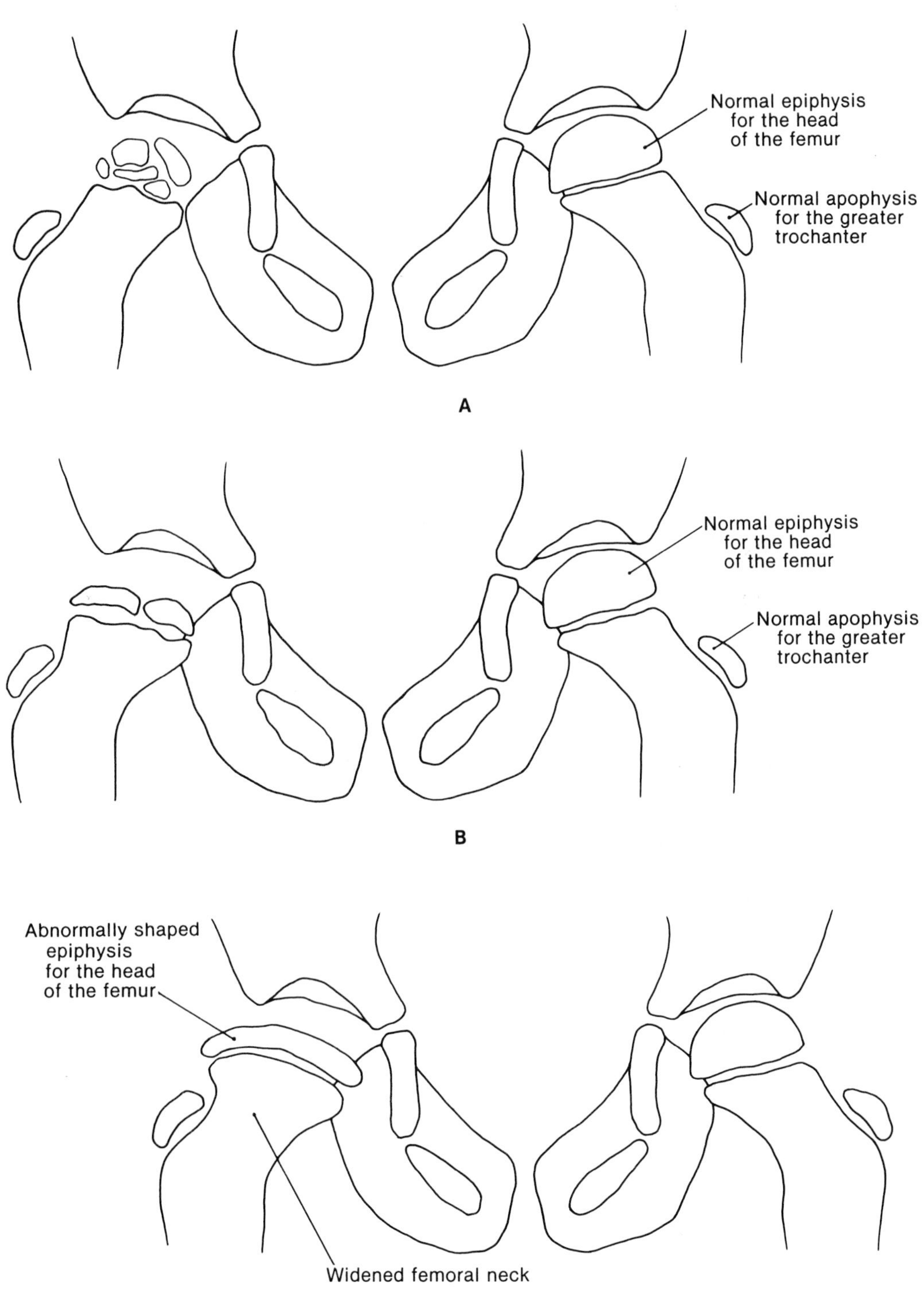

Figure 2-3. The characteristic outlines of AP pelvis radiographs of Legg-Perthes disease in the right femoral head taken (*A*) near the end of the degenerative phase, (*B*) early in the regenerative phase, and (*C*) late in the regenerative phase. The left femoral head is normal in each outline. (See section I C 5 c.)

b. Radiographic features

(1) The **superior joint space**, in particular, narrows in width as a consequence of **focal degeneration and thinning** of the articular cartilage surfaces. This focal thinning is commonly associated with a minor but distinct **superolateral displacement of the femoral head** within the acetabular cavity.

(2) The subchondral bone areas of the femoral head and acetabular cavity exhibit osteosclerosis.

(3) Osteophytes are formed mainly along the rim of the acetabular cavity and the margin of union between the femoral head and neck.

(4) Subchondral cysts may appear in the cancellous interior of the femoral head or the innominate bone about the acetabulum as a result of seepage of synovial fluid through minute fractures in the cortical bone of the femoral head or acetabular floor.

8. Rheumatoid arthritis of the hip joint

a. Clinical features. Flexion contractures at the hip joint may accompany progression of rheumatoid arthritis of the joint.

b. Radiographic features

(1) The **superior, axial, and medial joint spaces** all narrow in width as a consequence of **diffuse degeneration and thinning** of the articular cartilage surfaces. This diffuse thinning is commonly associated with a **medial displacement of the femoral head** within the acetabular cavity. The acetabulum itself may become so thin medially that the medial margin of the femoral head protrudes medial to the pelvic margin of the innominate bone (**acetabular protrusio**; Figure 2-4).

(2) The periarticular areas become osteopenic as a consequence of osteoporosis.

(3) The peripheral regions of subchondral bone exhibit erosions.

(4) Radiolucent cysts which communicate with the joint's synovial cavity may appear in the cancellous interior of the femoral head or the innominate bone about the acetabulum.

II. KNEE

A. Anatomy of the knee region

1. Bones

a. Distal end of the femur

(1) Longitudinal growth of the femoral shaft during childhood and adolescence occurs more actively at the distal end of the bone than at the proximal end.

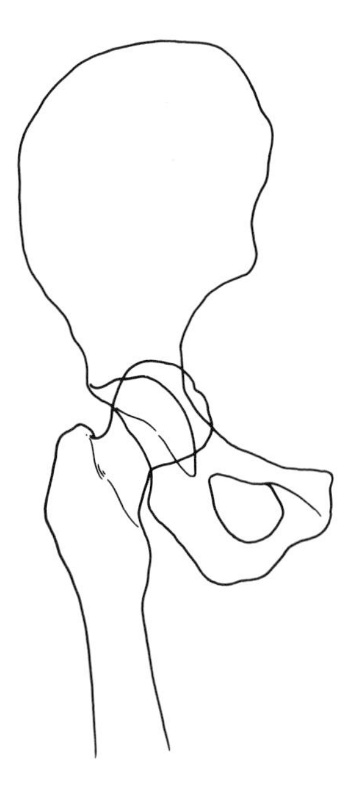

Figure 2-4. An outline of an AP radiograph of a hip joint with acetabular protrusio. [See section I C 8 b (1).]

(2) The distal end of the femur bears a single **secondary center of ossification** during childhood and adolescence.

(a) This center is the only secondary center of ossification among the long bones of the extremities that **always appears before birth**; specifically, it always appears by 36 to 37 weeks of gestation.

(b) Since this center is always present during the last 3 to 4 weeks of a normal gestational period, its presence in the lower limbs of an abandoned and deceased newborn forensically establishes that the child was viable at birth.

b. Patella. The patella is the largest sesamoid bone of the body. Ossification begins at the age of 3 years.

c. Proximal ends of the tibia and fibula

(1) The tibia and fibula each have a single **secondary center of ossification** at the proximal end during childhood and adolescence. The proximal tibial center appears at birth, and the proximal fibular center appears at 3 to 4 years of age.

(2) The **epiphysis** at the **proximal end of the fibula** is the first epiphysis of the fibula to fuse with its metaphysis during late adolescence; the epiphysis at the **proximal end of the tibia** is the last epiphysis of the tibia to fuse with its metaphysis.

2. Joints

a. Knee joint. The knee joint provides for flexion, extension, medial rotation, and lateral rotation of the leg.

(1) The joint consists of three **articulations**.

(a) The medial femoral condyle articulates with the medial tibial condyle and medial meniscus.

(b) The lateral femoral condyle articulates with the lateral tibial condyle and lateral meniscus.

(c) The patellar surface of the femur articulates with the posterior surface of the patella.

(2) Five major **ligaments** stabilize the integrity of the knee joint.

(a) The **anterior cruciate ligament** limits anterior displacement of the tibia within the knee joint during extension of the leg.

(b) The **posterior cruciate ligament** limits posterior displacement of the tibia within the knee joint during flexion of the leg.

(c) The **medial collateral and lateral collateral ligaments** together limit side-to-side movements of the leg at the knee joint.

(d) The **oblique popliteal ligament** strengthens the posterior part of the knee joint's fibrous capsule.

(3) Numerous **bursae** are encountered around the knee joint.

(a) Four bursae commonly communicate with the joint's synovial cavity.

(i) The **suprapatellar bursa** intervenes between the quadriceps femoris tendon and the anterior surface of the distal end of the femur. The suprapatellar bursa forms the most anterosuperior recess of the knee joint's synovial cavity.

(ii) The **popliteus bursa** is associated with the lateral aspect of the joint; it intervenes between popliteus and the lateral femoral condyle.

(iii) The **gastrocnemius bursa** is associated with the medial aspect of the joint; it intervenes between the medial head of gastrocnemius and the joint's capsule.

(iv) The **semimembranosus bursa** is associated with the medial aspect of the joint; it intervenes between semimembranosus's tendon of insertion and the medial head of gastrocnemius.

(b) Three bursae around the patella generally do not communicate with the joint's synovial cavity.

(i) The **prepatellar bursa** is a subcutaneous bursa that overlies the quadriceps femoris tendon where it envelops the patella.

(ii) The **superficial infrapatellar bursa** is a subcutaneous bursa that overlies the ligamentum patellae.

(iii) The **deep infrapatellar bursa** intervenes between the ligamentum patellae and the anterior surface of the proximal end of the tibia.

b. Proximal tibiofibular joint. The proximal tibiofibular joint articulates the head of the fibula with the lateral tibial condyle. The proximal and distal tibiofibular joints provide for only a small range of movement.

3. Muscles that move the leg

a. Extensors of the leg

(1) The four muscles of the **quadriceps femoris** (namely, **rectus femoris**, **vastus medialis**,

vastus intermedius, and **vastus lateralis**) are the sole extensors of the leg. All four muscles of the quadriceps femoris are innervated by the femoral nerve.

(2) The **quadriceps femoris tendon reflex test** is a phasic stretch reflex test of the integrity of the neuronal pathways at the L2, L3, and L4 spinal cord segment levels.

b. Flexors of the leg

(1) **Semitendinosus**, **semimembranosus**, and **biceps femoris** are the chief flexors of the leg when walking. Semitendinosus, semimembranosus, and the long head of biceps femoris (the **hamstring muscles**) are all innervated by the tibial portion of the sciatic nerve; the short head of biceps femoris is innervated by the common peroneal portion of the sciatic nerve.

(2) **Other flexors of the leg**

(a) **Sartorius** is innervated by the femoral nerve.

(b) **Gracilis** is innervated by the obturator nerve.

(c) **Gastrocnemius** is innervated by the tibial nerve.

c. Medial rotators of the leg. Popliteus, **semitendinosus**, **semimembranosus**, **sartorius**, and **gracilis** are the medial rotators of the leg. If the leg is fully extended, popliteus exerts its medial leg rotation action at the initiation of leg flexion to unlock the knee joint. Popliteus is innervated by the tibial nerve.

d. Lateral rotator of the leg. Biceps femoris is the sole lateral rotator of the leg.

4. Nerves, blood vessels, and lymphatics

a. The tibial and common peroneal nerves, popliteal artery, and popliteal vein are the major neurovascular structures of the knee region; they extend from the thigh to the leg by traversing the popliteal fossa.

(1) The **tibial nerve** and the **common peroneal nerve** emerge in the popliteal fossa upon extending distally beyond the diverging insertions of semitendinosus and biceps femoris. Both nerves extend through the popliteal fossa superficial to the popliteal vessels.

(a) The **tibial nerve** exits the popliteal fossa by passing deep to the converging heads of gastrocnemius.

(b) The **common peroneal nerve** exits the popliteal fossa by curving inferolaterally around the head and neck of the fibula.

(i) The nerve's relatively superficial course around the fibular head and neck renders it susceptible to damage from any trauma that crushes the tissues superficial to the head or neck of the fibula.

(ii) Irreversible damage to the common peroneal nerve as it curves around the fibula produces **footdrop**. In this paralysis, the walking gait is disturbed because the forefoot strikes the ground before the heel, due to the loss of the dorsiflexor actions of tibialis anterior, extensor hallucis longus, and extensor digitorum longus at the ankle joint (see also section III A 3 a).

(2) The **pulsations of the popliteal artery** can be felt upon deep palpation of the popliteal fossa with the leg partially flexed to about 45°.

(3) The **small saphenous vein** [see section III A 5 b (2)] generally ends in the popliteal fossa by uniting with the **popliteal vein**.

b. The most distal group of **lymph nodes** in the lower limb lie embedded in the fat of the popliteal fossa. These popliteal nodes receive lymph from the deep tissues of the foot and leg, and from the superficial tissues of the posterolateral aspect of the leg and the lateral aspect of the foot.

B. Major features of radiographs of the knee

1. AP radiograph. An AP radiograph of the knee has the following distinguishing features (Figure 2-5).

a. Femoral condyles

(1) The anteroinferior articular surfaces of the femoral condyles cast gently curved, convex profiles medial and lateral to the relatively shallow, concave profile cast by the anteroinferior border of the intercondylar notch.

(2) The distinct medial and lateral walls of the **intercondylar notch** project as faint vertical radiopaque lines at the distal end of the femur.

(3) The bony protuberance on the lateral surface of the lateral femoral condyle is the **lateral femoral epicondyle**, and the bony protuberance on the medial surface of the medial femoral condyle is the **medial femoral epicondyle**.

(4) The **adductor tubercle** casts a faintly radiopaque triangular image at the point where the medial supracondylar ridge meets the medial femoral condyle.

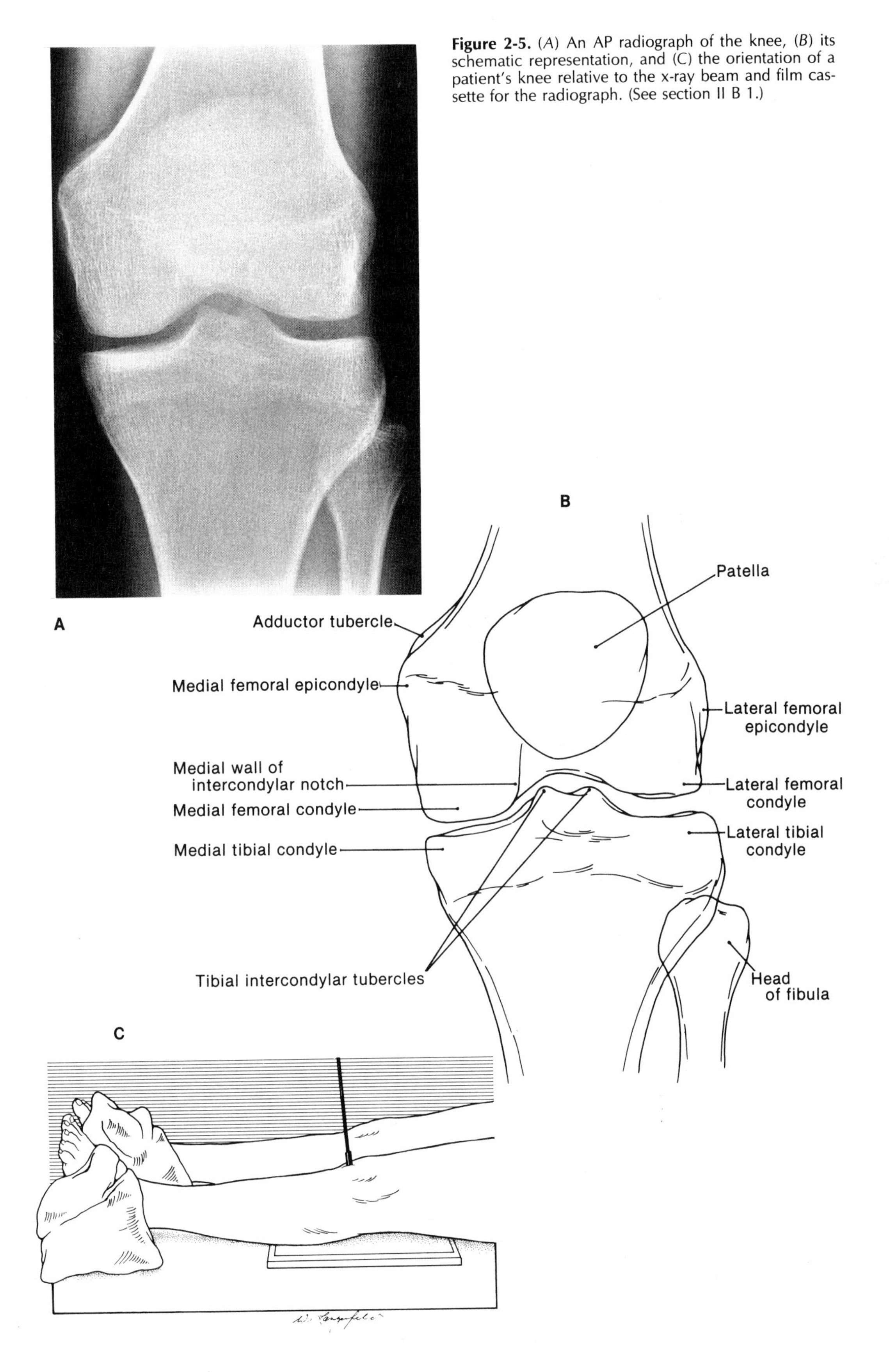

Figure 2-5. (*A*) An AP radiograph of the knee, (*B*) its schematic representation, and (C) the orientation of a patient's knee relative to the x-ray beam and film cassette for the radiograph. (See section II B 1.)

b. **Patella.** The image of the patella is superimposed upon the distal end of the femur; the center of the patellar shadow lies approximately at the level of the adductor tubercle when the leg is fully extended at the knee joint.

c. **Tibial condyles**

(1) The articular surfaces of the tibial condyles cast concave profiles medial and lateral to the profile of the **intercondylar eminence** and its pointed medial and lateral **intercondylar tubercles**. The articular surfaces of the medial and lateral tibial condyles are called, respectively, the **medial** and **lateral tibial plateaus**.

(2) The images of the **head of the fibula** and the **lateral tibial condyle** are partially superimposed.

(3) On both the medial and lateral sides of the knee, the radiolucent space between the femoral and tibial condyles represents the apposition of the **articular cartilages of the condyles** with each other and with the partially intervening **meniscus**.

(4) The radiolucent space bounded above by the concave profile of the anteroinferior part of the femoral intercondylar notch and below by the twin-peak profile of the tibial intercondylar tubercles bears the extracapsular **anterior and posterior cruciate ligaments**.

2. **Tunnel radiograph.** A tunnel radiograph of the knee provides an **angled PA projection** of the knee (Figure 2-6).

a. The tunnel and AP radiographs of the knee principally **differ** in that a tunnel radiograph

(1) Casts the highly curved, convex profiles of the posterosuperior articular surfaces of the medial and lateral femoral condyles

(2) Displays the relatively deep, concave profile of the intercondylar notch

(3) More clearly demonstrates the notch on the lateral surface of the lateral femoral condyle from which popliteus originates

(4) Does not show the patella en face

b. The tunnel and AP radiographs of the knee are **similar** in that each provides a low-angle sagittal projection of

(1) The articular surfaces of the medial and lateral tibial condyles

(2) The intervening intercondylar eminence with its pointed medial and lateral intercondylar tubercles

3. **Lateral radiograph.** A lateral radiograph of the knee has the following distinguishing features (Figure 2-7).

a. The **femoral condyles** each cast a knuckle-shaped profile. The images of the femoral condyles partially overlap each other; the contour of the medial condyle is more rounded than that of the lateral condyle.

b. The **patella** casts a quadrilateral-shaped radiopaque shadow.

(1) The **quadriceps femoris tendon** is seen as a **water-density band** (i.e., a band having a radiographic density characteristic of water) extending from the lower anterior thigh to the superior border of the patella.

(2) The poorly delineated fat-density zone posterior to the image of the quadriceps femoris tendon represents the **suprapatellar fat pad**, into which the **suprapatellar bursa** protrudes.

(3) The water-density band extending from the patella to the tibial tuberosity represents the **ligamentum patellae**.

(4) The poorly delineated fat-density zone posterior to the image of the ligamentum patellae represents the **infrapatellar (Hoffa's) fat pad**.

c. The images of the **tibial plateaus** overlap each other. The tibial bony prominence anterior and distal to the tibial plateaus is the **tibial tuberosity**, which is the attachment site of the ligamentum patellae.

d. The **head of the fibula** is partially overlapped by the tibial condyles; the view of the remainder of the fibular head and the proximal part of the fibular shaft is unobstructed.

e. About 10% to 20% of individuals have a small sesamoid bone, the **fabella**, embedded in the lateral head of gastrocnemius. When present, the fabella casts a sesame seed–shaped radiopaque shadow directly behind the femoral condyles.

4. **Axial radiograph.** An axial radiograph of the patella has the following distinguishing features (Figure 2-8).

a. The radiograph shows in profile the superior aspect of the grooved **patellar surface of the femur**. The **medial and lateral femoral condyles** form prominent shoulders on the sides of the patellar surface.

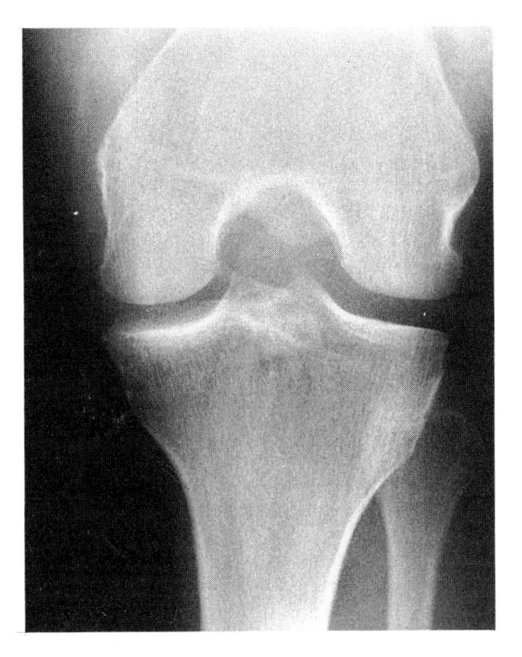

Figure 2-6. (*A*) A tunnel radiograph of the knee, (*B*) its schematic representation, and (C) the orientation of a patient's knee relative to the x-ray beam and film cassette for the radiograph. (See section II B 2.)

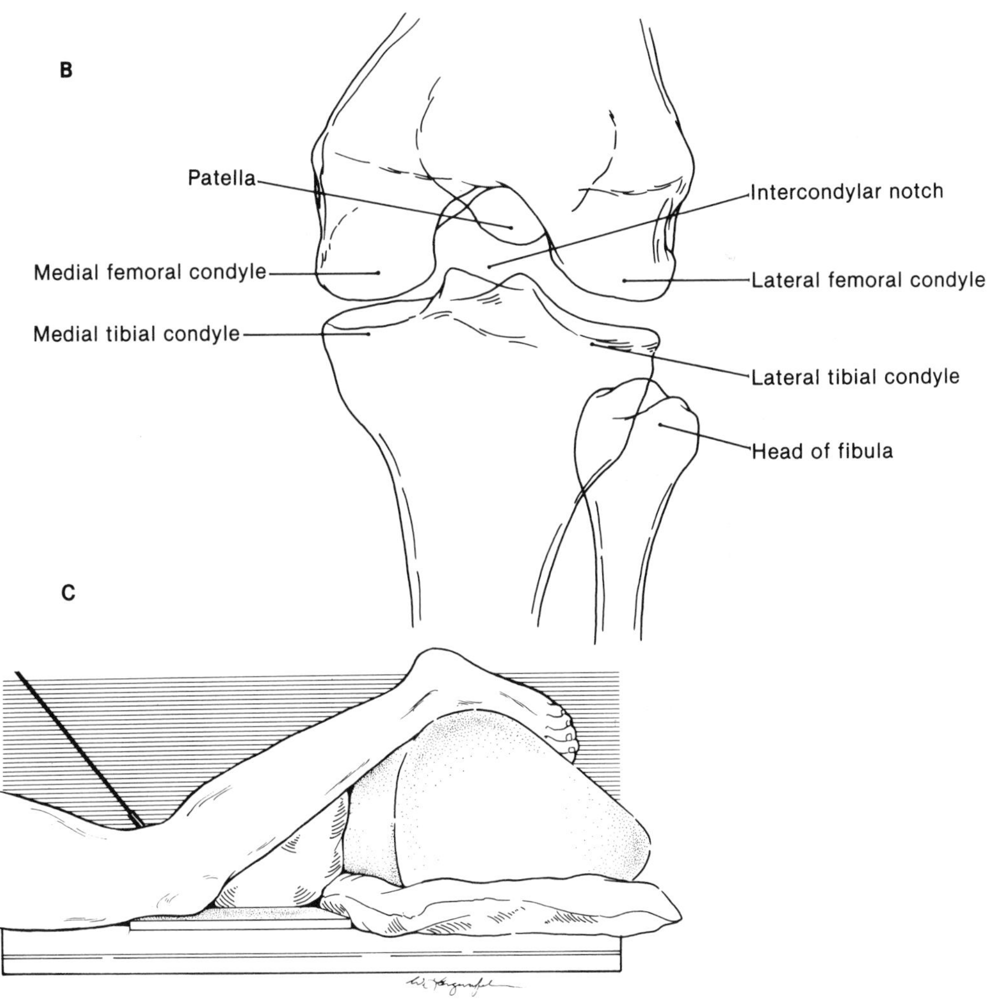

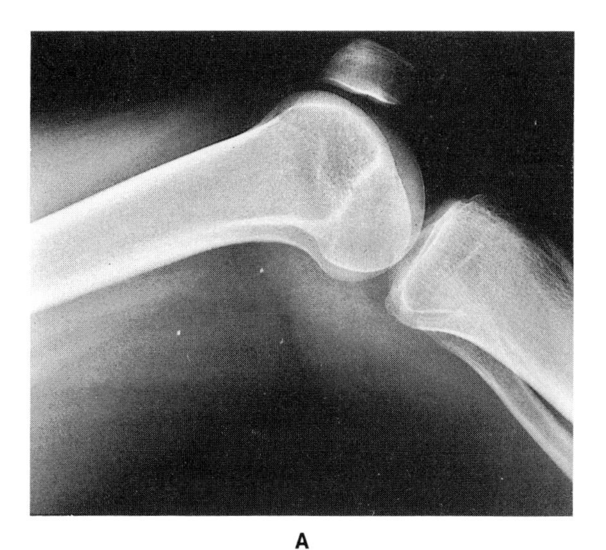

A

Figure 2-7. (*A*) A lateral radiograph of the knee, (*B*) its schematic representation and (*C*) the orientation of a patient's knee relative to the x-ray beam and film cassette for the radiograph. (See section II B 3.)

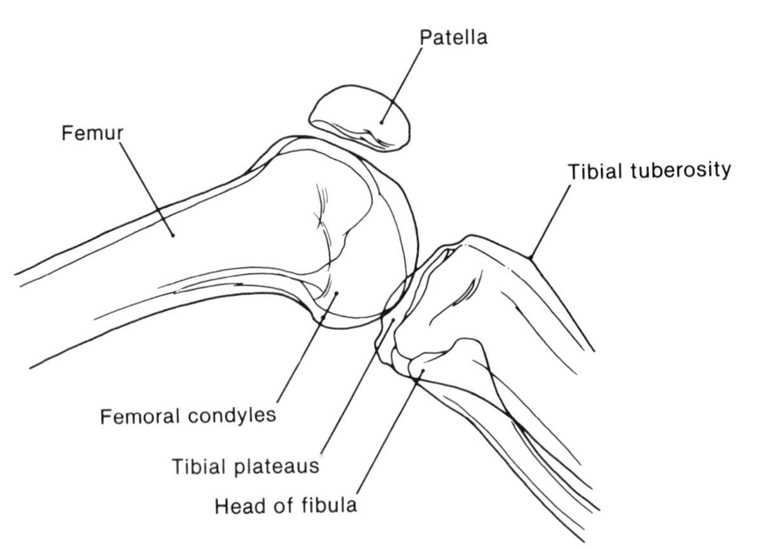

B

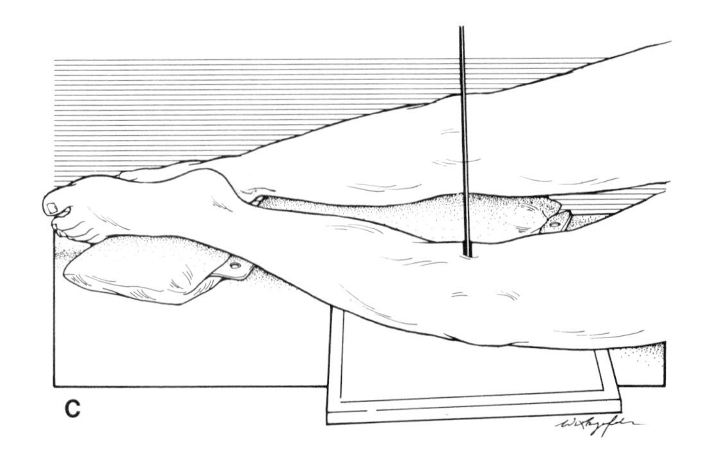

C

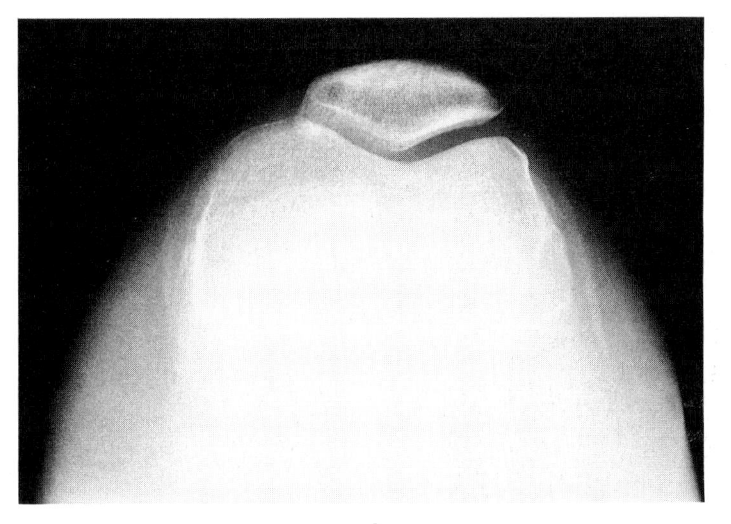

A

Figure 2-8. (*A*) An axial radiograph of the knee, (*B*) its schematic representation, and (*C*) a commonly selected orientation of the patient's knee relative to the x-ray beam and film cassette for the radiograph. (See section II B 4.) [Figure 2-8C is adapted with permission from Greenspan A: *Orthopedic Radiology*. Philadelphia, Lippincott, 1988, p. 6.5.]

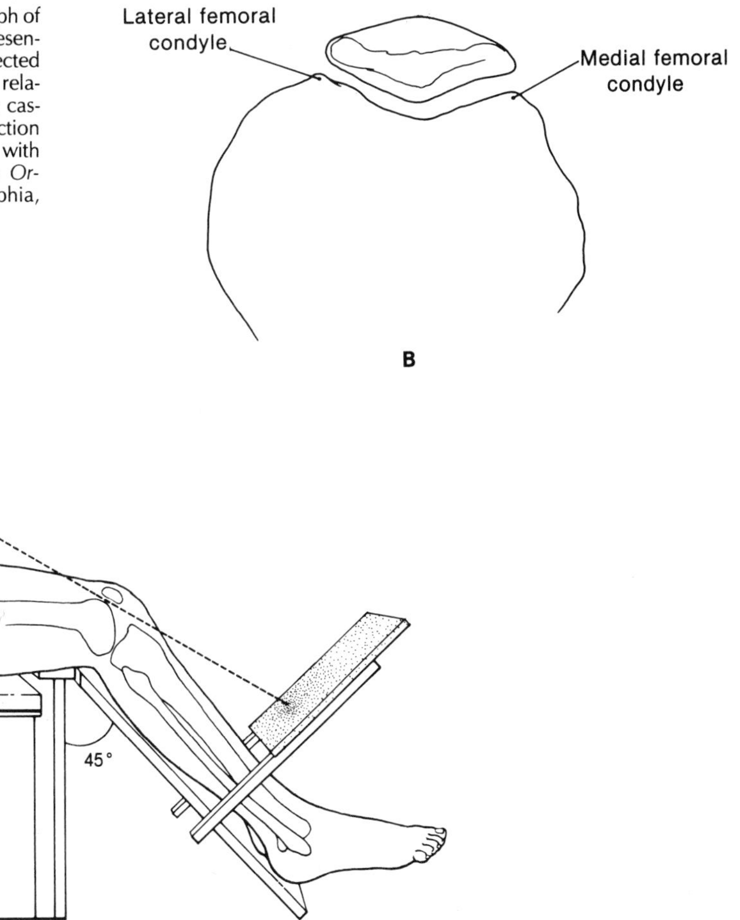

b. The radiograph provides a low-angle superoinferior projection of the **articular surface of the patella**. The lateral limb of the V-shaped articular surface of the patella is longer than the medial limb.

c. The lateral limbs of the patellar and femoral articular surfaces are parallel; the medial limbs diverge as they extend medially.

C. Major features of T1-weighted magnetic resonance (MR) images* of 3-mm-thick coronal sections of the knee

1. A coronal section through the patella exemplifies the characteristic appearance of **compact and cancellous bone** in T1-weighted images (Figure 2-9):

a. Compact (cortical) bone generates a very **weak signal**. The thin, dark perimeter of the patella thus delineates this sesamoid bone's cortex.

b. Fat generates a **high-intensity signal**. The patella's subcortical brightness is a measure of the fat content of its cancellous interior.

2. A coronal section 18 mm posterior to the patellar section shows the following features (Figure 2-10).

a. The **vastus lateralis and medialis muscles** generate signals of moderately low intensity on, respectively, the lateral and medial sides of the femoral shaft.

b. The **subcutaneous fat** on each side of the lower thigh appears as a high-intensity band superficial to the vastus muscle.

c. The remnant of the **epiphyseal growth plate** at the distal end of the **femur** appears as a tenuous band of low intensity.

d. The **infrapatellar fat pad** generates a high-intensity signal in the space anterior to the femoral and tibial condyles.

e. The **iliotibial tract** appears as a low-intensity band extending past the lateral side of the knee to merge with the dark band of cortical bone on the lateral surface of the lateral tibial condyle.

A

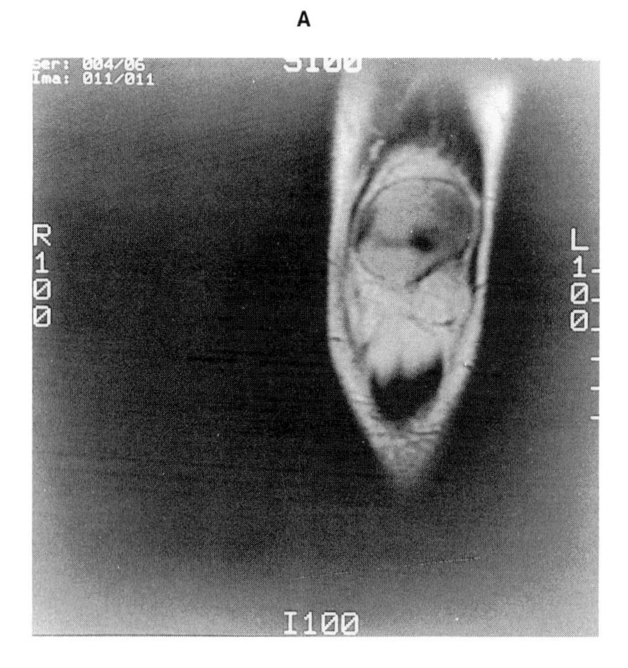

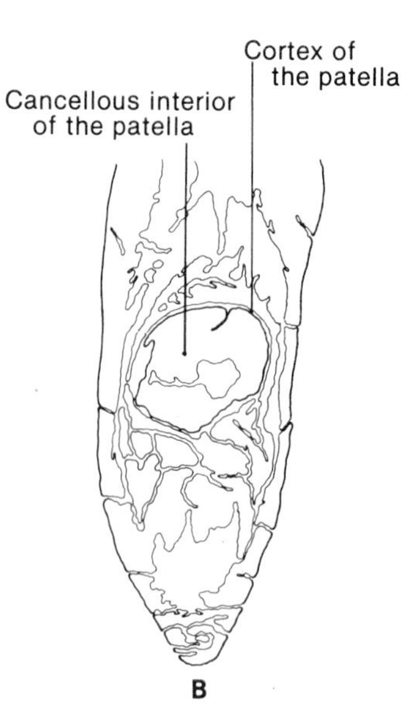

Figure 2-9. (*A*) A T1-weighted MR image of a coronal section through the patella and (*B*) its schematic representation. (See section II C 1.)

*Magnetic resonance images are produced by radiofrequency signals coming from the body following exposure to radio waves. Excited atomic nuclei (i.e., the nuclei producing the radiofrequency signals) return to lower-energy states via two processes, called T1 and T2 relaxation. T1-weighted images are images in which the differences in radiofrequency signal strength between different tissues primarily represent differences in T1 relaxation times.

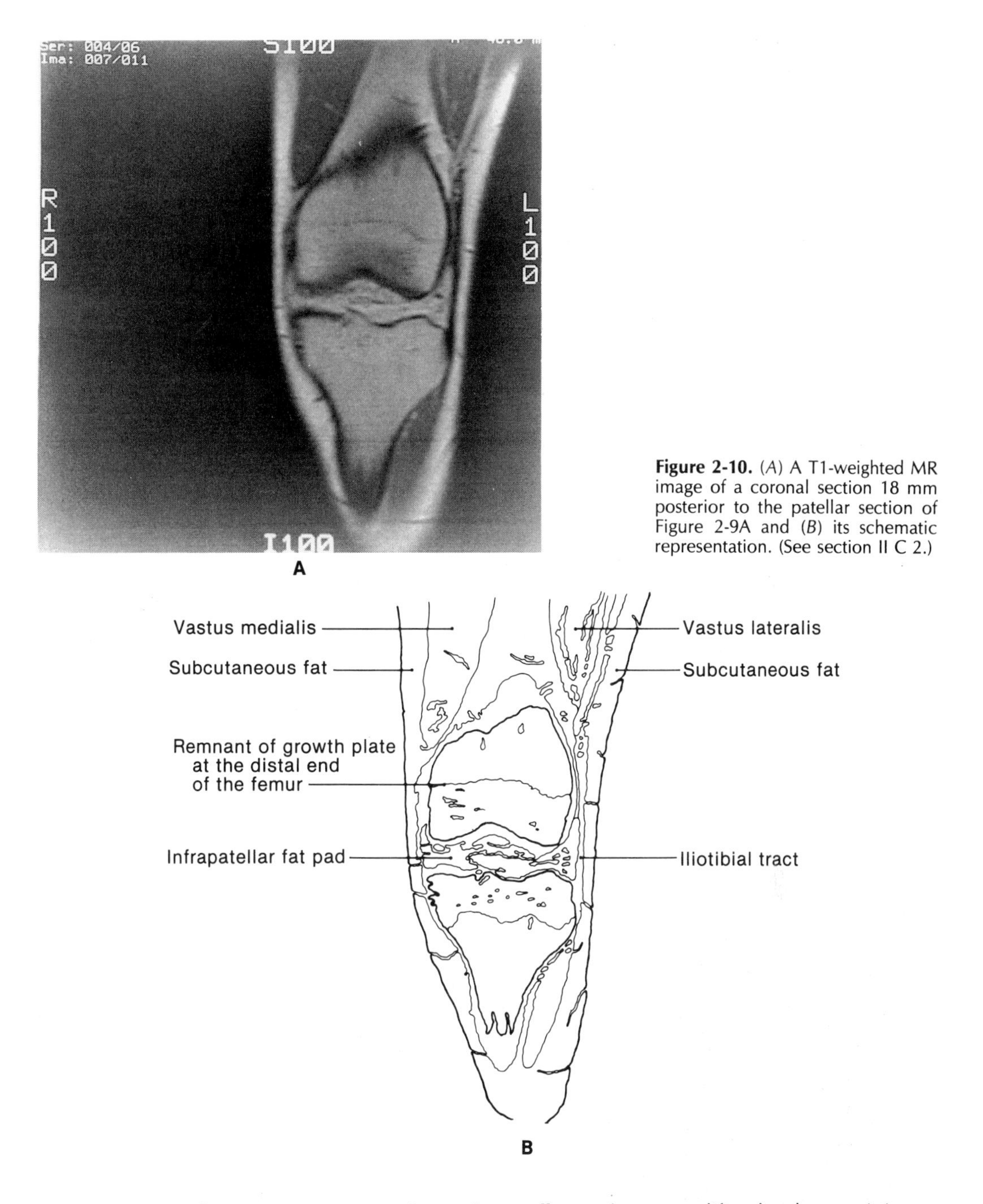

Figure 2-10. (*A*) A T1-weighted MR image of a coronal section 18 mm posterior to the patellar section of Figure 2-9A and (*B*) its schematic representation. (See section II C 2.)

3. **A coronal section 36 mm posterior to the patellar section** exemplifies the characteristic appearance of **ligaments and articular cartilage** in T1-weighted images (Figure 2-11):
   a. **Ligaments** generate a **low-intensity signal**. Thus, the **medial collateral ligament** of the knee joint appears as a low-intensity band merging
      (1) Superiorly with the dark band of cortical bone of the medial femoral epicondyle
      (2) Inferiorly with the dark band of cortical bone on the medial surface of the medial tibial condyle
   b. **Articular cartilage** generates an **intermediate-density signal**.
      (1) The **articular cartilages** covering the **medial condyles of the femur and tibia** generate an intermediate-density region between the condyles. The small triangular region of low intensity at the medial limit of the blended images of the articular cartilages represents the **medial meniscus**.

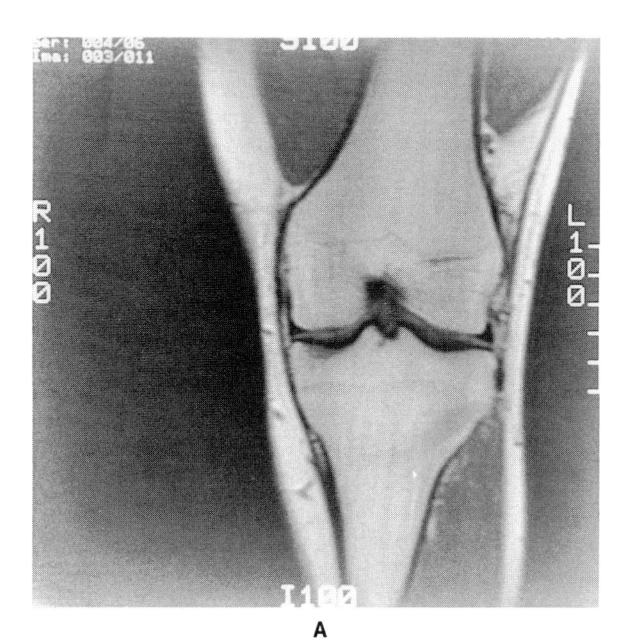

A

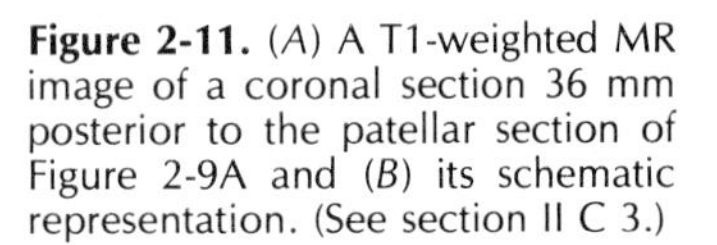

Figure 2-11. (*A*) A T1-weighted MR image of a coronal section 36 mm posterior to the patellar section of Figure 2-9A and (*B*) its schematic representation. (See section II C 3.)

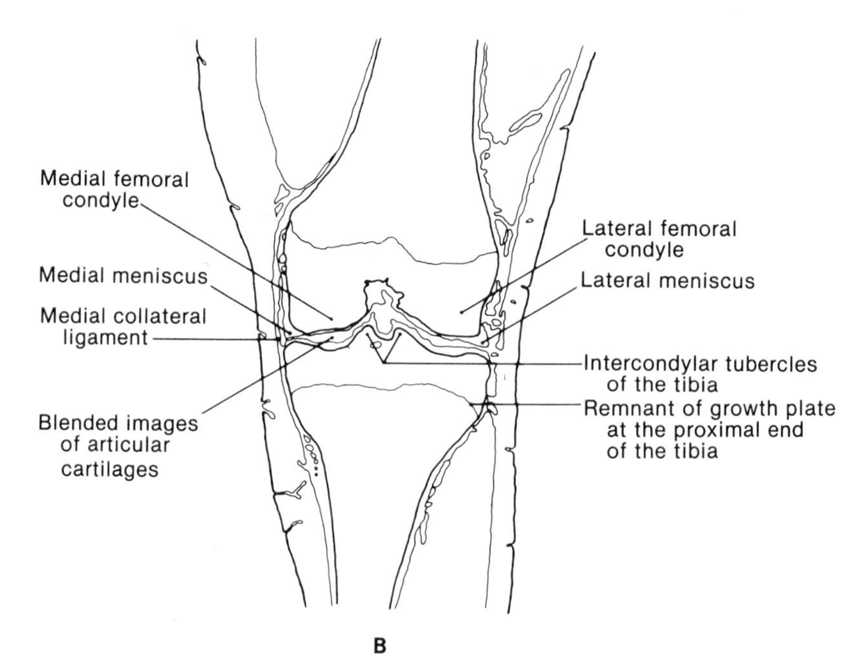

B

(2) As on the medial side of the joint, the **articular cartilages** covering the **lateral condyles of the femur and tibia** generate an intermediate-density region between the condyles. The small triangular region of low intensity at the lateral limit of the blended images of the articular cartilages represents the **lateral meniscus**.

c. The **cortical bone** of the **intercondylar tubercles of the tibia** caps the tubercles in dark outline just beneath the anterior part of the intercondylar notch of the femur.

d. The remnant of the **epiphyseal growth plate** at the proximal end of the **tibia** appears as a tenuous band of low intensity.

4. A coronal section 45 mm posterior to the patellar section shows the following features (Figure 2-12).

a. Some structures appear much as in the preceding (36 mm) coronal section:

(1) The **medial collateral ligament** appears as a low-intensity band extending from the dark band of cortical bone of the medial femoral epicondyle to the dark band of cortical bone on the medial surface of the medial tibial condyle.

(2) The images of the apposed femoral and tibial **articular cartilages** are blended on each side of the knee joint.

(3) The **medial and lateral menisci** appear as small triangular regions of low intensity.

b. The **lateral collateral ligament** of the knee joint appears as a low-intensity band extending from the dark band of cortical bone of the lateral epicondyle of the femur to the dark band of cortical bone on the head of the fibula.

c. The **posterior cruciate ligament** appears as a short, thick, low-intensity band extending inferolaterally from the lateral surface of the medial femoral condyle.

d. The section includes the notch on the lateral surface of the lateral condyle of the femur for the origin of popliteus.

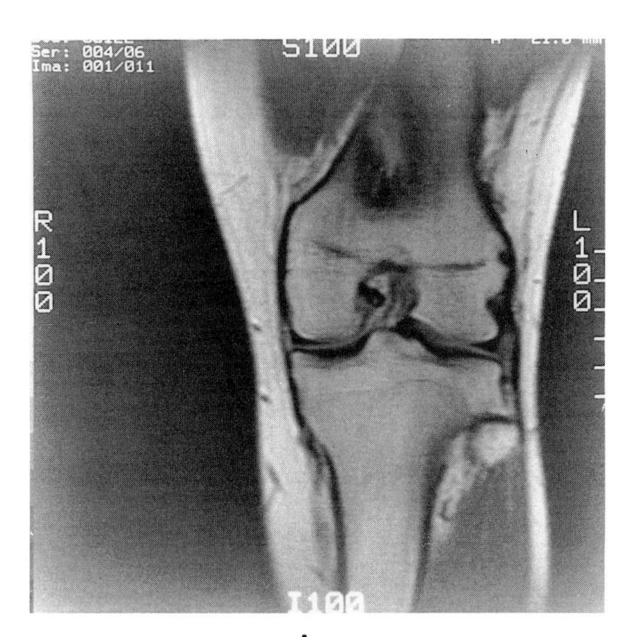

A

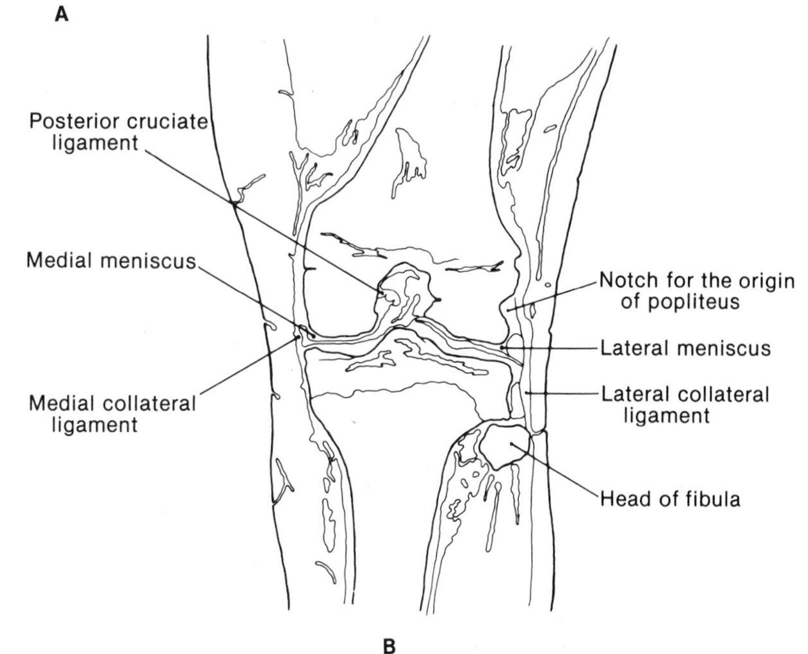

B

Figure 2-12. (*A*) A T1-weighted MR image of a coronal section 45 mm posterior to the patellar section of Figure 2-9A and (*B*) its schematic representation. (See section II C 4.)

5. **A coronal section 53.5 mm posterior to the patellar section** shows the following features (Figure 2-13).
   a. The **posterior cruciate ligament** appears as a thick, low-intensity band that tapers as it extends superomedially from its attachment to the posterior area of the tibial intercondylar surface.
   b. The **posterior horns of the medial and lateral menisci** each appear as a thick, low-intensity band sandwiched between the femoral condyle above and the articular cartilage of the tibial plateau below.

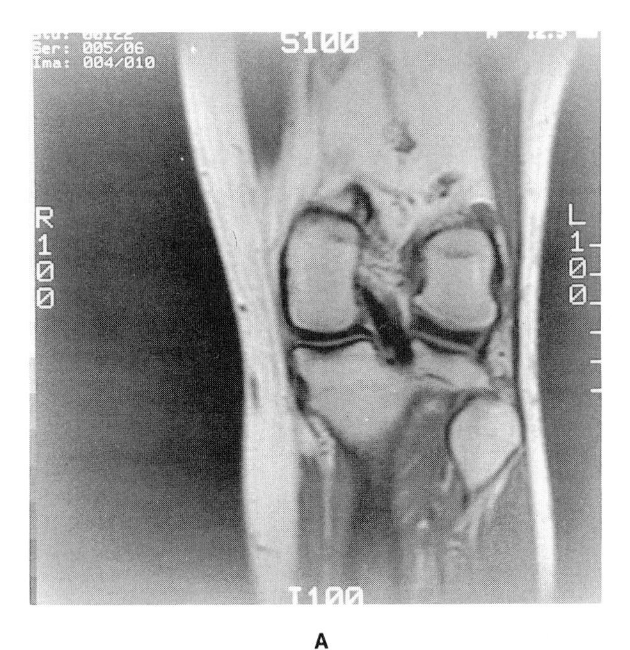

A

Figure 2-13. (*A*) A T1-weighted MR image of a coronal section 53.5 mm posterior to the patellar section of Figure 2-9A and (*B*) its schematic representation. (See section II C 5.)

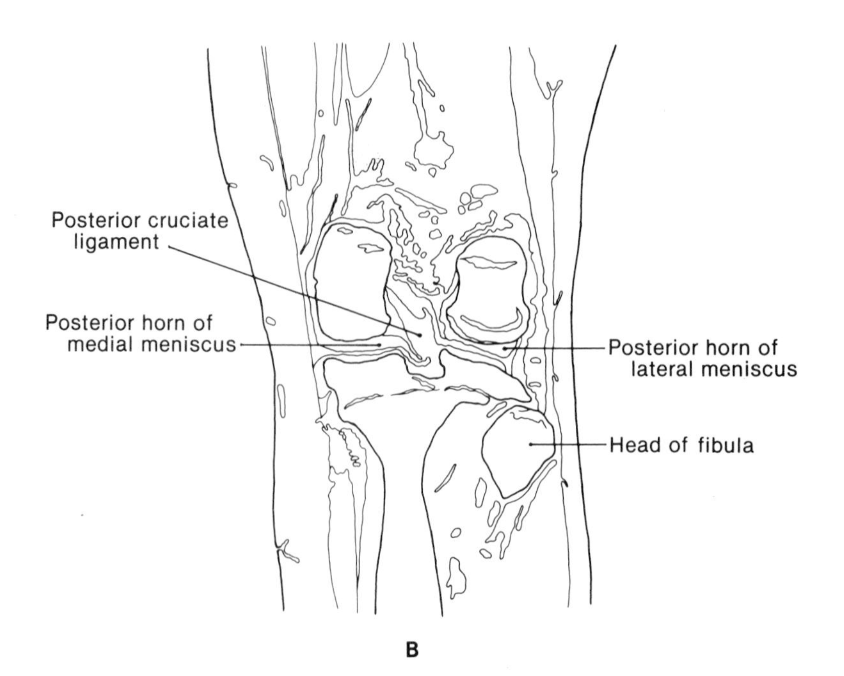

B

D. Major features of T1-weighted MR images of 3-mm-thick sagittal sections of the knee

1. **A sagittal section through the head of the fibula** shows the following features (Figure 2-14).
   a. The section passes through the most lateral aspects of the **lateral femoral and lateral tibial condyles**. The **articular cartilage** covering the **lateral tibial plateau** casts a thin, intermediate-density band atop the low-intensity cortical bone of the plateau.
   b. The **lateral meniscus** appears as a low-intensity band sandwiched between the lateral femoral condyle and the articular cartilage covering the lateral tibial plateau.

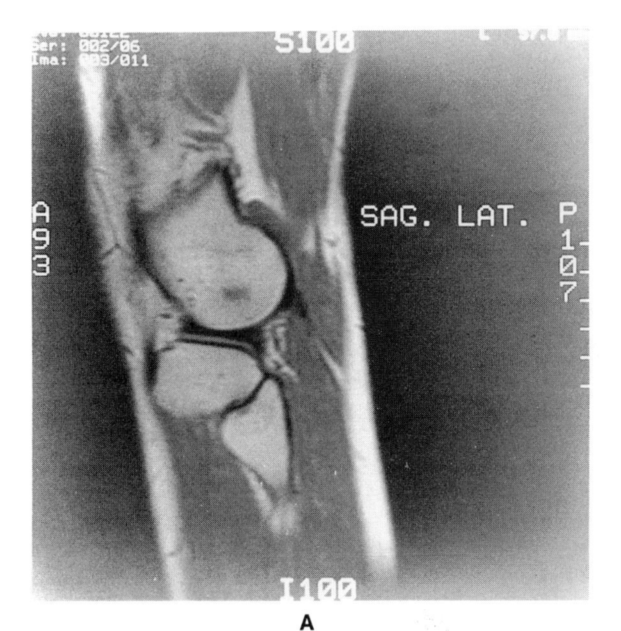

A

Figure 2-14. (*A*) A T1-weighted MR image of a sagittal section through the head of the fibula and (*B*) its schematic representation. (See section II D 1.)

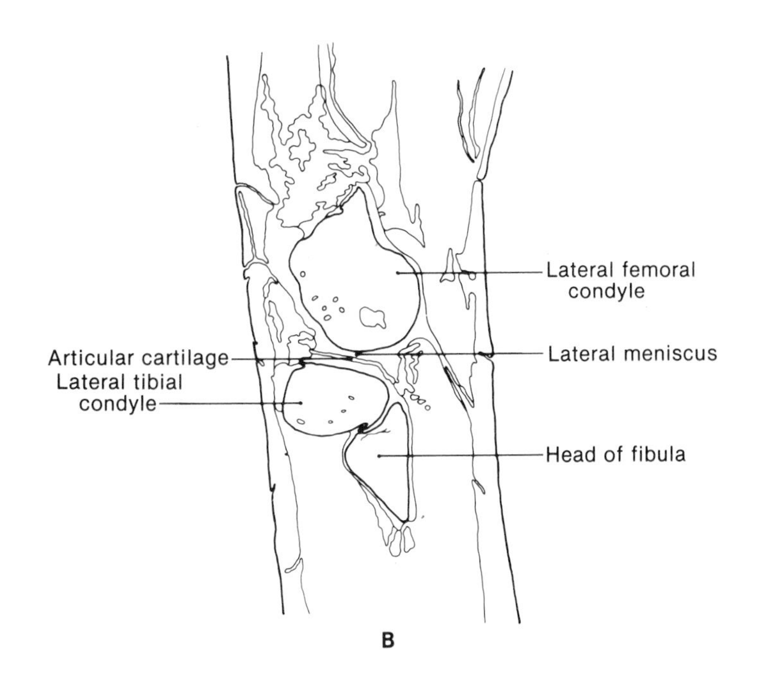

B

2. **A sagittal section 9 mm medial to the fibular head section** shows the following features (Figure 2-15).
   a. The high-intensity cancellous interior of the lateral aspect of the **patella** is embedded within the low-intensity **quadriceps femoris tendon**.
   b. The high-intensity **suprapatellar fat pad** lies in the space between the patella and the anterior margin of the lateral femoral condyle. The high-intensity **infrapatellar fat pad** fills in the space anteroinferior to the lateral femoral condyle and anterosuperior to the lateral tibial condyle.
   c. The remnant of the **epiphyseal growth plate** at the distal end of the **femur** appears as a tenuous band of low intensity.
   d. The intermediate-density images of the **articular cartilages** covering the **lateral femoral condyle** and **lateral tibial plateau** are blended along the margin of apposition between the

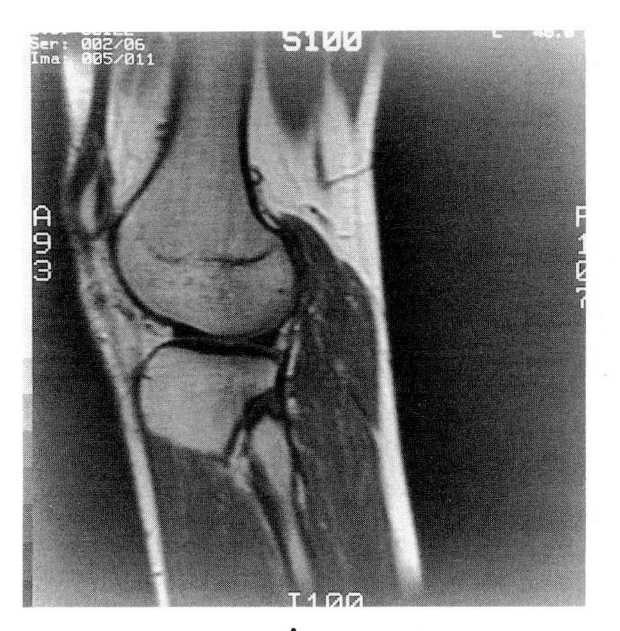

A

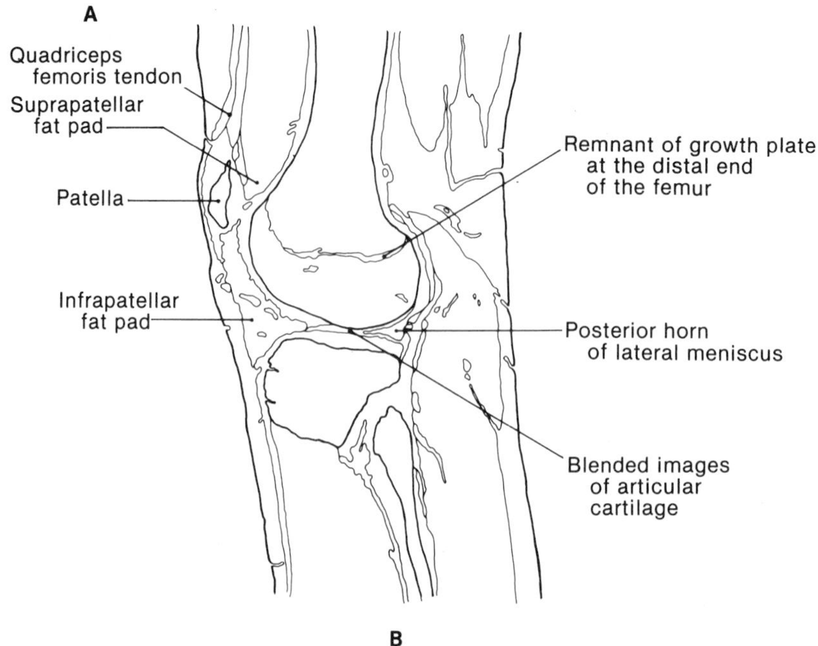

B

Figure 2-15. (*A*) A T1-weighted MR image of a sagittal section 9 mm medial to the fibular head section of Figure 2-14A and (*B*) its schematic representation. (See section II D 2.)

cartilages. The blended images intervene between the two low-intensity triangular regions generated by the **anterior and posterior horns of the lateral meniscus**.

e. The **lateral head of gastrocnemius** generates an image of moderately low intensity directly posterior to the lateral femoral condyle.

3. A sagittal section 22.5 mm medial to the fibular head section shows the following features (Figure 2-16).

a. A very fine low-intensity line marks the **margin of apposition** between the articular cartilages covering the posterior surface of the patella and the patellar surface of the femur. The low-intensity band that extends anterosuperiorly from this margin into the suprapatellar fat pad represents the **suprapatellar bursa**.

b. The **ligamentum patellae** appears as a thick, low-intensity band extending from the patella to the tibial tuberosity.

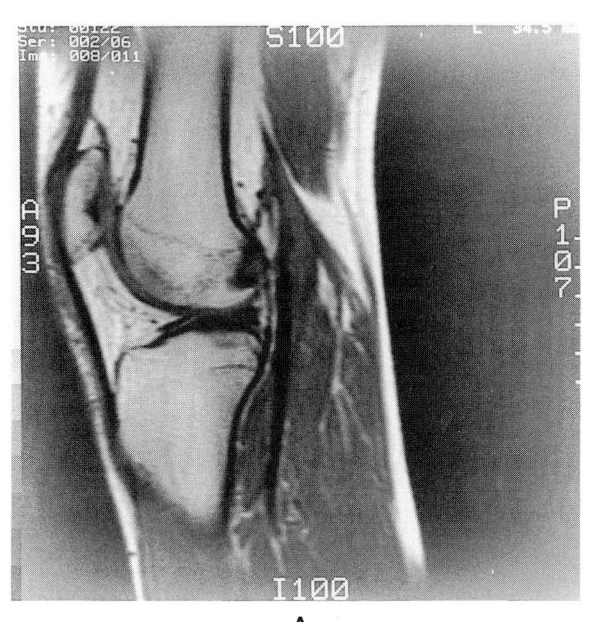

A

Figure 2-16. (*A*) A T1-weighted MR image of a sagittal section 22.5 mm medial to the fibular head section of Figure 2-14A and (*B*) its schematic representation. (See section II D 3.)

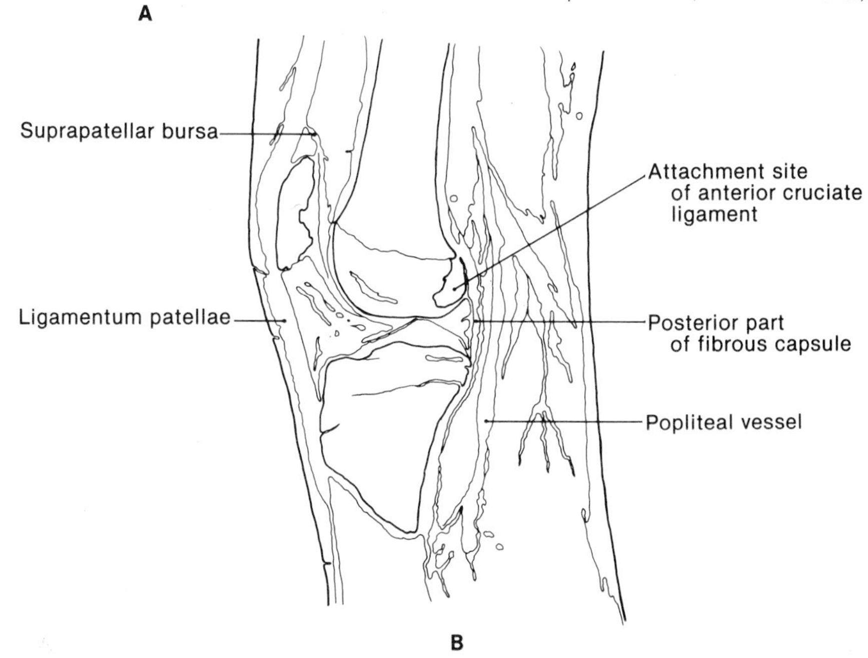

B

c. An irregular low-intensity region marks the attachment of the **anterior cruciate ligament** to the medial surface of the lateral femoral condyle.

d. The posterior part of the **fibrous capsule of the knee joint** appears as a low-intensity band extending between the lateral femoral condyle and lateral tibial condyle.

e. A popliteal vessel appears as a low-intensity band directly posterior to the posterior part of the knee joint's fibrous capsule.

4. A sagittal section 31.5 mm medial to the fibular head section shows the following features (Figure 2-17).

a. The **anterior cruciate ligament** appears as a thick, low-intensity band extending postero-superiorly from the anterior area of the tibial intercondylar surface.

b. The **posterior cruciate ligament** appears as a thick, low-intensity band extending anterosuperiorly from the posterior area of the tibial intercondylar surface.

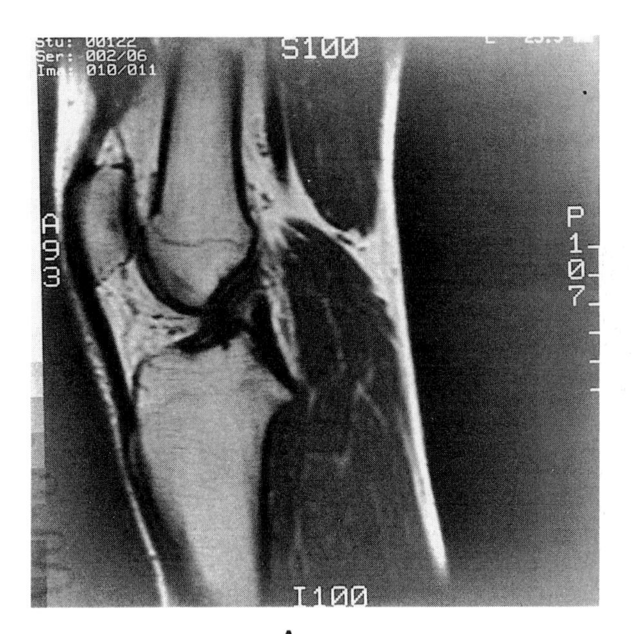

A

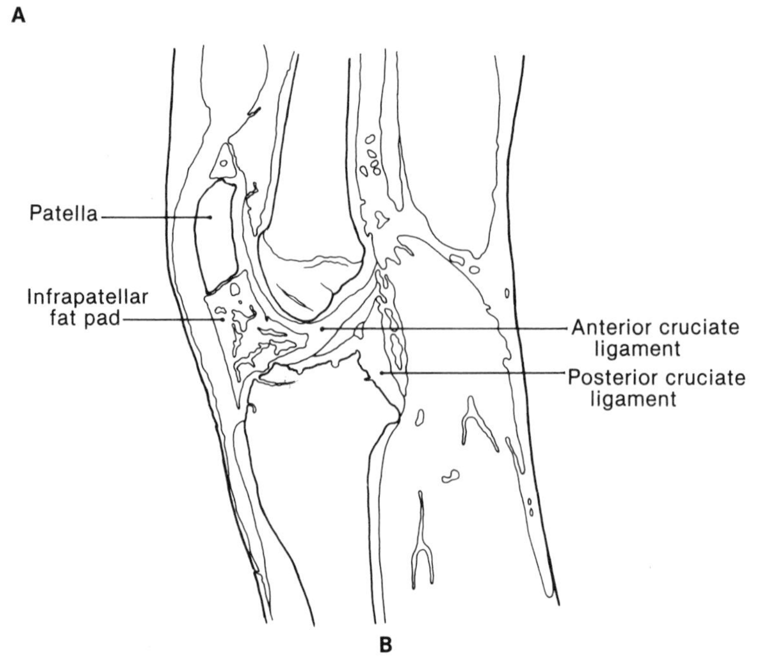

B

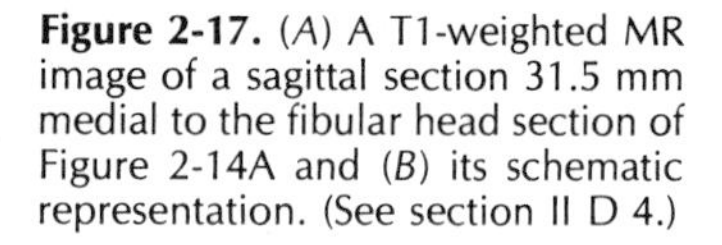

Figure 2-17. (*A*) A T1-weighted MR image of a sagittal section 31.5 mm medial to the fibular head section of Figure 2-14A and (*B*) its schematic representation. (See section II D 4.)

5. **A sagittal section 41.5 mm medial to the fibular head section** shows the following features (Figure 2-18).
   a. An irregular low-intensity region marks the attachment of the **posterior cruciate ligament** to the lateral surface of the medial femoral condyle.
   b. The **medial head of gastrocnemius** generates an image of moderately low intensity directly posterior to the medial femoral condyle.

6. **A sagittal section 55 mm medial to the fibular head section** shows the following features (Figure 2-19).
   a. The intermediate-density images of the **articular cartilages** covering the **medial femoral condyle** and **medial tibial plateau** are blended along the margin of apposition between the cartilages. The blended images intervene between the two low-intensity triangular regions generated by the **anterior and posterior horns of the medial meniscus**.

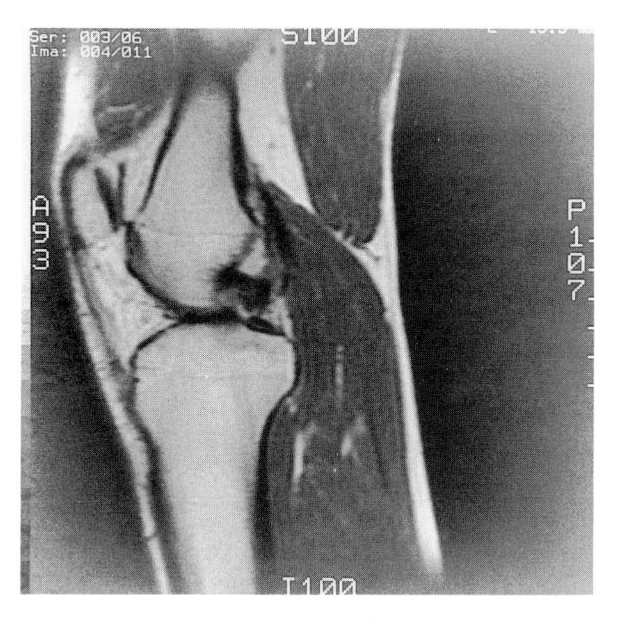

A

Figure 2-18. (A) A T1-weighted MR image of a sagittal section 41.5 mm medial to the fibular head section of Figure 2-14A and (B) its schematic representation. (See section II D 5.)

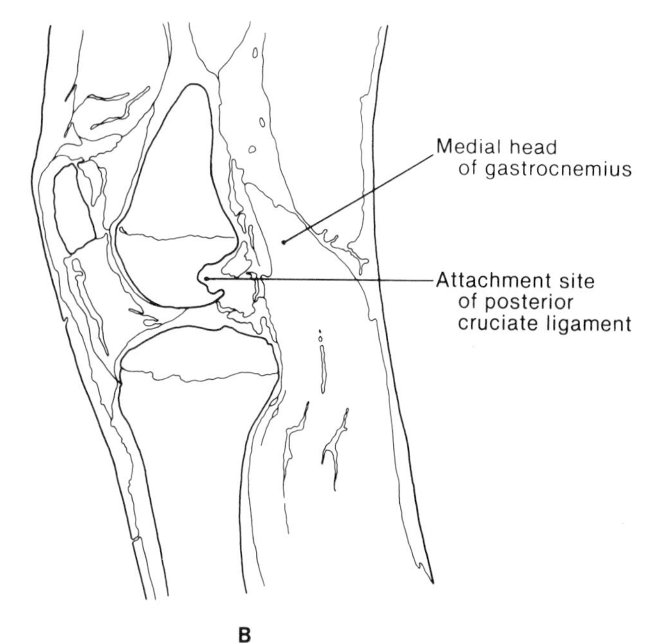

B

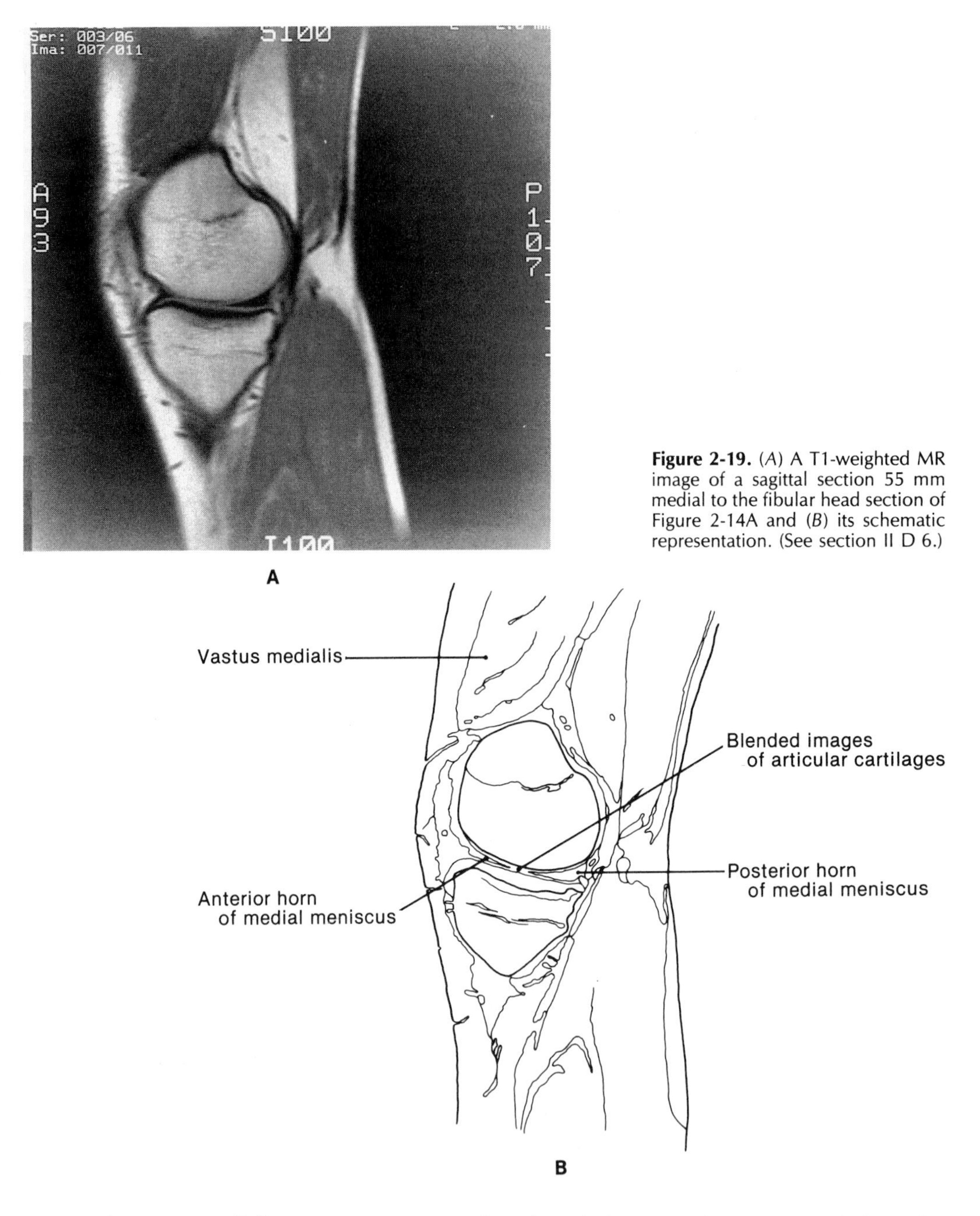

Figure 2-19. (*A*) A T1-weighted MR image of a sagittal section 55 mm medial to the fibular head section of Figure 2-14A and (*B*) its schematic representation. (See section II D 6.)

b. Vastus medialis generates an image of moderately low intensity anterosuperiorly to the medial femoral condyle.

E. Clinical and radiographic features of common traumatic injuries and diseases

1. Recurrent lateral patellar subluxation

a. Pathogenesis

(1) When the leg is extended at the knee joint, the vastus intermedius and lateralis muscles exert a laterally directed pull on the patella that is counteracted by the medially directed pull of vastus medialis and the interposition of the lateral femoral condyle. The patella is thus subject to recurrent lateral subluxation if vastus medialis is weakened or the lateral femoral condyle is congenitally underdeveloped.

(2) The patella is also subject to recurrent lateral subluxation if the ligamentum patellae is abnormally long—that is, if the length of the ligamentum patellae, as measured along its posterior margin with Hoffa's fat pad, is 1.2 or more times greater than the superoinferior dimension of the patella. Such an abnormally long ligamentum patellae is called **patella alta**.

b. Radiographic features. Recurrent lateral patellar subluxation is best assessed by an axial radiograph of the patella. Such a radiograph commonly documents the subluxation by showing the lateral edge of the patella displaced laterally to the lateral border of the lateral femoral condyle.

2. Fractures of the distal femur and proximal tibia

a. Etiology and clinical features

(1) Automobile accidents and falls from significant heights are the most common causes of **fractures of the distal femur**.

(2) Tibial plateau fractures are called "**bumper fractures**" or "**fender fractures**" because such fractures are commonly sustained when an individual is struck in the knee by an automobile. The forces which produce such fractures drive the femoral condyle down onto the corresponding tibial plateau.

b. Radiographic features. A cross-table lateral radiograph of a knee with an intracapsular fracture of the femur or a tibial plateau fracture generally shows a straight fat–fluid-density interface in the anterosuperior compartment of the joint cavity (see section II E 4 b and Figure 2-20).

3. Fractures of the patella

a. Etiology and clinical features. Patellar fractures can occur either from a direct blow to the patella or from indirect tension generated by sudden active contraction of quadriceps femoris. The fracture fragments are more likely to be displaced with the latter mechanism of injury.

b. Radiographic features. AP and lateral radiographs of the knee are generally adequate for the demonstration of patellar fractures. A cross-table lateral radiograph of the knee may show a straight fat–fluid-density interface in the anterosuperior compartment of the joint cavity.

c. A **multipartite patella** must be distinguished from a patellar fracture.

(1) A multipartite patella is a variant of the normal patella. The patella ossifies from a number of central and peripheral centers of ossification. The bone tissue masses generated from one or more of the peripheral centers in the superolateral patellar area occasionally do not fuse with the central mass; a patella so produced is a **multipartite patella**.

(2) Several criteria help to distinguish a multipartite patella from a fractured patella in an AP radiograph of the knee:

(a) Whereas the margins of the accessory bone tissue masses of a multipartite patella are completely outlined by cortical bone, the fragments of a fractured patella are not.

(b) The accessory bone tissue masses of a multipartite patella almost invariably border the superolateral margin of the patella.

(c) Whereas an imagined reconstruction of the fragments of a fractured patella will produce a normal patellar outline, similar reconstruction of the parts of a multipartite patella will not quite produce a normal patellar outline.

4. Knee joint effusions: radiographic features

a. The suprapatellar bursa always becomes distended with fluid whenever a moderate to marked effusion accumulates within the knee joint's synovial cavity.

(1) A lateral radiograph of a knee with moderate to marked joint effusion shows the water-density image of the quadriceps femoris tendon bordered posteriorly by the water-density image of the fluid-filled suprapatellar bursa. The border between the tendon and the fluid-filled bursa is radiographically imperceptible.

(2) The fat-density image of the suprapatellar fat pad is posteriorly displaced and less evident because the distended suprapatellar bursa has pressed the fat pad deeply against the femur.

b. The presence of fat in a knee joint effusion is pathognomonic of a patellar fracture or an intracapsular fracture of the femur or tibia at the knee.

(1) Such fractures always release both fat and blood-bearing fluid into the joint cavity (the fat is extravasated from the cancellous bone bordering the fracture site). The fat coalesces and floats atop the blood-bearing fluid within the joint cavity.

(2) The presence of fat within an effused knee is best documented by taking a cross-table lateral radiograph of the knee with the patient lying in the supine position. The floating coalesced fat and the underlying blood-bearing fluid together generate a distinct straight **fat–fluid-density interface** in the region between the quadriceps femoris tendon and patella above and the distal end of the femur below (Figure 2-20.)

5. Sinding Larsen–Johansson disease (Larsen-Johansson disease) and Osgood-Schlatter disease

a. Clinical features

(1) These two similar "diseases" are trauma-induced conditions which occur at opposite ends of the ligamentum patellae: Sinding Larsen–Johansson disease at the proximal end; Osgood-Schlatter disease at the distal end.

(2) Each condition occurs mainly among adolescents. Osgood-Schlatter disease occurs more often in boys than in girls, and is frequently bilateral.

(3) A diagnostic feature of each condition is soft tissue swelling at the appropriate end of the ligamentum patellae; palpation of the local area generally elicits tenderness.

b. Radiographic features. A lateral radiograph of a knee with either condition shows localized soft tissue swelling and, generally, bony fragmentation at the appropriate attachment site of the ligamentum patellae. Thus, Sinding Larsen–Johansson disease shows fragmentation of the patella, and Osgood-Schlatter disease exhibits fragmentation of the tibial tuberosity.

6. Osteochondritis dissecans in the knee

a. Clinical features

(1) Osteochondritis dissecans is predominantly encountered in the knee (the other common but secondary sites are the ankle and elbow). The condition occurs mainly among adolescents and young adults; the incidence in males is greater than that in females.

(2) The condition is believed to occur as a consequence of chronic physical insult to a segment of articular cartilage and the underlying subchondral bone; disruption of blood supply to the subchondral bone segment may also be involved in the etiology.

(3) Most osteochondritis dissecans lesions in the knee occur in the lateral aspect of the medial femoral condyle.

b. Radiographic features. AP, tunnel, and lateral radiographs of the knee are required to document the extent of the lesion.

(1) The lesion in the subchondral bone presents as a curved radiolucent band with a sclerotic margin, typically extending from the posterior, non–weight-bearing part of the medial femoral condyle that faces the intercondylar notch to the anterior, weight-bearing part of the condyle that apposes the medial tibial condyle.

(2) Extension of the lesion into the articular cartilage may result in detachment and dislodgement of an osteochondral body.

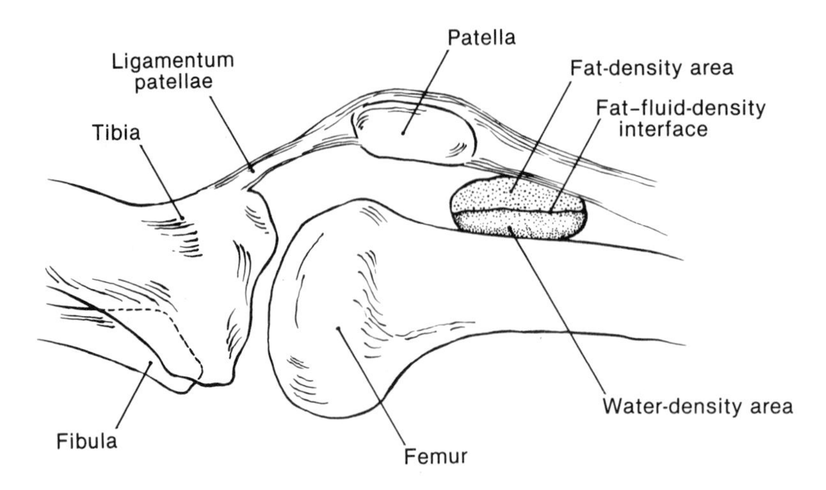

Figure 2-20. An outline of a cross-table lateral radiograph of a knee whose joint cavity is swollen with blood-bearing fluid and bone marrow fat as a result of an intracapsular fracture. The coalescence and flotation of the bone marrow fat atop the blood-bearing fluid account for the straight fat–fluid-density interface in the anterosuperior part of the joint cavity. [See sections II E 2 b and 4 b (2).]

7. Acute hematogenous osteomyelitis of the distal femur or proximal tibia

a. Clinical features and pathogenesis

(1) Most cases of bacterial bone infection occur in children and adolescents. In this population, hematogenous spread is the most common mode of acquisition; trauma to a bone region appears to be a major predisposing factor for the seeding of bacteria in the region from a distant site of infection.

(2) The most common sites of acute hematogenous osteomyelitis in children and adolescents are the metaphyses of the distal femur and proximal tibia. The sluggish and turbulent blood flow through the metaphyses of developing long bones renders these sites susceptible to the deposition and proliferation of blood-borne bacteria, especially following trauma-induced occlusion of the microvasculature at these sites.

(3) When pediatric patients can describe their condition, the complaint is constant and severe pain. Localized warmth and soft tissue swelling may also be present.

b. Radiographic features

(1) The initial radiographic signs of acute hematogenous osteomyelitis are edema and loss of fascial plane definition of the overlying soft tissues; these signs occur within 24 to 48 hours.

(2) If untreated, lytic lesions of the infected metaphysis occur within 7 to 10 days, followed by endosteal sclerosis due to new periosteal bone formation.

8. Primary osteoarthritis of the knee joint

a. Clinical features

(1) The knee joint is a common site of primary osteoarthritis; the medial femorotibial and patellofemoral articulations are more commonly affected than the lateral femorotibial articulation.

(2) Marked degeneration of the medial femorotibial articulation can produce a varus deformity at the knee. (The term **varus** indicates that the distal bone points toward the midline of the body; the term **valgus** indicates that the distal bone points away from the midline.)

b. Radiographic features. The principal findings are similar to those of primary osteoarthritis of the hip joint, namely, narrowing of the joint space, subchondral osteosclerosis, osteophyte formation, and subchondral cyst formation.

9. Rheumatoid arthritis of the knee joint

a. Clinical features. The knee joint is commonly affected in individuals with rheumatoid arthritis.

b. Radiographic features. The principal findings are similar to those of rheumatoid arthritis of the hip joint, namely, narrowing of all the joint spaces, periarticular osteopenia, subchondral erosions, and subchondral cyst formation.

III. ANKLE AND FOOT

A. Anatomy of the ankle and foot

1. Bones

a. Distal ends of the tibia and fibula

(1) The **shaft of the tibia** has three **surfaces**: anteromedial, anterolateral, and posterior.

(a) The **anteromedial surface** is subcutaneous from the medial tibial condyle to the medial malleolus. Many tibial shaft fractures are open because of the subcutaneous lie of the anteromedial surface.

(b) The distinct **bony ridge** between the anteromedial and anterolateral surfaces is colloquially called the **shin**.

(c) The upper half of the **posterior surface** bears the opening for the nutrient artery to the shaft of the tibia. Fractures through the distal shaft may be complicated by delayed union of the fragments following reduction.

(2) The **medial and lateral malleoli** form subcutaneous bony prominences on, respectively, the medial and lateral sides of the ankle. The tip of the lateral malleolus is more distal than the tip of the medial malleolus.

b. Tarsals

(1) The **calcaneus** is palpable in the heel, and the **sustentaculum tali** is palpable on the medial side of the foot immediately distal to the medial malleolus.

(2) The **ossification centers** for the calcaneus and talus are present at birth.

(3) The **lateral cuneiform** begins to ossify in the first year, the **medial cuneiform** in the second year, and the **intermediate cuneiform** in the third year.

c. Metatarsals

(1) The heads of the metatarsals lie embedded in the foot pad at the bases of the toes.

(2) Each metatarsal generally bears only a single **epiphysis** during childhood and adolescence. Whereas the epiphysis of the first metatarsal resides at the bone's base, the epiphyses of the second to fifth metatarsals reside at the heads of the bones.

d. Phalanges. Each phalanx bears only a single **epiphysis** during childhood and adolescence. The epiphysis of each phalanx resides at the bone's base.

2. Joints

a. Distal tibiofibular joint. The distal tibiofibular joint unites the distal end of the fibula with the fibular notch of the tibia; it is a **syndesmosis** (a fibrous joint in which the bones are united by a sheet of fibrous tissue).

b. Ankle joint. The ankle joint articulates the talus with the distal ends of the tibia and fibula. It provides for dorsiflexion and plantar flexion of the foot.

c. Joints of foot inversion and eversion. Inversion and eversion of the foot occur primarily at a group of articulations that anatomists distinguish as three anatomic joints but that physicians distinguish as two functional joints.

(1) Anatomic joints

(a) The **anatomic subtalar joint** articulates the posterior ends of the talus and calcaneus.

(b) The **talocalcaneonavicular joint** consists of the talocalcaneal articulation at the sustentaculum tali and the articulation of the anterior end of the talus with the posterior surface of the navicular.

(c) The **calcaneocuboid joint** articulates the anterior surface of the calcaneus with the posterior surface of the cuboid.

(2) Functional joints

(a) The **functional subtalar joint** consists of the anatomic subtalar joint and the talocalcaneal articulation at the sustentaculum tali.

(b) The **transverse tarsal (Chopart's) joint** consists of the calcaneocuboid joint and the articulation of the anterior end of the talus with the posterior surface of the navicular.

d. Metatarsophalangeal and interphalangeal joints

(1) The head of the metatarsal articulates with the base of the proximal phalanx within each **metatarsophalangeal joint**. Each metatarsophalangeal joint provides for abduction, adduction, flexion, and extension of the proximal phalanx of the toe.

(2) Each **interphalangeal joint** provides for only flexion and extension of the more distal phalanx.

3. Muscles

a. Muscles that move the foot

(1) There are four leg muscles whose tendons extend into the foot by passing **anterior to the ankle joint** (where they are held in position by the extensor retinacula).

(a) These muscles represent all the dorsiflexors of the foot, and they are all innervated by the deep peroneal nerve.

(i) Tibialis anterior is the chief dorsiflexor of the foot and the second most powerful invertor of the foot.

(ii) Extensor hallucis longus can extend the phalanges of the big toe; it is also a minor invertor of the foot.

(iii) Extensor digitorum longus can extend the phalanges of the four most lateral toes.

(iv) Peroneus tertius is a minor evertor of the foot.

(b) Loss of nerve supply to these muscles causes **footdrop** [see section II A 4 a (1) (b) (ii)].

(2) There are two muscles whose tendons extend into the foot by passing **posterior to the lateral malleolus** (where they are held in position by the peroneal retinacula). Both muscles are innervated by the superficial peroneal nerve.

(a) Peroneus longus is the chief evertor of the foot; it can also plantar flex the foot.

(b) Peroneus brevis is the second most powerful evertor of the foot; it can also plantar flex the foot.

(3) There are three muscles whose tendons contribute to the **tendo calcaneus (Achilles tendon)**.

(a) These muscles are all plantar flexors of the foot, and they are all innervated by the tibial nerve.

(i) **Gastrocnemius** is the most powerful plantar flexor of the foot; it can also flex the leg at the knee joint.
(ii) **Soleus** is the second most powerful plantar flexor of the foot.
(iii) **Plantaris** is a relatively weak plantar flexor of the foot. Its tendon of insertion is often sacrificed in reconstructive repair of tendons of functionally important muscles.

(b) The **Achilles tendon reflex test** is a phasic stretch reflex test of the integrity of the neuronal pathways at the S1 and S2 spinal cord segment levels.

(4) There are three muscles whose tendons extend into the foot by passing **posterior to the medial malleolus** (where they are held in position by the flexor retinaculum). The three muscles are all innervated by the tibial nerve.
(a) **Tibialis posterior** is the chief invertor of the foot; it can also plantar flex the foot.
(b) **Flexor hallucis longus** can flex the phalanges of the big toe and plantar flex the foot.
(c) **Flexor digitorum longus** can flex the phalanges of the four most lateral toes and plantar flex the foot.

b. Intrinsic muscles of the foot

(1) The foot bears three short muscles of the big toe.
(a) **Abductor hallucis** abducts and flexes the big toe at its metatarsophalangeal joint.
(b) **Flexor hallucis brevis** flexes the big toe at its metatarsophalangeal joint.
(c) **Adductor hallucis** adducts and flexes the big toe at its metatarsophalangeal joint.

(2) **Extensor digitorum brevis** serves all but the little toe.
(a) It extends the proximal phalanx of the big toe.
(b) It extends the phalanges of the second, third, and fourth toes.

(3) **Flexor digitorum brevis** flexes the proximal and middle phalanges of the four most lateral toes.

(4) **Quadratus plantae** assists flexor digitorum longus in flexing the phalanges of the four most lateral toes.

(5) The **lumbricals** serve in large measure to prevent the four most lateral toes from buckling under the foot when they are flexed during the stance phase of the walking gait.

(6) The **plantar and dorsal interossei** are prime adductors and abductors of the toes.
(a) **Adductors**
(i) The first plantar interosseous adducts the third toe.
(ii) The second plantar interosseous adducts the fourth toe.
(iii) The third plantar interosseous adducts the fifth toe.
(b) **Abductors**
(i) The first dorsal interosseous abducts the second toe.
(ii) The second dorsal interosseous abducts the second toe.
(iii) The third dorsal interosseous abducts the third toe.
(iv) The fourth dorsal interosseous abducts the fourth toe.

(7) The foot bears two short muscles of the little toe.
(a) **Abductor digiti minimi** abducts and flexes the little toe at its metatarsophalangeal joint.
(b) **Flexor digiti minimi brevis** flexes the little toe at its metatarsophalangeal joint.

4. Nerves

a. The **tibial nerve** extends into the foot by passing posterior to the medial malleolus and deep to the flexor retinaculum.
(1) The tibial nerve divides in the sole of the foot into the medial and lateral plantar nerves.
(2) The **medial and lateral plantar nerves** together innervate:
(a) All the intrinsic muscles of the foot except for extensor digitorum brevis
(b) Most of the skin on the sole of the foot

b. The **deep peroneal nerve** extends into the foot by passing anterior to the ankle joint and deep to the extensor retinacula. In the foot, the deep peroneal nerve innervates extensor digitorum brevis and the skin on the adjacent sides of the big and second toes.

c. Cutaneous branches of the **superficial peroneal nerve** supply most of the dorsum of the foot.

5. Blood vessels and lymphatics

a. The plantar arterial arch. The plantar arterial arch derives from the posterior tibial artery and dorsalis pedis.
(1) The pulsations of the **posterior tibial artery** can be palpated posteroinferiorly to the

medial malleolus. The posterior tibial artery divides in the foot into two terminal branches, the **medial and lateral plantar arteries**. The plantar arterial arch is a direct continuation of the **lateral plantar artery**.

(2) The **anterior tibial artery** ends anterior to the ankle joint as the origin of the **dorsalis pedis**. The pulsations of the dorsalis pedis can be palpated on the dorsum of the foot immediately lateral to the tendon of extensor hallucis longus. The **deep plantar artery**, which is a branch of the dorsalis pedis, joins the lateral plantar artery in the foot to form the **plantar arterial arch**.

b. Venous and lymphatic drainage

(1) Blood and lymph from the superficial tissues on the **medial side** of the foot are primarily drained by the **great saphenous vein** and its **accompanying lymphatics**. The great saphenous vein ascends to the leg from the foot by passing anterior to the medial malleolus.

(2) Blood and lymph from the superficial tissues on the **lateral side** of the foot are primarily drained by the **small saphenous vein** and its **accompanying lymphatics**. The small saphenous vein ascends to the leg from the foot by passing posterior to the lateral malleolus.

B. Major features of radiographs of the ankle and foot

1. Mortise radiograph. A mortise radiograph of the ankle provides an AP projection of the ankle of an internally rotated foot, and has the following distinguishing features (Figure 2-21).

a. The mortise radiograph is so named because it best displays the tenon-and-mortise configuration of the ankle joint, in which the **body of the talus** forms the **tenon**, and the **medial malleolus, tibial plafond**, and **lateral malleolus** form the slot-shaped **mortise**. (The inferiorly directed articular surface at the distal end of the tibia is called the **tibial plafond** because it represents the plafond, or **ceiling**, of the ankle joint.)

b. The radiograph shows the **radiolucent joint spaces** separating the body of the talus from the lateral malleolus, tibial plafond, and medial malleolus. These joint spaces are uniform in width in a normal ankle joint.

c. The **floor of the fibular notch of the tibia** presents as a vertical radiopaque line at the distal end of the tibia. The lateral margin of the **body of the talus** is colinear with the floor of the fibular notch.

d. The **posterior malleolus** of the ankle joint overlaps the superior margin of the body of the talus and is seen as a blunt, stout process that projects inferiorly from the posterior margin of the distal end of the tibia.

2. Lateral radiograph. A lateral radiograph of the foot has the following distinguishing features (Figure 2-22).

a. Ankle

(1) The **tibial plafond** casts a concave profile opposite the convex profile cast by the superior articular surface of the **body of the talus**. The **intervening joint space** has a uniform width between its anterior and posterior limits.

(a) The images of the medial and lateral malleoli overlap the joint space.

(b) Fat-density areas bracket the anterior and posterior limits of the joint space. These fat-density areas represent the **fat pads** which directly abut the anterior and posterior parts of the ankle joint's fibrous capsule.

(2) The images of the **medial and lateral malleoli** are superimposed upon the body of the talus; the medial malleolus is the shorter of the two processes. The radiograph provides an unobstructed profile view of the **posterior malleolus** of the ankle joint.

b. Foot

(1) The radiograph displays major features of the **calcaneus**, namely:

(a) The articular surface for the anatomic subtalar joint

(b) The sustentaculum tali

(c) The anterior horn

(d) The articular surface for the calcaneocuboid joint

(e) The posterior tuberosity

(2) An angle called **Boehler's angle** measures the angular relationship between segments of the calcaneus. The most superior point of the calcaneus's articular surface for the anatomic subtalar joint marks the vertex of Boehler's angle; the angle is plotted by drawing one line from the posterosuperior edge of the calcaneus through the vertex and a second line from the vertex to the anterior horn of the calcaneus (Figure 2-23). Boehler's angle is the anterior angle between the two lines, and its normal range is 20° to 40°.

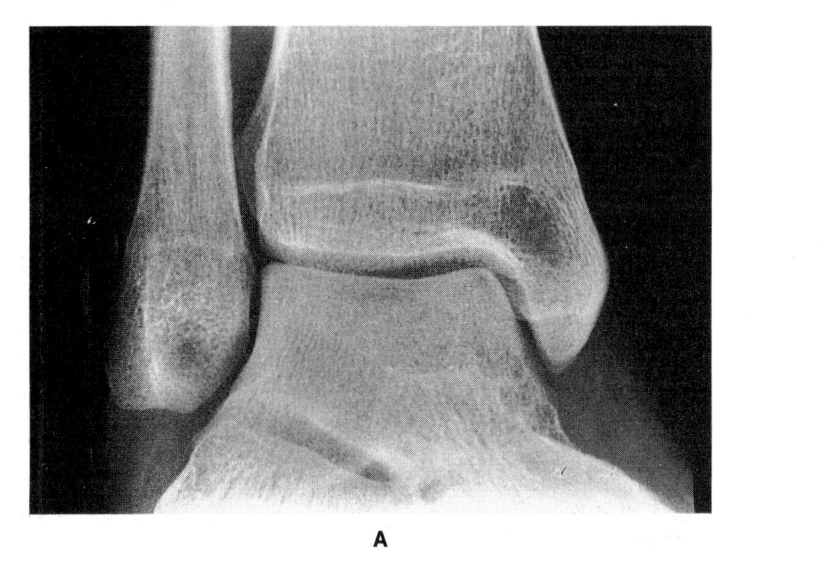

A

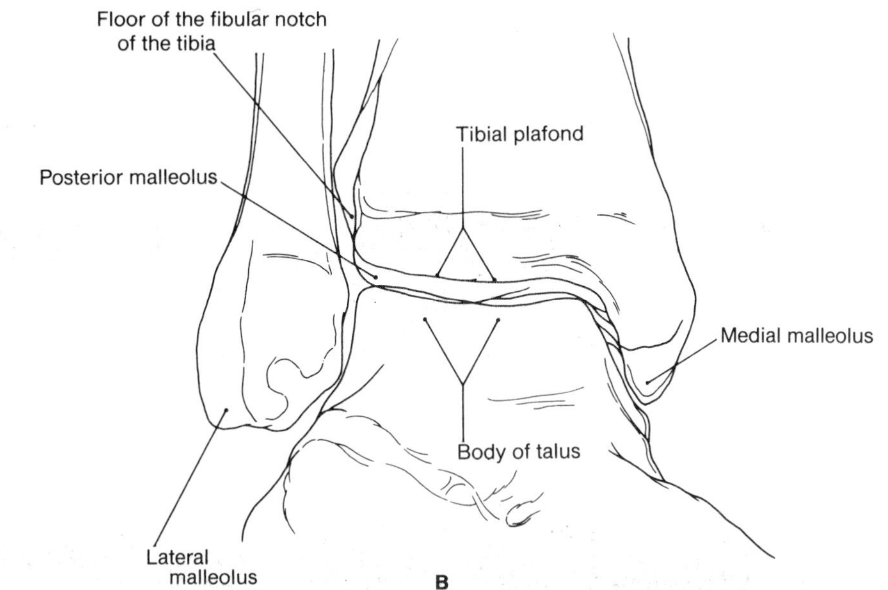

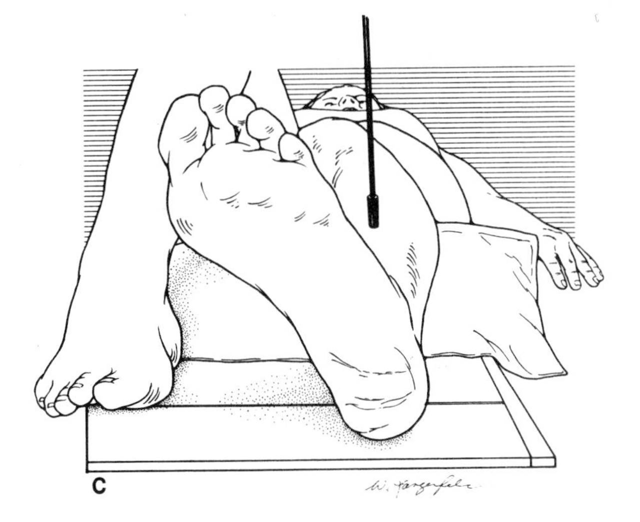

Figure 2-21. (*A*) A mortise radiograph of the ankle, (*B*) its schematic representation, and (*C*) the orientation of a patient's foot relative to the x-ray beam and film cassette for the radiograph. Note that the foot is internally rotated to render the line between the medial and lateral malleoli perpendicular to the path of the x-ray beam. (See section III B 1.)

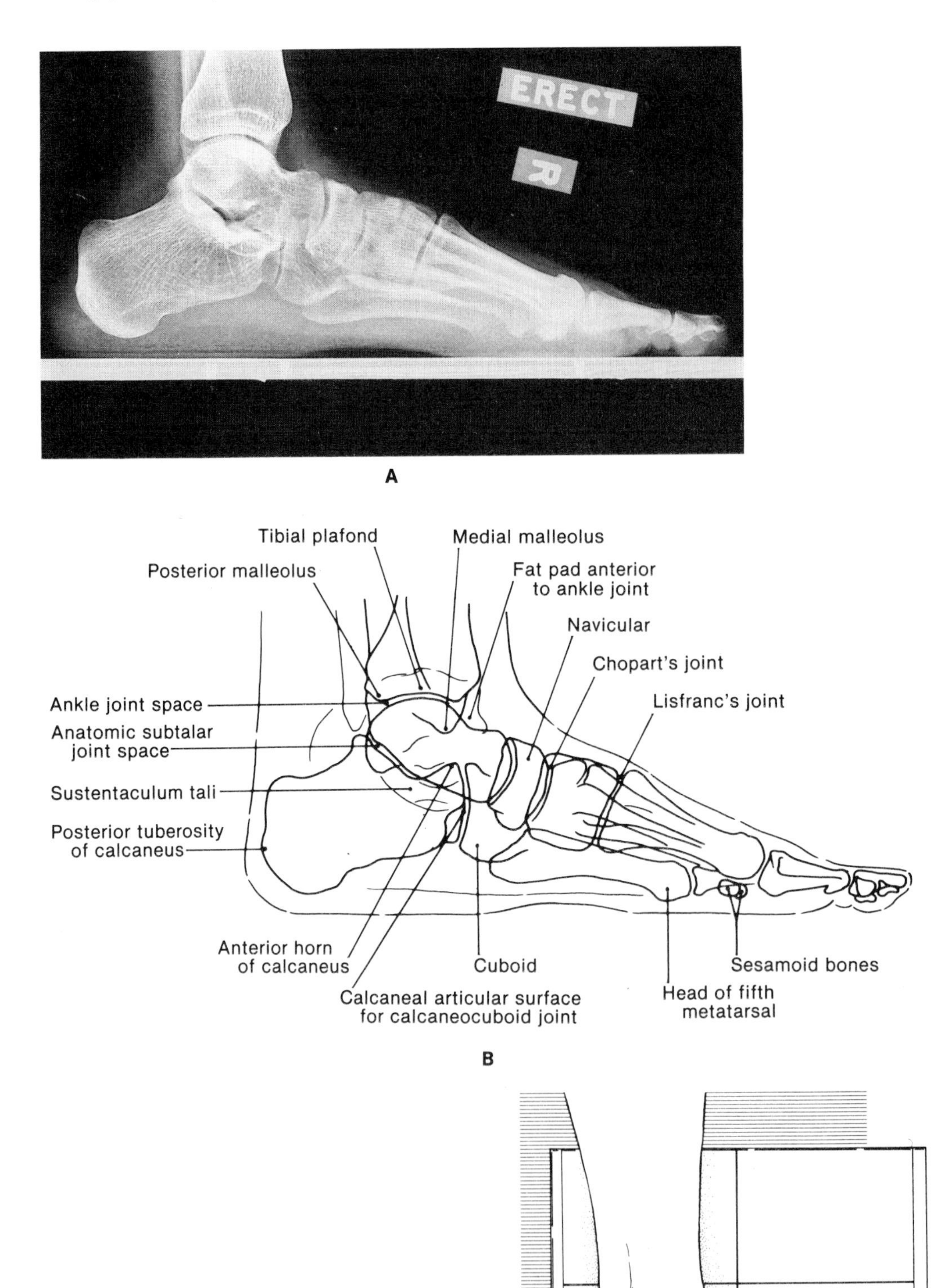

Figure 2-22. (*A*) A lateral radiograph of the foot, (*B*) its schematic representation, and (*C*) the orientation of a patient's foot relative to the x-ray beam and film cassette for the radiograph. (See section III B 2.)

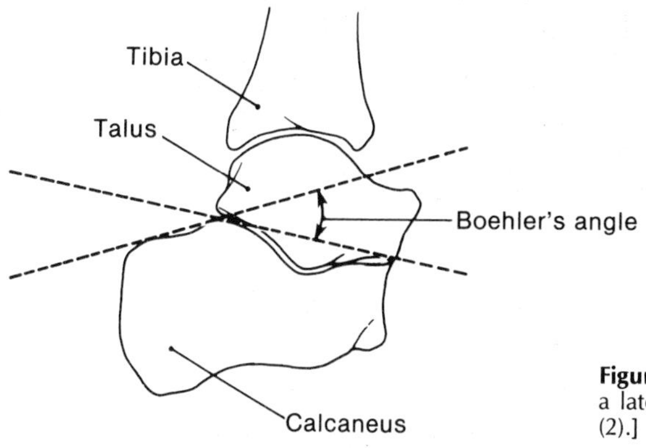

Figure 2-23. An outline of the plot of Boehler's angle on a lateral radiograph of the foot. [See section III B 2 b (2).]

(3) The presence of fat layers anterior and posterior to the **tendo calcaneus (Achilles tendon)** permits delineation of the tendon down to its attachment to the posterior surface of the calcaneus.

(4) The radiograph shows much of the joint spaces in **Chopart's joint** and **Lisfranc's joint**.

(a) **Chopart's joint** is the eponym for the **transverse tarsal joint**, which consists of the calcaneocuboid joint and the talonavicular articulation in the talocalcaneonavicular joint.

(b) **Lisfranc's joint** is the eponym for the **five synovial joints** which collectively articulate the cuneiforms and cuboid with the bases of the five metatarsals.

(5) The radiograph shows the pair of **sesamoid bones** that underlie the head of the first metatarsal.

3. Oblique radiograph. An oblique radiograph of the foot has the following distinguishing features (Figure 2-24).

a. The radiograph shows part of the joint space of the **talocalcaneal articulation** at the sustentaculum tali.

b. The radiograph shows most of the joint spaces in **Chopart's joint** and **Lisfranc's joint**.

c. The radiograph provides, for the most part, unobstructed views of

(1) The **metatarsophalangeal and interphalangeal joints** of the toes

(2) The **metatarsals** and the **phalanges** of the toes

d. The perspective of the radiograph superimposes the heads of the **first and second metatarsals** on the pair of sesamoid bones that underlie the head of the first metatarsal.

4. AP radiograph. An AP radiograph of the foot has the following distinguishing features (Figure 2-25).

a. The radiograph shows some of the joint spaces in **Chopart's and Lisfranc's joints**.

b. The radiograph provides, for the most part, unobstructed views of

(1) The **metatarsophalangeal and interphalangeal joints** of the toes

(2) The **metatarsals** and the **phalanges** of the toes

c. The perspective of the radiograph superimposes the head of the **first metatarsal** on the underlying pair of sesamoid bones.

C. Clinical and radiographic features of common traumatic injuries

1. Fractures about the ankle joint

a. General considerations

(1) The ankle region should be regarded structurally as a united ring of bones and ligaments that encircles the talus (Figure 2-26). This **osseoligamentous ring** consists of:

(a) The **ligaments of the distal tibiofibular joint**, namely, the anterior tibiofibular, posterior tibiofibular, inferior transverse, and interosseous ligaments

(b) The **tibial plafond** and **medial malleolus** at the distal end of the tibia

(c) The **medial collateral ligament** of the ankle joint (i.e., the **deltoid ligament**)

(d) The **calcaneus**

(e) The **lateral collateral ligament** of the ankle joint, which consists of the anterior talofibular, calcaneofibular, and posterior talofibular ligaments

(f) The **lateral malleolus**

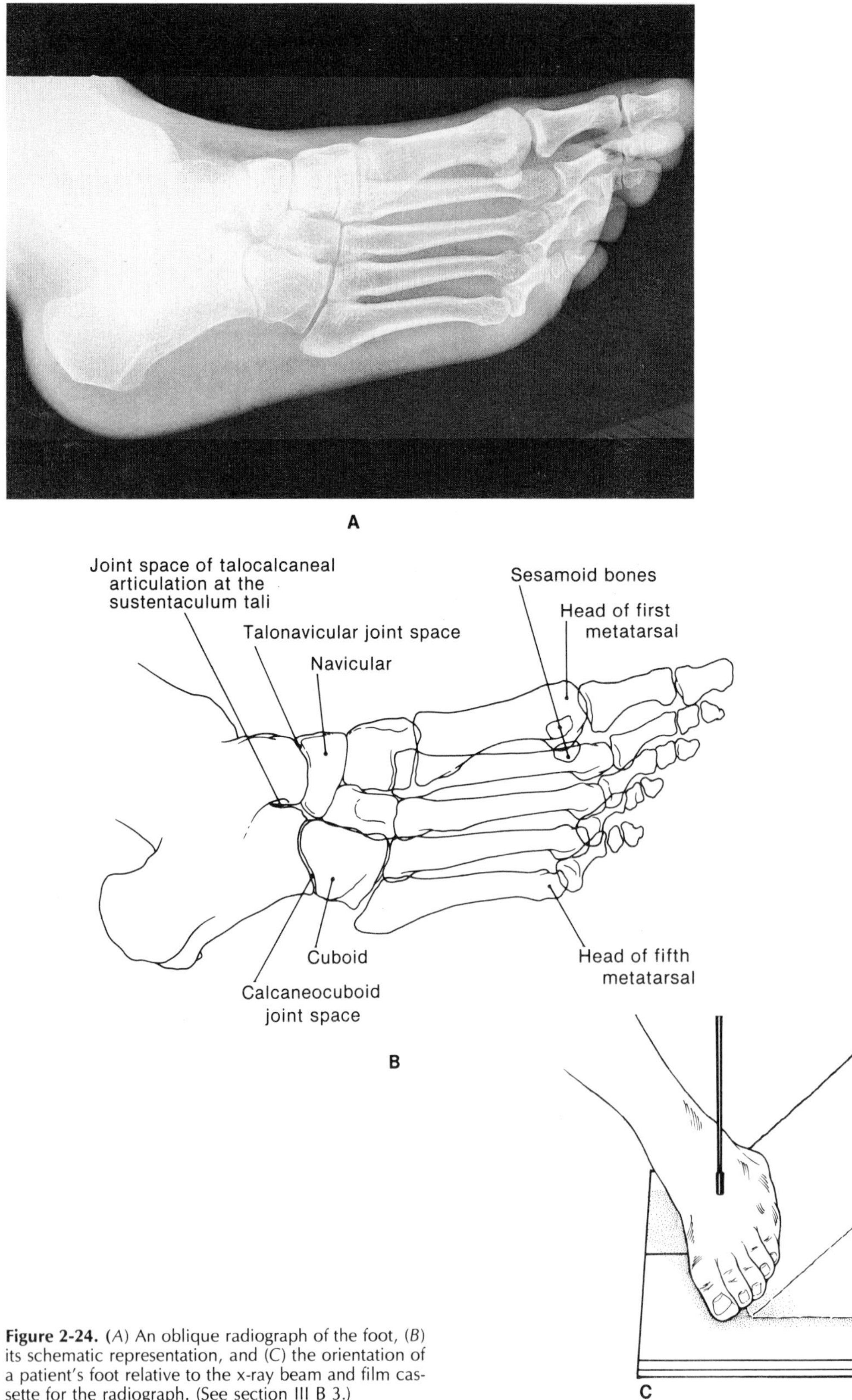

Figure 2-24. (*A*) An oblique radiograph of the foot, (*B*) its schematic representation, and (*C*) the orientation of a patient's foot relative to the x-ray beam and film cassette for the radiograph. (See section III B 3.)

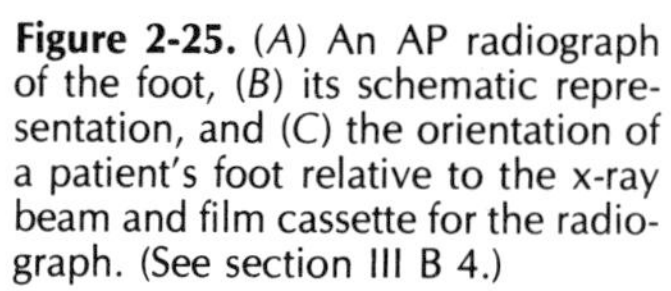

Figure 2-25. (*A*) An AP radiograph of the foot, (*B*) its schematic representation, and (*C*) the orientation of a patient's foot relative to the x-ray beam and film cassette for the radiograph. (See section III B 4.)

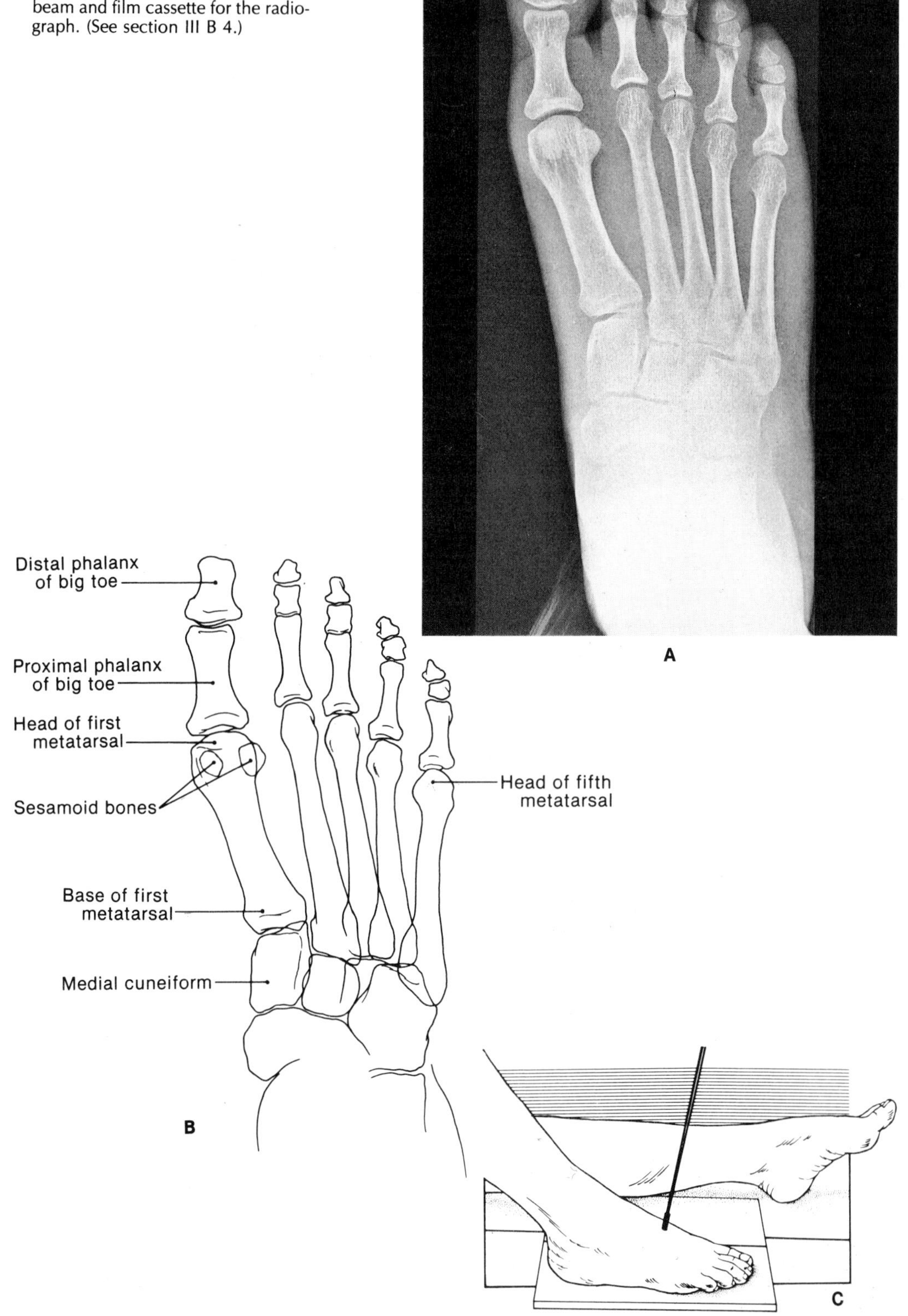

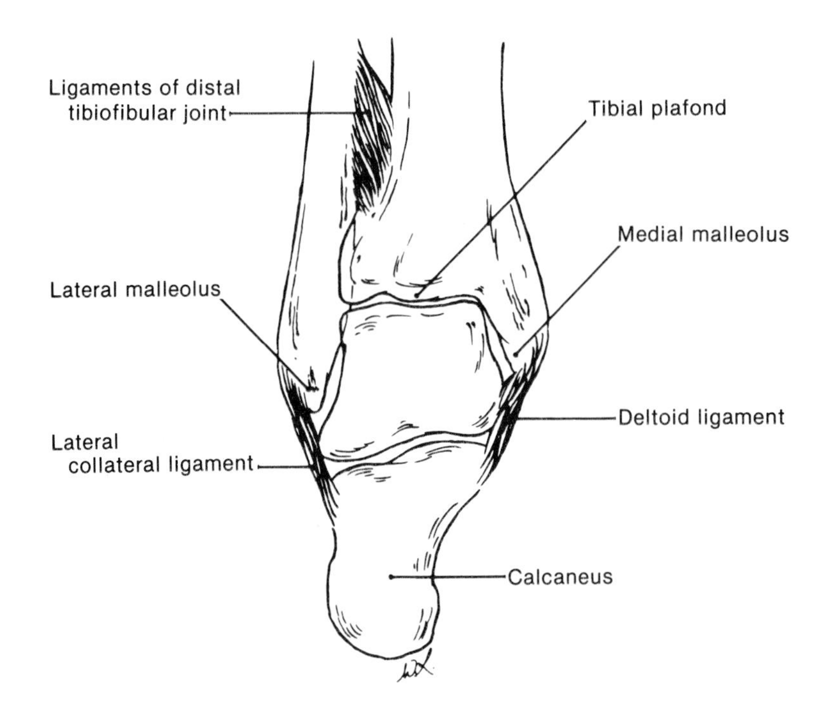

Figure 2-26. A diagram of the ring of bones and ligaments that encircles the talus in the ankle region. (See section III C 1 a.)

(2) **Breaks within the osseoligamentous ring** generally occur in pairs.
  (a) In most instances, a pair of breaks consists of a **fracture** of either the medial or lateral malleolus plus a **ruptured ligament**.
  (b) **Medial or lateral displacement of the talus** is pathognomonic of a pair of breaks within the ring; such displacement is documented in a mortise radiograph of the ankle by portrayal of a nonlinear relationship between the lateral margin of the body of the talus and the floor of the fibular notch of the tibia.

(3) A fracture of either the medial or lateral malleolus is called a **unimalleolar fracture**. An injury in which both malleoli are fractured is called a **bimalleolar fracture**. The term **trimalleolar fracture** is applied to injuries in which the medial, lateral, and posterior malleoli are all fractured.

b. Types of fractures

(1) Forces which produce a break in the **medial aspect of the osseoligamentous ring** around the talus more commonly produce avulsion of the medial malleolus rather than rupture of the deltoid ligament, because the deltoid ligament can bear greater tensile forces than the medial malleolus can.

(2) Forces which produce a break in the **lateral aspect of the osseoligamentous ring** around the talus more commonly produce a rupture of one of the component ligaments of the lateral collateral ligament rather than a fracture of the lateral malleolus.

(3) Forces which fracture the **distal end of the fibula** at a site above the level of the ligaments of the distal tibiofibular joint almost always produce a complete rupture of these ligaments and also of the interosseous membrane up to the level of the fracture site.

2. Fractures of the calcaneus

a. Clinical features. A fall from a significant height is a common cause of fractures of the calcaneus. Compression fractures of the calcaneus which occur as a consequence of such a fall are commonly accompanied by one or more compression fractures of thoracic or lumbar vertebral bodies.

b. Radiographic features. A marked decrease of Boehler's angle is indicative of a compression fracture of the calcaneal bone mass underlying the anatomic subtalar joint.

3. **Avulsion fractures of the base of the fifth metatarsal (Jones' fractures)**
   a. **Clinical features.** Jones' fractures occur as a result of forceful inversion of the foot concurrent with contraction of peroneus brevis. Consequently, the fracture line almost always extends transversely or obliquely through the base of the fifth metatarsal.
   b. **Radiographic features.** Children and adolescents may bear a secondary center of ossification at the base of the fifth metatarsal. The radiolucent space representative of the apophyseal plate extends longitudinally through the base of the fifth metatarsal. A normal apophyseal plate is distinguished from a Jones' fracture by the difference in orientation through the base of the fifth metatarsal.

4. **Ankle joint effusions**
   a. **Clinical features**
      (1) A person suffering from a painful ankle effusion is most comfortable when the foot is slightly dorsiflexed and inverted.
      (2) Soft tissue swelling both medial and lateral to the Achilles tendon is generally indicative of intracapsular ankle joint effusion. Soft tissue swelling only medial or only lateral to the Achilles tendon is indicative of extracapsular edema.
   b. **Radiographic features**
      (1) A lateral radiograph of the ankle provides the most sensitive indicators of ankle joint effusion because the anterior and posterior parts of the joint capsule are the parts most readily displaced by an effusion.
      (2) A fluid-filled bulge of the anterior part of the capsule displaces the anterior fat pad, so that a water-density area replaces the usual fat-density area at the anterior limit of the joint space.
      (3) The posterior tibiofibular ligament of the distal tibiofibular joint limits fluid-filled bulges of the capsule's posterior part to the regions above and below the ligament, creating a doublet of water-density areas in place of the fat-density area at the posterior limit of the joint space.

STUDY QUESTIONS

Directions: Each question below contains five suggested answers. Choose the **one best** response to each question.

1. A slipped capital femoral epiphysis is a displaced Salter-Harris

(A) Type I fracture
(B) Type II fracture
(C) Type III fracture
(D) Type IV fracture
(E) Type V fracture

2. The most superior point of the iliac crest lies at the level of the spinous process of the

(A) first lumbar vertebra
(B) second lumbar vertebra
(C) third lumbar vertebra
(D) fourth lumbar vertebra
(E) fifth lumbar vertebra

3. Which of the following muscles is innervated by the common peroneal portion of the sciatic nerve?

(A) Long head of biceps femoris
(B) Short head of biceps femoris
(C) Hamstring portion of adductor magnus
(D) Semimembranosus
(E) Semitendinosus

4. The safest site for an intramuscular injection in the buttock is the

(A) upper medial quadrant
(B) upper lateral quadrant
(C) lower lateral quadrant
(D) lower medial quadrant
(E) central area

5. The Achilles tendon reflex test assesses the integrity of the neuronal pathways at which of the following spinal cord segment levels?

(A) L1 and L2
(B) L2 and L3
(C) L3 and L4
(D) S1 and S2
(E) S3 and S4

6. The horizontal group of superficial inguinal lymph nodes drains all of the following tissues EXCEPT

(A) the urethra
(B) superficial tissue of the buttock
(C) the testes
(D) the vagina below the hymen
(E) the lower half of the anal canal

7. Which of the following secondary centers of ossification is present in a full-term newborn?

(A) The center for the head of the femur
(B) The center for the greater trochanter of the femur
(C) The center for the distal end of the femur
(D) The center for the proximal tibia
(E) The center for the proximal fibula

8. A young football player sustains a severe blow to the lateral aspect of his left knee. After the swollen knee joint is aspirated, physical examination reveals that the left tibia can be pulled anteriorly at the knee to a significantly greater extent than the right tibia can. This finding suggests a torn

(A) anterior cruciate ligament
(B) posterior cruciate ligament
(C) medial collateral ligament
(D) lateral collateral ligament
(E) oblique popliteal ligament

9. Inversion and eversion of the foot occur at two functional joints. All of the following bones contribute an articular surface to these two functional joints EXCEPT

(A) talus
(B) calcaneus
(C) cuboid
(D) navicular
(E) medial cuneiform

10. All of the following statements concerning the femoral triangle are true EXCEPT

(A) the inguinal ligament forms the superior border of the femoral triangle
(B) adductor longus, pectineus, psoas, and iliacus form the floor of the femoral triangle
(C) the femoral artery lies medial to the femoral vein in the femoral triangle
(D) the femoral nerve lies lateral to the femoral artery in the femoral triangle
(E) a femoral hernia may protrude onto the floor of the femoral triangle

Directions: Each question below contains four suggested answers. Choose the **one best** response to each question.

11. Which of the following radiographic signs in an AP radiograph of the pelvis would indicate a slipped capital femoral epiphysis?

(A) The medial edge of the growth plate for the capital femoral epiphysis abuts the lower rim of the acetabular cavity at an abnormally low point
(B) A line drawn along the superior margin of the femoral neck projects proximally above the level of the capital epiphysis
(C) Both signs
(D) Neither sign

12. True statements regarding hip joint effusions include which of the following?

(A) A person suffering from a painful hip joint effusion is most comfortable standing erect
(B) The most sensitive indicator of hip joint effusion in an AP radiograph is lateral displacement of the gluteal line
(C) Both statements
(D) Neither statement

13. The integrity of neuronal pathways at the L2, L3, and L4 spinal cord segment levels can be tested by a reflex test of

(A) the adductor portion of adductor magnus
(B) quadriceps femoris
(C) both muscles
(D) neither muscle

14. True statements regarding tibial fractures include which of the following?

(A) Many tibial shaft fractures are open
(B) Tibial plateau fractures may be complicated by delayed union of the fragments following reduction
(C) Both statements
(D) Neither statement

15. True statements regarding a multipartite patella include which of the following?

(A) The accessory bone tissue masses are not completely outlined by cortical bone
(B) Mental reconstruction of the component parts of a multipartite patella produces a normal patellar outline
(C) Both statements
(D) Neither statement

16. True statements regarding osteochondritis dissecans include which of the following?

(A) The most common sites of this lesion are the shoulder and hip joints
(B) The lesion may result in detachment and dislodgement of an osteochondral body
(C) Both statements
(D) Neither statement

17. True statements regarding acute hematogenous osteomyelitis include which of the following?

(A) Most cases occur in the distal femur and proximal tibia in an elderly person
(B) Plain radiographs do not show lytic lesions until 7 to 10 days after the onset of the infection
(C) Both statements
(D) Neither statement

18. AP and lateral radiographs are taken after injection of a radiopaque solution into the synovial cavity of a normal knee joint. The solution should appear in

(A) the suprapatellar bursa
(B) the deep infrapatellar bursa
(C) both bursae
(D) neither bursa

19. True statements regarding relationships about the medial malleolus include which of the following?

(A) The pulsations of the posterior tibial artery can be palpated posteroinferiorly to the medial malleous
(B) The great saphenous vein ascends from the foot to the leg by passing anterior to the medial malleolus
(C) Both statements
(D) Neither statement

Directions: Each question below contains four suggested answers of which **one or more** is correct. Choose the answer

A if **1, 2, and 3** are correct
B if **1 and 3** are correct
C if **2 and 4** are correct
D if **4** is correct
E if **1, 2, 3, and 4** are correct

20. The quadriceps femoris consists of which of the following muscles?

(1) Vastus lateralis
(2) Rectus femoris
(3) Vastus medialis
(4) Sartorius

21. An AP radiograph of a normal pelvis typically shows that

(1) the symphysis pubis aligns with the midline of the sacrum
(2) the neck of the femur is foreshortened if the lower limb is internally rotated at the hip joint by 10° to 15°
(3) the curved, superior margin of the obturator foramen is continuous with the curved, inferior margin of the neck of the femur
(4) the superior, axial, and medial joint spaces of the hip joint are approximately equal in width

22. Posterior hip dislocations show which of the following features?

(1) The lower limb is abducted and externally rotated
(2) An AP radiograph of the pelvis shows the dislocated femoral head displaced superiorly from its normal alignment with the acetabular cavity
(3) Shenton's line remains continuous on both sides in an AP radiograph of the pelvis
(4) The sciatic nerve commonly is compressed by the dislocated femoral head

23. True statements regarding femoral neck fractures in the elderly include which of the following?

(1) Most of the fractures occur at the distal end of the femoral neck
(2) External rotation of the foot is limited to 90° following intracapsular fracture of the femoral neck
(3) Avascular necrosis of the femoral head rarely occurs following reduction of the fracture
(4) Osteoporosis contributes to the genesis of the fractures

24. True statements regarding Legg-Perthes disease include which of the following?

(1) The child may initially present with just knee pain
(2) The disease is bilateral in most patients
(3) Radiographs generally are normal early in the initial phase of the disease
(4) The regenerative phase of the disease restores the femoral head to its normal shape

25. True statements regarding AP and tunnel radiographs of the knee include which of the following?

(1) An AP radiograph shows the profiles of the anteroinferior articular surfaces of the femoral condyles
(2) An AP radiograph shows the patella en face
(3) A tunnel radiograph shows the profiles of the posterosuperior articular surfaces of the femoral condyles
(4) A tunnel radiograph shows the patella en face

26. True statements regarding T1-weighted magnetic resonance images of musculoskeletal tissues about the knee include which of the following?

(1) Cortical bone generates a high-intensity signal
(2) Fat generates a low-intensity signal
(3) Fibrous cartilage generates a high-intensity signal
(4) Hyaline cartilage generates an intermediate-density signal

27. Which of the following fractures would release fat into the knee joint cavity?

(1) A fracture through the articular surface of the lateral femoral condyle
(2) A patellar fracture
(3) A tibial plateau fracture
(4) A fracture through the head of the fibula

28. Which of the following radiographic features would be characteristic of both primary osteoarthritis and rheumatoid arthritis of the knee joint?

(1) Narrowing of joint spaces
(2) Periarticular osteopenia
(3) Subchondral cyst formation
(4) Subchondral erosions

29. Medial rotators of the leg include which of the following muscles?

(1) Semitendinosus
(2) Sartorius
(3) Gracilis
(4) Popliteus

30. Which of the following muscles would be susceptible to paralysis following a crushing injury to the lateral aspect of the head and neck of the fibula?

(1) Extensor digitorum longus
(2) Extensor digitorum brevis
(3) Tibialis anterior
(4) Peroneus longus

31. The popliteal nodes receive lymph from

(1) the soleus muscle
(2) the skin covering the lateral aspect of the heel
(3) the talus
(4) the skin covering the medial aspect of the big toe

32. A mortise radiograph of a normal ankle typically shows

(1) the lateral margin of the body of the talus colinear with the floor of the fibular notch of the tibia
(2) the joint space between the talus and medial malleolus equal in width to that between the talus and lateral malleolus
(3) the posterior malleolus overlapping the superior margin of the talus
(4) the joint space between the talus and medial malleolus twice as wide as that between the talus and the tibial plafond

33. A lateral radiograph of a normal foot typically shows

(1) a Boehler's angle of 10° to 15°
(2) the tip of the medial malleolus lying distal to the tip of the lateral malleolus
(3) a water-density area directly abutting the anterior limit of the ankle joint space
(4) a fat-density area directly abutting the posterior limit of the ankle joint space

Directions: The groups of questions below consist of lettered choices followed by several numbered items. For each numbered item, select the one lettered choice with which it is most closely associated. Each lettered choice may be used once, more than once, or not at all. Choose the answer

A if the item is associated with **(A) only**
B if the item is associated with **(B) only**
C if the item is associated with **both (A) and (B)**
D if the item is associated with **neither (A) nor (B)**

Questions 34–36

For each movement listed below, select the gluteal muscle or muscles that act as prime movers of the movement.

(A) Gluteus maximus
(B) Gluteus medius
(C) Both muscles
(D) Neither muscle

34. Extending the thigh during walking

35. Balancing the upper body over the non-weight-bearing lower limb during walking

36. Extending the trunk relative to the thigh when rising from a seated position

Questions 37 and 38

For each movement listed below, select the thigh muscle or muscles that can exert the movement.

(A) Sartorius
(B) Gracilis
(C) Both muscles
(D) Neither muscle

37. Flexion of the thigh

38. Flexion of the leg

Questions 39 and 40

For each movement listed below, select the leg muscle or muscles that act as prime movers of the movement.

(A) Tibialis anterior
(B) Tibialis posterior
(C) Both muscles
(D) Neither muscle

39. Dorsiflexion of the foot

40. Inversion of the foot

ANSWERS AND EXPLANATIONS

1. The answer is A. [*I C 4 a (2); Chapter 1 II C 2 c (1)*] A slipped capital femoral epiphysis is a Salter-Harris Type I fracture because the fracture extends through only the growth plate for the femoral head. Although the injury does not lead to avascular necrosis of the femoral head, it predisposes the hip joint to premature osteoarthritis.

2. The answer is D. [*I A 1 a (2) (a)*] The most superior point of the iliac crest lies at the level of the spinous process of the fourth lumbar vertebra. This relationship is used to identify the L3–L4 and L4–L5 interspinous process spaces for the site of needle entry when performing procedures such as lumbar puncture or lumbar epidural anesthesia. In an adult, the conus medullaris (i.e., the tapered, lower end of the spinal cord) lies at the level of the lower border of the body of L1; in a child, the conus medullaris can lie as low as the level of L3. Accordingly, either the L3–L4 or L4–L5 interspinous process space can be chosen for needle entry in an adult patient, whereas only the latter space is appropriate in a pediatric patient.

3. The answer is B. [*I A 3 a (3); II A 3 b (1)*] The short head of biceps femoris is the only muscle of the lower limb innervated by the common peroneal portion of the sciatic nerve. The long head of biceps femoris, the hamstring portion of adductor magnus, the semimembranosus, and the semitendinosus are all innervated by the tibial portion of the sciatic nerve.

4. The answer is B. [*I A 4 b, c*] The sciatic nerve follows a curved inferolateral course through the lower medial quadrant of the gluteal region. Therefore, the upper lateral quadrant is the safest site for an intramuscular injection because this is the quadrant furthest removed from the course of the sciatic nerve through the gluteal region.

5. The answer is D. [*III A 3 a (3) (b)*] The muscles that contribute to the Achilles tendon (gastrocnemius, soleus, and plantaris) all receive most of their innervation from the S1 and S2 spinal cord segments. Another test of neuronal pathways at levels including the S1 and S2 levels is the medial hamstring tendon reflex test; this test assesses neuronal pathways at the L4, L5, S1, and S2 levels through the collective response of semitendinosus, semimembranosus, gracilis, and sartorius to a phasic stretch of their tendons of insertion.

6. The answer is C. [*I A 5 b (3) (c) (i)*] The gonads of both sexes are drained by para-aortic nodes lying near the origin of the gonadal arteries from the abdominal aorta. The lateral members of the horizontal group of superficial inguinal nodes receive lymph from the superficial buttock tissues. The medial members of the horizontal group receive lymph from the anterolateral abdominal wall up to the level of the umbilicus, the urethra, the lower half of the anal canal, and the external genitalia of both sexes (which includes the vagina below the hymen in a female but not the testes in a male). The medial members are thus among the first lymph nodes to react and enlarge in response to lymphatogenous dissemination of cancer of the lower half of the anal canal or to lymphatogenous dissemination of syphilitic infections of the external genitalia.

7. The answer is C. [*II A 1 a (2)*] The secondary center of ossification for the distal end of the femur is the only secondary center among the long bones of the extremities that consistently appears before a full-term birth; specifically, it always appears by 36 to 37 weeks of gestation. The presence of this center in the lower limbs of an abandoned and deceased newborn constitutes forensic evidence that the newborn was viable at birth.

8. The answer is A. [*II A 2 a (2) (a)*] The anterior cruciate ligament restricts the tibia from being pulled too far forward during extension of the leg. A tear or rupture of the anterior cruciate ligament is an injury that is especially common among football players, in whom the injury often results from a severe blow delivered to the lateral side of the knee at a moment when the knee is partially flexed and the foot is firmly planted on the ground. The forces that tear the anterior cruciate ligament under these conditions almost always also tear or rupture the medial collateral ligament and the medial meniscus.

The anterior drawer test can ascertain the integrity of the anterior cruciate ligament. After any trauma-induced hemorrhagic effusion of the knee joint's synovial cavity has been aspirated, the patient lies supine on an examination table with the injured lower limb flexed 25° to 30° at the knee joint and the foot resting on the table. The examiner grasps the upper end of the leg with one hand and the lower end of the thigh with the other hand, requests the patient to relax the muscles, and then pulls the leg forward. The anterior cruciate ligament is ruptured if the tibial condyles can be pulled more than 1 cm forward underneath the femoral condyles; such a finding is called a positive anterior drawer sign. A positive anterior drawer sign on the injured knee should always be compared with test results on the contralateral knee.

9. The answer is E. [*III A 2 c (2)*] The functional subtalar joint and Chopart's joint are the two functional joints at which inversion and eversion of the foot occur. The functional subtalar joint consists of the anatomic subtalar joint (which is a joint between the talus and calcaneus) and the talocalcaneal articulation in the talocalcaneonavicular joint. Chopart's joint consists of the calcaneocuboid joint and the talonavicular articulation in the talocalcaneonavicular joint. Thus, the talus, calcaneus, cuboid, and navicular all contribute to the two functional joints at which inversion and eversion of the foot occur, whereas the medial cuneiform does not.

10. The answer is C. [*I A 5 a, b (1), (2) (b)*] The femoral triangle is bordered superiorly by the inguinal ligament, medially by the medial border of adductor longus, and laterally by the medial border of sartorius. The femoral sheath envelops, from lateral to medial, the proximal segment of the femoral artery, the terminal segment of the femoral vein, and the deep inguinal nodes of the femoral canal. The femoral nerve extends onto the floor of the femoral triangle lateral to the femoral sheath.

The neck of a femoral hernia lies at the femoral ring, which is inferolateral to the pubic tubercle. The sac of a femoral hernia and its contents may protrude through the femoral canal, onto the floor of the femoral triangle, and even through the saphenous opening in the fascia lata of the thigh. If a femoral hernia extends through the saphenous opening, the sharp lower border of the opening commonly turns the sac and its contents superiorly into the superficial fascia of the thigh, a condition that can quickly lead to an acute abdomen due to constriction of the blood supply to the contents of the sac (which generally is a segment of small intestine).

11. The answer is C. [*I C 4 c*] A slipped capital femoral epiphysis is a Salter-Harris Type I fracture; it occurs most commonly during early adolescence. In addition to the two radiographic signs listed in the question, a slipped capital femoral epiphysis may also be indicated by an abnormally widened growth plate.

12. The answer is D. [*I C 6 b, c (1)*] A person suffering from a painful hip joint effusion is most comfortable when seated with the painful thigh slightly abducted and externally rotated at the hip joint. Inferolateral displacement of the femoral head is the most sensitive indicator of hip joint effusion in an AP radiograph. Whereas displacements of the fat lines about the hip joint are unreliable indicators of hip joint effusion in adults, medial displacement of the psoas line or the obturator line is a sensitive indicator in pediatric patients.

13. The answer is C. [*I A 3 d (3); II A 3 a (2)*] The adductor portion of adductor magnus is innervated by the obturator nerve, and quadriceps femoris is innervated by the femoral nerve. Both nerves are derived from the L2, L3, and L4 roots of the lumbar plexus.

14. The answer is A. [*II E 2 a (2); III A 1 a (1) (a), (c)*] Many tibial shaft fractures are open because of the subcutaneous lie of the shaft's anteromedial surface. Tibial shaft fractures may be complicated by delayed union of the reduced fragments if the fracture occurs distal to the foramen for the nutrient artery to the tibial shaft; the foramen is located in the upper half of the posterior surface of the shaft. Tibial plateau ("bumper") fractures are generally confined to just the tibial condyles and thus are located proximal to the foramen for the nutrient artery to the tibial shaft. Tibial plateau fractures are often called "bumper fractures" because such fractures are commonly sustained when a person is struck in the knee by an automobile bumper.

15. The answer is D. [*II E 3 c*] A multipartite patella is a variant of the normal patella in which the bone tissue masses generated from one or more peripheral centers of ossification do not fuse with the central bone mass. The accessory bone tissue masses of a multipartite patella are completely outlined by cortical bone, and they generally border the superolateral margin of the patella. Mental reconstruction of the parts of a multicomponent patella produces a normal patellar outline if the parts are fragments of a fractured patella; such an exercise does not produce a completely normal outline if the parts are components of a multipartite patella.

16. The answer is B. [*II E 6 a (1), b (2)*] Osteochondritis dissecans occurs mainly in adolescents and young adults. The most common site of the lesion is the knee; most knee lesions occur in the lateral aspect of the medial femoral condyle. Detachment and dislodgement of an osteochondral body may occur if the lesion extends into the articular cartilage. The segment of the lesion extending through the subchondral bone is not always detectable in plain film radiographs early in the course of the condition.

17. The answer is B. [*II E 7 a (1), (2), b*] About 80% of all cases of hematogenous osteomyelitis occur in children and adolescents; the most common sites of bacterial bone infection are the metaphyses of the distal femur and proximal tibia. The principal radiographic findings during the first 24 to 48 hours are edema and loss of fascial plane definition of the overlying soft tissues. If the condition continues untreated, lytic lesions of the infected metaphysis occur within 7 to 10 days, followed by sclerosis due to new periosteal bone formation.

18. The answer is A. [*II A 2 a (3) (a) (i), (b) (iii)*] The suprapatellar bursa is the most anterosuperior recess of the knee joint's synovial cavity; it lies between the quadriceps femoris tendon and the anterior surface of the distal femur, embedded within the suprapatellar fat pad. Since the suprapatellar bursa communicates with the joint's synovial cavity, it should fill with radiopaque solution injected into the synovial cavity. The popliteal, gastrocnemius, and semimembranosus bursae should also be filled with the radiopaque solution, as these bursae commonly communicate with the joint's synovial cavity. The deep infrapatellar bursa does not communicate with the joint's synovial cavity; it lies between the ligamentum patellae and the anterior surface of the proximal tibia, embedded within the infrapatellar fat pad.

19. The answer is C. [*III A 5 a (1), b (1)*] The great saphenous vein is commonly selected for prolonged intravenous administration of fluids and drugs. It is also commonly used for coronary artery bypass surgery because (1) it can be readily resected, (2) its diameter closely approximates that of the coronary arteries and their major branches, and (3) its wall bears a comparatively high content of elastic tissue. If the vein is not visible in a patient's lower limb, it can be reliably accessed surgically by an incision in front of the medial malleolus.

The pulsations of the posterior tibial artery can be palpated posteroinferiorly to the medial malleolus of the tibia. Additionally, the pulsations of the dorsalis pedis can be palpated on the dorsum of the foot immediately lateral to the tendon of extensor hallucis longus.

20. The answer is A (1, 2, 3). [*II A 3 a (1)*] Vastus lateralis, vastus intermedius, vastus medialis, and rectus femoris are the four muscles of the quadriceps femoris. These four muscles are the only extensors of the leg. Rectus femoris can also flex the thigh.

21. The answer is B (1, 3). [*I B 1 b (2) (a), c, 3 b (3), 4 a; Figure 2-1*] In an AP radiograph of the pelvis, alignment of the symphysis pubis with the midline of the sacrum helps establish the absence of pelvic rotation. Internal rotation of the lower limb at the hip joint by 10° to 15° provides for almost maximum projection of the femoral neck. A continuous curve can be drawn from the superior margin of the obturator foramen to the inferior margin of the neck of the femur; this curve is called Shenton's line. The medial joint space is approximately twice as wide as the superior and axial joint spaces.

22. The answer is C (2, 4). [*I C 1 a (1), (2), c*] Posterior hip dislocations account for most hip joint dislocations. The person presents with a shortened, adducted, and internally rotated limb. The dislocated femoral head commonly compresses the sciatic nerve. An AP radiograph of the pelvis shows the femoral head displaced superiorly from its normal alignment with the acetabular cavity; this displacement breaks the continuity of Shenton's line.

23. The answer is D (4). [*I C 3 a*] Femoral neck fractures are especially common among the elderly; osteoporosis contributes to the genesis of such fractures. Most of the fractures are subcapital fractures; that is, they occur at the proximal end of the femoral neck. The accompanying rupture of the circumflex femoral arterial branches to the femoral head generally leads to avascular necrosis of the femoral head. External rotation of the foot is limited to 45° following intracapsular fracture of the femoral neck; external rotation can be as great as 90° following extracapsular fracture.

24. The answer is B (1, 3). [*I C 5 b (2), (3), c (1), (3) (a)*] The hip joint and knee joint are both innervated by the femoral and obturator nerves; disease of either joint may thus elicit referred pain in the other joint. That is why Legg-Perthes disease (idiopathic avascular necrosis of the head of the femur) can cause knee pain alone. The disease is rarely bilateral, and when it is bilateral, it is almost never in the same stage on both sides. Radiographic evidence for the initial phase of Legg-Perthes disease, such as wider superior, axial, and medial joint spaces or a subchondral radiolucency, generally does not appear until late in the initial phase. The femoral head reossifies during the regenerative phase but does not regain its normal shape. The regenerative phase produces an abnormally flattened femoral head.

25. The answer is A (1, 2, 3). [*II B 1 a (1), b, 2 a (1), (4)*] The AP and tunnel radiographs principally differ in that a tunnel radiograph casts the posterosuperior articular surfaces of the femoral condyles, displays the intercondylar notch, shows the notched origin of popliteus more clearly, and does not show the patella en face. Both radiographs are similar in that each shows a low-angle anteroposterior projection of the tibial plateaus.

26. The answer is D (4). [*II C 1, 3 b*] The suprapatellar and infrapatellar fat pads and cancellous bone about the knee exhibit high values (i.e., light shades) of grey in T1-weighted magnetic resonance images, because fat generates a high-intensity signal. The hyaline cartilage plates covering the articular surfaces of the femoral condyles and tibial plateaus exhibit intermediate values of grey. Ligaments, cortical bone, and the fibrous cartilage of the menisci all generate low-intensity signals, and thus are portrayed in dark shades of grey.

27. The answer is A (1, 2, 3). [*II E 2 b, 3 b, 4 b*] A fracture at the knee will release fat into the knee joint cavity if the fracture extends from a bone's articular surface within the knee joint to the bone's cancellous interior. The presence of fat is documented if a cross-table lateral radiograph shows a fat–fluid-density interface in the anterosuperior compartment of the joint cavity. The bony articular surfaces of the knee joint are provided by the femoral condyles, tibial plateaus, and patella. The head of the fibula contributes an articular surface to the proximal tibiofibular joint but not to the knee joint.

28. The answer is B (1, 3). [*II E 8 b, 9 b*] Joint space narrowing, periarticular osteopenia, and subchondral cysts and erosions all are characteristic features of rheumatoid arthritis of any large synovial joint. Features characteristic of primary osteoarthritis include, in addition to narrowing of the joint spaces and subchondral cyst formation, subchondral osteosclerosis and osteophyte formation. The knee joint is a common site of primary osteoarthritis.

29. The answer is E (all). [*II A 3 c*] Five muscles can medially rotate the leg: popliteus, semitendinosus, semimembranosus, sartorius, and gracilis. Popliteus's capacity to rotate the leg medially serves to unlock the knee joint at the commencement of flexion of a fully extended leg. Semitendinosus, sartorius, and gracilis all insert onto the upper part of the medial surface of the tibial shaft; their insertion tendons are collectively called the pes anserinus (goose's foot) because their configuration suggests the imprint of a goose's foot.

30. The answer is E (all). [*II A 4 a (1) (b); III A 3 a (1), (2) (a), 4 b*] The common peroneal nerve's relatively superficial course around the head and neck of the fibula renders it susceptible to damage by a crushing injury to the lateral aspect of the fibular head and neck. Such damage may paralyze the five muscles innervated by the deep peroneal nerve (tibialis anterior, extensor hallucis longus, extensor digitorum longus, peroneus tertius, and extensor digitorum brevis) and the two muscles innervated by the superficial peroneal nerve (peroneus longus and peroneus brevis). Paralysis of the major dorsiflexors of the foot (i.e., tibialis anterior, extensor hallucis longus, and extensor digitorum longus) produces footdrop.

31. The answer is A (1, 2, 3). [*II A 4 b*] Lymph from the soleus muscle, the skin on the lateral aspect of the heel, and the talus would drain into the popliteal nodes. This is because the popliteal nodes receive lymph from the deep tissues of the foot and leg and the superficial tissues of the posterolateral aspect of the leg and the lateral aspect of the foot. The remainder of the superficial tissues of the lower limb (except for those of the buttock) are drained by the vertical group of superficial inguinal nodes. Therefore, these nodes would receive lymph from the skin on the medial aspect of the big toe. The deep tissues of the thigh are drained by the deep inguinal and external iliac nodes.

32. The answer is A (1, 2, 3). [*III B 1 b–d; Figure 2-21*] A mortise radiograph of the ankle shows the tenon-and-mortise configuration of the joint. One important characteristic of this configuration is the uniformity of the joint space's width at all sites. Malalignment of the lateral margin of the body of the talus with the floor of the fibular notch of the tibia is pathognomonic of a pair of breaks within the osseoligamentous ring of the ankle region. The posterior malleolus overlaps the superior margin of the talus in a mortise radiograph. A lateral radiograph of the ankle provides an unobstructed view of the posterior malleolus.

33. The answer is D (4). [*III B 2 a (1) (b), (2), b (2); Figure 2-22*] Boehler's angle measures the angular relationship between segments of the calcaneus; its normal range is 20° to 40°. The medial malleolus is shorter than the lateral malleolus; both malleoli overlap the ankle joint space and body of the talus in the radiograph. Fat-density areas bracket both the anterior and posterior limits of the joint space.

34–36. The answers are: 34-D, 35-B, 36-A. [*I A 3 a (1), (2), c (1)*] The chief extensors of the thigh when a person is walking are the hamstring muscles: semitendinosus, semimembranosus, and the long head of biceps femoris. Gluteus maximus is the chief extensor of the trunk relative to the thigh when a person rises from a seated position.

Gluteus medius and gluteus minimus are the muscles chiefly responsible for supporting and steadying the upper body over the non–weight-bearing limb during walking. The capacity of these two gluteal muscles to exert this action can be examined by the Trendelenburg test: The patient stands in front of the examiner, with his or her back to the examiner, and alternately raises each foot off the ground. If gluteus medius and gluteus minimus on (let us say) the right side can adequately support and steady the upper body, the left side of the pelvis becomes very slightly elevated when the left foot is raised off the ground. Observation of such a normal reaction is reported as a negative Trendelenburg test for the right lower limb. If, however, the capacity of the right gluteus medius and gluteus minimus to support the upper body is compromised, the left side of the pelvis tilts, or sags, downward as the left foot is raised off the ground. Observation of such an abnormal reaction is reported as a positive Trendelenburg test for the right lower limb. The three most common conditions which produce a positive Trendelenburg test are (1) paralysis or weakness of the gluteus medius and gluteus minimus, (2) dislocation of the hip joint, and (3) an abnormal angle between the neck and shaft of the femur.

37 and 38. The answers are: 37-A, 38-C. [*I A 3 b (2); II A 3 b (2) (a), (b)*] Sartorius is an active flexor of the thigh when one is walking. Sartorius and gracilis assist the chief flexors of the leg (semitendinosus, semimembranosus, and biceps femoris) during walking. Sartorius is the only muscle of the lower limb that can flex both the thigh and the leg.

39 and 40. The answers are: 39-A, 40-C. [*III A 3 a (1) (a) (i), (4) (a)*] Tibialis posterior is the chief invertor of the foot, and tibialis anterior is the second most powerful invertor of the foot. The invertor action of the two tibialis muscles pulls the leg medially during the stance phase of the walking gait and thus serves to counteract any lateral overbalancing of the body caused by the actions of gluteus medius and gluteus minimus at the hip joint. Whereas tibialis anterior is the chief dorsiflexor of the foot, tibialis posterior is a plantar flexor of the foot. Tibialis anterior exerts its foot dorsiflexor action twice during walking: Pulling forward on the leg from the foot, it acts through most of the flat-foot period of the stance phase to help propel the body forward over the limb; pulling upward on the foot from the leg, it helps raise the forefoot above the surface below just after toe-off.

3 Thorax

I. ANATOMY OF THE THORAX

A. Chest wall

1. Skeletal and cartilaginous framework

a. Thoracic vertebrae

(1) The spinous process of the first thoracic vertebra is the second highest palpable spinous process in the vertebral column (that of the seventh cervical vertebra being the highest).

(2) The tip of the spinous process of each thoracic vertebra rests at about the level of the body of the vertebra immediately below.

b. Sternum

(1) The **sternal angle**, or **angle of Louis**, is the posterior angle between the manubrium and the body of the sternum at the manubriosternal joint.

(2) The costal cartilage of the second rib articulates with the sternum at the level of the sternal angle.

(3) In adults, the body of the sternum may be selected for needle biopsy of hematopoietic bone marrow.

c. Costal cartilages

(1) The costal cartilages are bars of hyaline cartilage.

(2) The synovial articulations between the costal cartilages of the seventh to tenth ribs form, on each side, the **costal margin** of the rib cage.

d. Ribs

(1) A typical rib has three segments, called the **head**, **neck**, and **body**; the **tubercle** of the rib marks the origin of the body of the rib.

(2) The **angle** of a rib is the segment of the body which has the greatest curvature.

(3) The **costal groove** of a rib is the shallow groove on the inner surface of the rib's inferior border.

(4) A typical rib forms two synovial joints with vertebrae.

(a) The **head** of the rib forms a **costovertebral joint** with the body of the thoracic vertebra at the same level and the body of the thoracic vertebra immediately above.

(b) The **tubercle** of the rib forms a **costotransverse joint** with the transverse process of the thoracic vertebra at the same level.

2. Intercostal muscles

a. Three overlapping muscles extend along most of the length of each intercostal space: the **external intercostal muscle**, the **internal intercostal muscle**, and the **deepest intercostal muscle layer.**

b. The intercostal muscles contribute to the respiratory movements of the ribs. They also serve to prevent the intercostal spaces from bellowing inward during inspiration and bulging outward during expiration.

c. The intercostal muscles in each intercostal space are innervated by the space's intercostal nerve.

3. Neurovascular elements

a. The major neurovascular bundle in each intercostal space lies between the two innermost intercostal muscle layers and partially under cover of the costal groove of the rib immediately above; within the bundle, the vein is the highest element and the nerve is the lowest element. When it is necessary to insert a needle through an intercostal space, insertion should occur along the upper border of the rib immediately below, so as to avoid the major neurovascular bundle.

b. The eleven pairs of **intercostal nerves** are derived from the anterior rami of the first eleven thoracic spinal nerves.

c. Each intercostal space is supplied by two anterior intercostal arteries (except for the two lowest spaces) and a single posterior intercostal artery.

(1) The **anterior intercostal arteries** of the five or six upper spaces are branches of the internal thoracic artery; the anterior intercostal arteries of the next four or three lower spaces are branches of the musculophrenic artery.

(2) The **posterior intercostal arteries** of the two uppermost spaces are branches of the superior intercostal artery; the posterior intercostal arteries of the nine lowest spaces are branches of the descending thoracic aorta.

d. The **venae comitantes** of the anterior intercostal arteries and the two uppermost posterior intercostal arteries drain toward the brachiocephalic veins; the venae comitantes of the nine lowest posterior intercostal arteries are tributaries of the azygos system of veins.

B. Diaphragm. The diaphragm is the chief muscle of inspiration; it can account for about two-thirds of the lungs' volumetric increase during inspiration. It is the most effective respiratory muscle when a person is supine.

1. Innervation

a. The **phrenic nerves** provide motor innervation of the diaphragm. They provide sensory innervation for the parietal pleura overlying the central tendon of the diaphragm and for the parietal peritoneum underlying the central tendon. The phrenic nerves also provide sensory innervation for the mediastinal pleura of the pleural cavities.

b. The lowest five **intercostal nerves** and the **subcostal nerves** (i.e., the anterior rami of spinal nerves T7 to T12) provide sensory innervation for the parietal pleura and parietal peritoneum lining the peripheral surfaces of the diaphragm.

2. Openings. The diaphragm has three major openings.

a. The **caval opening** lies at the level of the body of the eighth thoracic vertebra, and transmits

(1) The inferior vena cava

(2) The right phrenic nerve

b. The **esophageal opening** lies at the level of the body of the tenth thoracic vertebra, and transmits

(1) The esophagus

(2) The anterior and posterior vagal trunks

(3) The esophageal branches of the left gastric artery

(4) The esophageal tributaries of the left gastric vein

c. The **aortic opening** lies at the level of the body of the twelfth thoracic vertebra, and transmits

(1) The aorta

(2) The azygos vein

(3) The thoracic duct

C. Lungs and pleural cavities

1. Surface projections of the lungs and the pleural cavities

a. Apex. The apex of each lung projects above the medial third of the clavicle.

b. Interlobar fissures

(1) The surface projection of each lung's **oblique fissure** begins posteriorly in the upper thoracic region, crosses the fifth and sixth ribs as it curves laterally to the midaxillary line, and then courses along the lower border of the sixth rib to the lateral border of the sternum.

(2) The surface projection of the right lung's **horizontal fissure** courses along the lower border of the fourth rib from the midaxillary line to the lateral border of the sternum.

c. Margins

(1) At midinspiration in quiet breathing, the **lower margin** of each lung lies at the level of

(a) The sixth rib anteriorly at the midclavicular line

(b) The eighth rib laterally at the midaxillary line

(c) The tenth rib posteriorly at the lateral border of the vertebral column

(2) The surface projection of the **costodiaphragmatic margin** of each pleural cavity passes through
(a) The eighth rib anteriorly at the midclavicular line
(b) The tenth rib laterally at the midaxillary line
(c) The eleventh or twelfth rib posteriorly at the lateral border of the vertebral column
(3) At midinspiration in quiet breathing, the **costodiaphragmatic recess** is the recess two rib spaces high in each pleural cavity between the costodiaphragmatic margins of the lung and the pleural cavity.

2. **Bronchopulmonary segments of the lungs.** These segments are the basic functional units of the lung.
a. The numbering and nomenclature of the bronchopulmonary segments are given in Table 3-1.
b. Each pyramid-shaped segment is
(1) Enveloped by a connective tissue sheath
(2) Supplied by a single segmental bronchus and a single pulmonary arterial branch
(3) Oriented so that its apex projects toward the hilum of the lung
c. The segmental bronchus for the apical segment of each lung's lower lobe is the segmental bronchus which arises most directly and posteriorly from the main stem bronchus. Consequently, when a supine person accidentally aspirates a small object into either lung, the object will most likely lodge in the lower lobe's apical segment.

3. The **root of the lung** is the bundle of structures extending between the lung and the mediastinum.

D. **Divisions of the mediastinum.** The mediastinum is the median region of the thorax; it is bounded above by the thoracic inlet and below by the diaphragm.

1. The **superior mediastinum** is the part of the mediastinum which lies above the level of the sternal angle.

2. The **inferior mediastinum** is the part of the mediastinum which lies below the level of the sternal angle. The inferior mediastinum has three subdivisions.
a. The **anterior mediastinum** is the region which lies between the sternum and the pericardial sac.
b. The **middle mediastinum** is the region which contains the heart and its pericardial sac.
c. The **posterior mediastinum** is the region which lies between the pericardial sac and the vertebral column.

E. **Heart**

1. **Anatomic surfaces**
a. The **apex** of the heart is formed by the left ventricle.
b. The **sternocostal surface** of the heart is formed, from right to left, by the right atrium, right ventricle, and left ventricle.

Table 3-1. Names and Numbers of the Bronchopulmonary Segments of the Lungs

Segments of the Right Lung	Segments of the Left Lung
Upper Lobe	**Upper lobe**
1. Apical	1–3. Apical posterior
2. Anterior	2. Anterior
3. Posterior	
Middle lobe	
4. Lateral	4. Superior lingular
5. Medial	5. Inferior lingular
Lower lobe	**Lower lobe**
6. Apical	6. Apical
7. Medial basal	7–8. Anteromedial basal
8. Anterior basal	
9. Lateral basal	9. Lateral basal
10. Posterior basal	10. Posterior basal

c. The **diaphragmatic surface** of the heart is formed by the right and left ventricles.
d. The **base** of the heart is formed largely by the left atrium.
e. The **right border** of the heart is formed by the right atrium.
f. The **left border** of the heart is formed mainly by the left ventricle; the uppermost part of the heart's left border is defined by the auricle of the left atrium.

2. Vasculature of the heart
a. Right coronary artery
(1) Route
(a) The right coronary artery emerges from the sinus of the right cusp of the aortic valve.
(b) It descends on the heart's sternocostal surface in the atrioventricular groove, giving rise to the **right marginal artery** near the heart's inferior border.
(c) It continues its course in the atrioventricular groove as it extends on the diaphragmatic surface of the heart.
(d) At the **crux** of the heart (i.e., at the point where the atrioventricular groove meets the inferior interventricular groove), in 90% of individuals, the artery enters the posterior interventricular groove, and here is called the **posterior descending artery,** or the **posterior interventricular artery**.
(2) Distribution
(a) The right coronary artery supplies all of the right atrium, much of the right ventricle, and variable parts of the left atrium and left ventricle.
(b) The nutrient artery for the sinoatrial node is a branch of the right coronary artery in 55% of individuals.
(c) The nutrient artery for the atrioventricular node is a branch of the right coronary artery in those 90% of individuals for whom the right coronary artery becomes the posterior descending artery.
(3) Of the heart's major arteries, the right coronary artery is the second most commonly occluded.
b. Left coronary artery
(1) Route
(a) The left coronary artery emerges from the sinus of the left cusp of the aortic valve.
(b) The left coronary artery emerges on the surface of the heart by extending between the auricle of the left atrium and the pulmonary trunk.
(c) Upon reaching the atrioventricular groove, the left coronary artery divides into two major **branches**.
(i) One major branch, called the **left anterior descending artery** or the **anterior interventricular artery**, descends on the heart's sternocostal surface in the anterior interventricular groove and then arches over the apex of the heart to meet the posterior descending artery in the posterior interventricular groove.
(ii) The other major branch, the **circumflex artery**, extends within the atrioventricular groove to the diaphragmatic surface, where it meets a branch of the right coronary artery.
(d) The circumflex artery gives rise to lateral and posterolateral branches near the left border of the heart. In 10% of individuals, the circumflex artery enters the posterior interventricular groove to become the **posterior descending artery**.
(2) Distribution
(a) The left anterior descending artery supplies both ventricles; it is the major source of the arterial supply to the interventricular septum.
(b) The circumflex artery supplies much of the left atrium and left ventricle.
(c) The nutrient artery for the sinoatrial node is a branch of the circumflex artery in 45% of individuals.
(d) The nutrient artery for the atrioventricular node is a branch of the circumflex artery in those 10% of individuals for whom the circumflex artery becomes the posterior descending artery.
(3) Of the heart's major arteries, the circumflex and left anterior descending arteries are, respectively, the most commonly and the third most commonly occluded.
c. Cardiac veins
(1) The **coronary sinus** is the largest of the cardiac veins. Throughout its length, it lies within the atrioventricular groove on the diaphragmatic surface. It terminates at its opening into the posterior floor region of the right atrium.
(2) The **great cardiac vein** is the second largest vein of the heart. It arises near the apex and

ascends on the sternocostal surface within the anterior interventricular groove. Upon reaching the atrioventricular groove, it turns and extends to the left within this groove until it gives rise to the coronary sinus at the left border of the heart.

(3) The **middle cardiac vein** arises near the apex and ascends on the diaphragmatic surface within the posterior interventricular groove to join the coronary sinus at the crux.

(4) The **anterior cardiac veins** emanate from the right ventricle and extend to the right on the heart's sternocostal surface, passing over the atrioventricular groove. The veins penetrate the anterior wall of the right atrium to open directly into the chamber.

3. Conducting system of the heart

a. The **sinoatrial (SA) node** extends from the superior vena caval opening in the right atrium into the upper end of the crista terminalis.

b. The **internodal tracts** extend from the SA node through the walls of the right atrium, and terminate in the atrioventricular node.

c. The **atrioventricular (AV) node** is located in the posteroinferior region of the interatrial septum, immediately adjacent to the fibrous anulus of the tricuspid valve.

d. The **atrioventricular (AV) bundle (bundle of His)** originates from the AV node, passes through an opening in the fibrous anulus of the tricuspid valve, and then extends through the membranous part of the interventricular septum. At the border between the membranous and muscular parts of the septum, the AV bundle divides into its left and right bundle branches.

(1) The **right bundle branch** reaches the anterior wall of the right ventricle via the moderator band before it ramifies into smaller tracts.

(2) The **left bundle branch** ramifies near its origin into smaller tracts.

e. The **Purkinje fibers** are the terminal cells of the conducting system in both ventricles. The terminal processes of the Purkinje fibers terminate in the subendocardial myocardium.

4. Auscultation sites for heart sounds

a. In a normal adult, the left fifth intercostal space at the midclavicular line is the site of the **apex beat**; that is, the site at which the heart's apex beats against the anterior chest wall.

b. The heart produces two sounds during each cardiac cycle.

(1) The **first heart sound** occurs just after the beginning of systole and is produced by the near-simultaneous closure of the tricuspid and mitral valves.

(a) The **mitral component** of the first heart sound is best heard on the chest wall region overlying the apex beat.

(b) The **tricuspid component** of the first heart sound is best heard over the anterior end of the left fifth intercostal space.

(2) The **second heart sound** marks the end of systole and is produced by the near-simultaneous closure of the aortic and pulmonary valves. The aortic and pulmonary components of the second heart sound are best heard over the anterior ends of the right and left second intercostal spaces, respectively.

F. Major vessels of the mediastinum

1. Thoracic aorta

a. The **ascending aorta** is the segment of the aorta that is enveloped by the pericardial sac, and hence lies in the middle mediastinum. The ascending aorta gives off **two branches**: the left and right coronary arteries.

b. The **aortic arch** is the segment which lies in the superior mediastinum.

(1) The aortic arch begins anterior to the right pulmonary artery, arches upward and backward over the bifurcation of the pulmonary trunk, and ends posterior to the left pulmonary artery.

(2) The space between the curved undersurface of the aortic arch and the upper surface of the T-shaped pulmonary trunk bifurcation is called the **aortic–pulmonary window**. The aortic–pulmonary window contains a few tracheobronchial lymph nodes and is crossed by the ligamentum arteriosum; it is also traversed by the left recurrent laryngeal nerve.

(3) The aortic arch has **three branches**: the brachiocephalic artery, left common carotid artery, and left subclavian artery.

c. The **descending thoracic aorta** is the segment which descends in the posterior mediastinum. It ends as it enters the abdomen through the aortic opening in the diaphragm.

(1) The descending thoracic aorta lies throughout much of its course directly anterior to the vertebral column, just left of the midline.

(2) **Branches** of the descending thoracic aorta include nine pairs of posterior intercostal arteries, one or two bronchial arteries, and esophageal arteries to the middle third of the esophagus.

2. **Superior vena cava and its tributaries**
   a. **Right brachiocephalic vein.** From its origin at the union of the right subclavian and right internal jugular veins, the right brachiocephalic vein extends almost directly inferior through the superior mediastinum.
   b. **Left brachiocephalic vein.** From its origin at the union of the left subclavian and left internal jugular veins, the left brachiocephalic vein assumes a course in the superior mediastinum which extends it both downward and to the right, directly anterior to the aortic arch.
   c. **Superior vena cava.** At a level just above that of the sternal angle, the right and left brachiocephalic veins unite to form the superior vena cava. The superior vena cava descends vertically to its opening into the posterior roof region of the right atrium.
   d. **Azygos vein.** The azygos vein joins the superior vena cava just above the latter's opening into the right atrium. The azygos vein passes behind the root of the right lung and then arches forward over it before joining the superior vena cava.

3. **Inferior vena cava.** The inferior vena cava enters the thorax by passing through the caval opening of the diaphragm. It then almost immediately opens into the posterior floor region of the right atrium.

G. Other mediastinal viscera

1. **Trachea and main stem bronchi**
   a. **Trachea**
      (1) **Route**
         (a) The trachea begins in the neck as an airway continuous with the lower border of the cricoid cartilage of the larynx.
         (b) The trachea occupies a midline position in the body as it descends through first the neck and then the superior mediastinum to its termination in the posterior mediastinum at the **carina**, the prominent ridge that marks the internal margin between the origins of the left and right primary bronchi.
         (c) The trachea passes behind the aortic arch as it descends in the superior mediastinum.
         (d) In the posterior mediastinum, the trachea lies directly behind the pericardial sac.
      (2) The trachea moves downward during inspiration and upward during expiration. Upon deep inspiration, the carina can be displaced inferiorly as far as the level of the body of the seventh thoracic vertebra. At the conclusion of expiration, it can rebound superiorly to just above the level of the sternal angle.
   b. **Main stem (primary) bronchi**
      (1) The main stem bronchi lie exclusively in the posterior mediastinum; they extend from the tracheal bifurcation to the roots of the lungs.
      (2) The right main stem bronchus is more vertical, larger, and shorter than the left main stem bronchus. Consequently, if a small object is accidentally aspirated into the trachea when a person is standing or seated upright, the object is more likely to pass into the right main stem bronchus than into the left one.

2. **Esophagus**
   a. **Route**
      (1) The esophagus begins in the neck as a muscular tube continuous with the laryngopharynx (hypopharynx). The esophagus lies directly anterior to and slightly to the left of the vertebral column as it descends through the superior mediastinum and then the posterior mediastinum.
         (a) In the superior mediastinum and upper part of the posterior mediastinum, the esophagus lies directly behind the trachea.
         (b) In the lower part of the posterior mediastinum, the esophagus lies directly behind the part of the pericardial sac that covers the base of the heart.
      (2) The esophagus exits the thorax by passing through the esophageal opening in the diaphragm.
   b. **Restricted segments**
      (1) Three segments of the esophagus are physically restricted from fully expanding during

the peristaltic transport of food boli because each segment is in contact with a structure that resists displacement by the food bolus as it passes down the esophagus.

(a) The aortic arch restricts the uppermost segment.

(b) The left main stem bronchus restricts the middle segment.

(c) The muscular border of the esophageal opening of the diaphragm restricts the lowest segment.

(2) These three esophageal segments are the most common sites of stricture after the swallowing of caustic agents, and are also the most common primary sites of esophageal carcinoma.

3. Thoracic duct

a. The thoracic duct begins in the abdomen as a continuation of the cisterna chyli. The thoracic duct enters the thorax via the aortic opening of the diaphragm.

b. As the thoracic duct ascends within the posterior mediastinum, its course takes it from behind and to the right of the esophagus to a position directly to the left of the esophagus at the level of the sternal angle.

c. As the thoracic duct then ascends within the superior mediastinum, it courses along the left side of the esophagus to the base of the neck, where it finally curves laterally and empties into the origin of the left brachiocephalic vein.

4. Phrenic nerves (see also section I B 1 a)

a. The phrenic nerves arise in the neck from the cervical plexus, generally receiving fibers from spinal nerves C3, C4, and C5. They descend through the superior and then the middle mediastinum, and finally end upon passing through the diaphragm.

b. In their descent through the middle mediastinum, the phrenic nerves course alongside the pericardial sac and pass in front of the roots of the lungs.

c. The **right phrenic nerve** exits the middle mediastinum via the caval opening of the diaphragm; the **left phrenic nerve** exits the middle mediastinum by piercing the left dome of the diaphragm.

5. Vagus nerves

a. The vagus nerves are the tenth pair of cranial nerves, and are the cranial nerves with the greatest field of distribution: they innervate structures in the head, neck, thorax, and abdomen.

(1) In the thorax, the vagus nerves provide all the parasympathetic innervation of its viscera.

(2) Specifically, they provide the preganglionic parasympathetic fibers which course through the autonomic plexuses of the thoracic viscera.

b. In passing from the neck to the abdomen, the vagus nerves descend through first the superior mediastinum and then the posterior mediastinum.

(1) Descent through the superior mediastinum

(a) In their descent through the superior mediastinum, the vagus nerves assume opposite anteroposterior relations with the aortic arch: whereas the right vagus nerve passes behind the beginning of the aortic arch, the left vagus nerve passes in front of the terminal part of the aortic arch.

(b) As the left vagus nerve descends in front of the terminal part of the aortic arch, it gives rise to the **left recurrent laryngeal nerve**. (The right recurrent laryngeal nerve arises from the right vagus nerve in the base of the neck.)

(2) Descent through the posterior mediastinum

(a) Each vagus nerve begins its descent through the posterior mediastinum by passing behind the root of the lung. Whereas the right vagus nerve then assumes a position on the posterior surface of the esophagus, the left vagus nerve assumes a position on the anterior surface of the esophagus.

(b) Upon assuming positions on the anterior and posterior esophageal surfaces, the vagus nerves progressively give rise to a **plexus** of nerve fibers which envelops the esophagus. It is in this dispersed configuration that the vagus nerves approach the esophageal opening of the diaphragm.

(c) Just before exiting the thorax via this opening, nerve fibers from both vagus nerves coalesce on the anterior and posterior surfaces of the esophagus to form nerve trunks called, respectively, the **anterior and posterior vagal trunks.**

6. Thymus. The thymus is a bilobar, lymphoid organ which degenerates by late adolescence. It is largely located in the anterior part of the superior mediastinum; the inferior poles of its lobes extend into the anterior mediastinum.

II. CHEST FILMS

A. PA chest film. The normal PA chest film is a composite of the images cast by the bones and soft tissues of the chest wall, the diaphragm, the viscera of the upper abdomen, the viscera of the mediastinum, and the major blood vessels and airways of the lungs (Figure 3-1).

1. Bones and soft tissues of the chest wall

a. Clavicles. The radiograph shows the entire or almost entire length of the clavicles.

(1) The medial ends of the clavicles should lie equidistant from the midline of the body of the fourth or fifth thoracic vertebra. If the medial end of either clavicle overlaps the body of the fourth or fifth thoracic vertebra, it signifies that the coronal plane of the patient's body was not oriented perpendicular to the path of the x-ray beam (i.e., the projection is oblique).

(2) A water-density band (i.e., a band with a radiographic density of water) may extend along the superior border of each clavicle; the band is called the **companion shadow of the clavicle**, and it represents the shadow cast by the soft tissues of the **supraclavicular fossa**.

b. Thoracic vertebrae

(1) The radiopaque bodies of the thoracic vertebrae should be discernible within the cardiovascular shadow (see section II A 3 a). The elliptic outlines superimposed upon the superolateral aspects of each vertebral body represent the vertebra's **pedicles**.

(2) Failure to see the thoracic vertebral bodies and pedicles indicates inadequate x-ray penetration. The radiograph is unacceptable since it does not permit visualization of any retrocardiac masses (i.e., of any radiopaque masses in the posterior mediastinum).

c. Ribs. The radiograph shows the **heads and necks** of most of the ribs and the **bodies** of the upper eight to ten ribs.

(1) Each of the upper eight ribs can generally be traced from the articulation of its head with the vertebral column to the union of the body of the rib with its costal cartilage.

(2) The posterior segments of the bodies of the third to eighth ribs project almost horizontally; the anterior segments of these bodies slope downward as they extend medially. The anterior segments slope downward less markedly in PA chest films of **neonates and children** (Figure 3-2) than in PA chest films of adults (see Figures 3-1A and 3-1B).

(3) A band parallels the apparent inferior border of the posterior body segment of most ribs. Each band is called the **companion shadow** of its rib, and it represents the shadow cast by the inferior part of the rib that borders the rib's costal groove.

d. Scapulae. The scapulae project lateral to the superolateral regions of the lung fields, because the scapulae become protracted and laterally rotated when the patient places the hands on the hips and pulls the shoulders forward into contact with the x-ray film cassette (see Figure 3-1C).

e. Soft tissues of the chest wall

(1) In an adult woman, the soft tissues of the **breasts** cast water-density shadows in the lower part of each lung field. The **nipples** may be well outlined.

(2) The **pectoralis major muscles** of many individuals cast a water-density shadow in the superolateral part of each lung field. The inferolateral margin of the shadow is continuous with the inferior margin of the water-density shadow cast by the soft tissues of the **anterior axillary fold**.

2. Diaphragm and underlying abdominal viscera

a. The **liver** and **right dome of the diaphragm** cast a domed water-density shadow at the base of the right lung field; the **liver**, the fundus of the **stomach**, **spleen**, and **left dome of the diaphragm** cast a domed water-density shadow at the base of the left lung field.

b. Both domes generally lie immediately below the body of the tenth thoracic vertebra; the downward thrust of the heart generally places the left dome slightly lower than the right dome.

c. A **gas bubble** in the **fundus of the stomach** will appear as a radiolucent area beneath the left dome of the diaphragm.

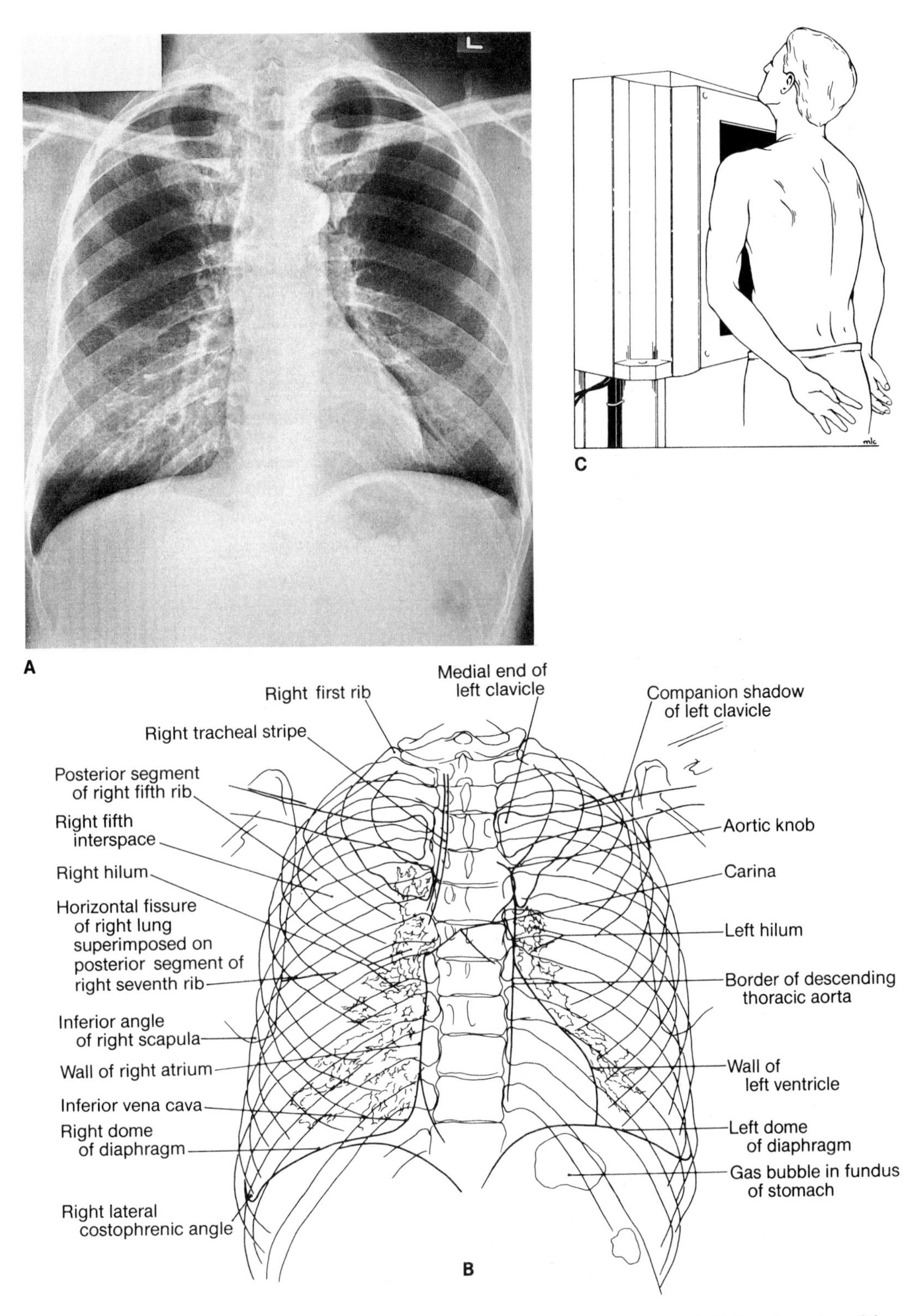

Figure 3-1. (*A*) PA chest film of a 54-year-old male, (*B*) its schematic representation, and (*C*) the orientation of the patient's thorax relative to the x-ray beam and film cassette for the radiograph. (See section II A.)

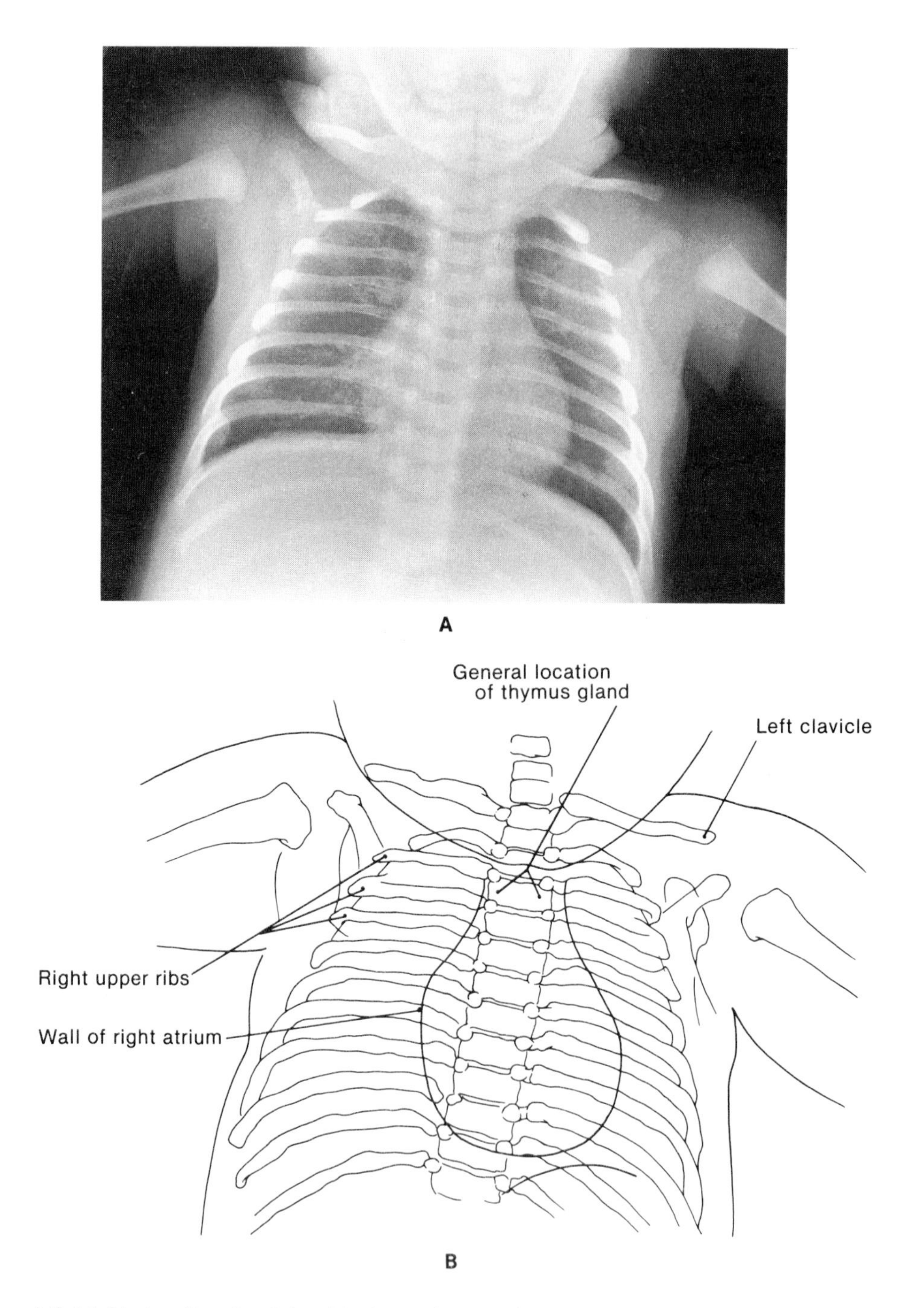

Figure 3-2. (*A*) PA chest film of an 8-day-old infant and (*B*) its schematic representation. [See section II A 1 c (2).] The infant's thymus gland is not prominent, and therefore does not significantly contribute to the upper parts of the left and right borders of the cardiovascular shadow.

3. Mediastinal viscera

a. In PA chest films of **adults**, the **heart** and the **major vessels** attached to it cast almost all of the central mediastinal shadow (the vertebral column and sternum also contribute to the shadow). Therefore, this central mediastinal shadow can be called the **cardiovascular shadow.**

(1) The curved water-density outlines of four sets of structures define the **right border** of the cardiovascular shadow (Figure 3-3; compare with Figure 3-1B). Proceeding from the uppermost to the lowermost, these structures are:

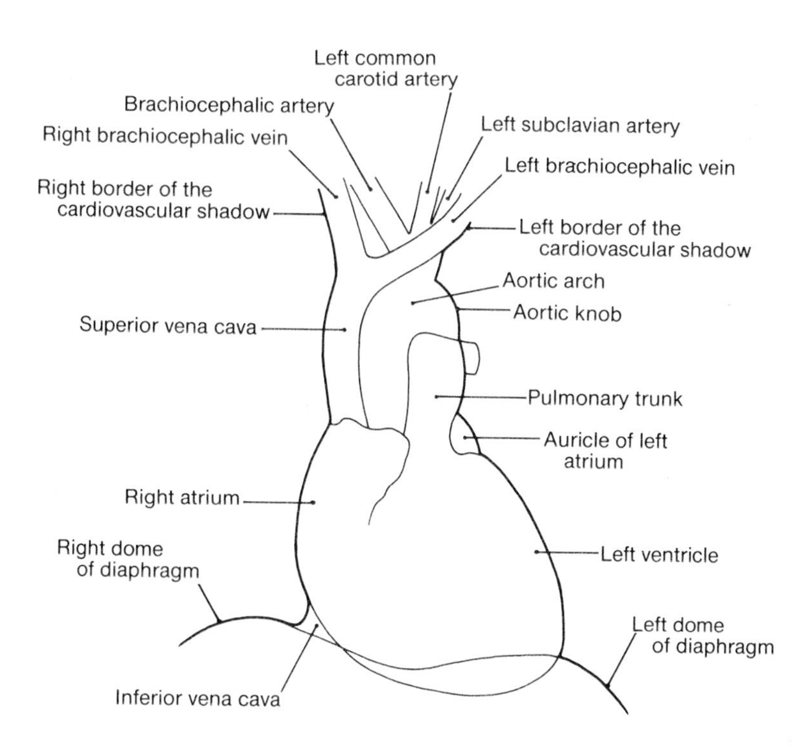

Figure 3-3. A schematic drawing of the outlines of the mediastinal viscera that define the left and right borders of the cardiovascular shadow of a PA chest film. (See section II A 3.)

(a) The brachiocephalic artery and right brachiocephalic vein together
(b) The superior vena cava and ascending aorta together
(c) The right atrium
(d) The inferior vena cava

(2) The curved water-density outlines of five sets of structures define the **left border** of the cardiovascular shadow (compare Figures 3-1B and 3-3). Proceeding from the uppermost to the lowermost, these structures are:
(a) The left subclavian artery and left brachiocephalic vein together
(b) The terminal part of the aortic arch (the prominent, rounded outline cast by the terminal part of the aortic arch is called the **aortic knob**)
(c) The pulmonary trunk
(d) The auricle of the left atrium
(e) The left ventricle

b. In PA chest films of **neonates and young children**, the outline of the comparatively prominent **thymus gland** may define the upper parts of the left and right borders of the cardiovascular shadow (see Figure 3-2).

c. In both adults and children, the **tracheal lumen** appears as a vertical radiolucent band in the midline of the neck and upper chest (the trachea in the upper chest may lie slightly to the right).

(1) The tracheal lumen is bordered on the right in most PA chest films by a water-density stripe, called the **right tracheal stripe**, that extends inferiorly to the origin of the right main stem bronchus. The right tracheal stripe represents the **right tracheal wall**; its normal width in adults is 4 to 5 mm.

(2) The **bifurcation of the trachea** at the carina into the **left and right main stem bronchi** is generally visible in the upper part of the cardiovascular shadow. Since a PA chest film is taken at full or deep inspiration, the **carina** lies in adults at about the level of the body of the sixth or seventh thoracic vertebra.

(3) The inferior **angle between the main stem bronchi** at the carina measures 60° to 75°.

d. The slightly curved left border of the **descending thoracic aorta**, from its origin at the end of the aortic arch through most of its descent in the posterior mediastinum, is commonly discernible in the cardiovascular shadow.

e. A fine, slightly bowed vertical line that overlaps the images of the thoracic vertebral bodies is generally visible in the cardiovascular shadow. This line is called the **azygoesophageal line** because its upper part represents the curved right border of the **azygos vein** and its lower part represents the curved right border of the **esophagus** in the inferior mediastinum.

4. Markings of the lung fields

a. The lungs appear as radiolucent fields whose only prominent markings are water-density bands which branch and radiate into the lung fields from about the midregion of the left and right borders of the cardiovascular shadow. The central area on each side is referred to as the **hilum** of the lung field.

(1) The **pulmonary artery** and its major branches and the **pulmonary veins** and their immediate tributaries in each lung cast the water-density bands of each hilum. The pulmonary artery casts the largest and most medial water-density band, and roughly two-thirds of the hilar area lies below the level of this band.

(2) The left hilum is higher than the right hilum in more than 95% of individuals.

(a) The hila are at the same level in the remainder of individuals. Thus, the left hilum is almost never lower than the right hilum in a normal individual.

(b) The left pulmonary artery has a more superior lie in the thorax than the right pulmonary artery as a result of the ascent of the left pulmonary artery and the descent of the right pulmonary artery from the bifurcation of the pulmonary trunk; the more superior lie of the left pulmonary artery is the basis for the more superior lie of the left hilum.

b. The walls of most of the **lobar and segmental bronchi** are too obliquely oriented to cast distinct shadows in the lung fields.

c. The pulmonary and bronchopulmonary **lymph nodes** are too small to cast distinct shadows in the lung fields.

d. The strips of area in each lung field between adjacent rib body segments are called **interspaces**.

e. The **apex of each lung field** projects above the medial third of the clavicle. The lateral margin of the lung apex may be bordered by a fat-density band. In such instances, the medial margin of the band represents the apposed **parietal and visceral pleura** at the lung apex; the band itself represents the **fat layer** superficial to the parietal pleura.

f. The **inferolateral corner of each lung field** is called the **lateral costophrenic angle**. The sharply acute angle represents the projection of the lateral aspect of the lung's **costodiaphragmatic margin** into the costodiaphragmatic recess.

g. The **inferomedial corner of each lung field** is called the **cardiophrenic angle**.

(1) The juxtaposed **apex of the heart and left dome of the diaphragm** define the cardiophrenic angle of the left lung field, and the juxtaposed **inferior vena cava and right dome of the diaphragm** define the cardiophrenic angle of the right lung field.

(2) Fat depositions around the margin of adhesion between the pericardial sac and the central tendon of the diaphragm may obscure the acuity of the cardiophrenic angles.

h. The **horizontal fissure of the right lung** may be visible as a thin water-density line extending medially from the most lateral edge of the right sixth rib.

B. Lateral chest film

1. General considerations. Lateral chest films are commonly taken to allow better visualization of a lesion or abnormality confined to one side of the thorax. A **left lateral chest film** (Figures 3-4A and 3-4B) is taken if a lateral view of the thorax is desired. The film cassette is placed against the left side of the chest, and the x-ray beam is directed toward the right side of the chest (Figure 3-4C).

2. Bones and soft tissues of the chest wall

a. The radiograph shows the **manubrium** and body of the **sternum** in profile. The radiolucent space between the manubrium and body of the sternum represents the apposed articular cartilages in the **manubriosternal joint.**

b. The radiograph shows the bodies of most of the **thoracic vertebrae;** the images of the paired pedicles of each vertebra are superimposed. The radiolucent space between adjacent vertebral bodies represents the **intervertebral disk** intervening between the bodies. The radiolucent space between the pedicles of adjacent vertebrae represents the superimposed outlines of the **intervertebral foramina** between the vertebrae.

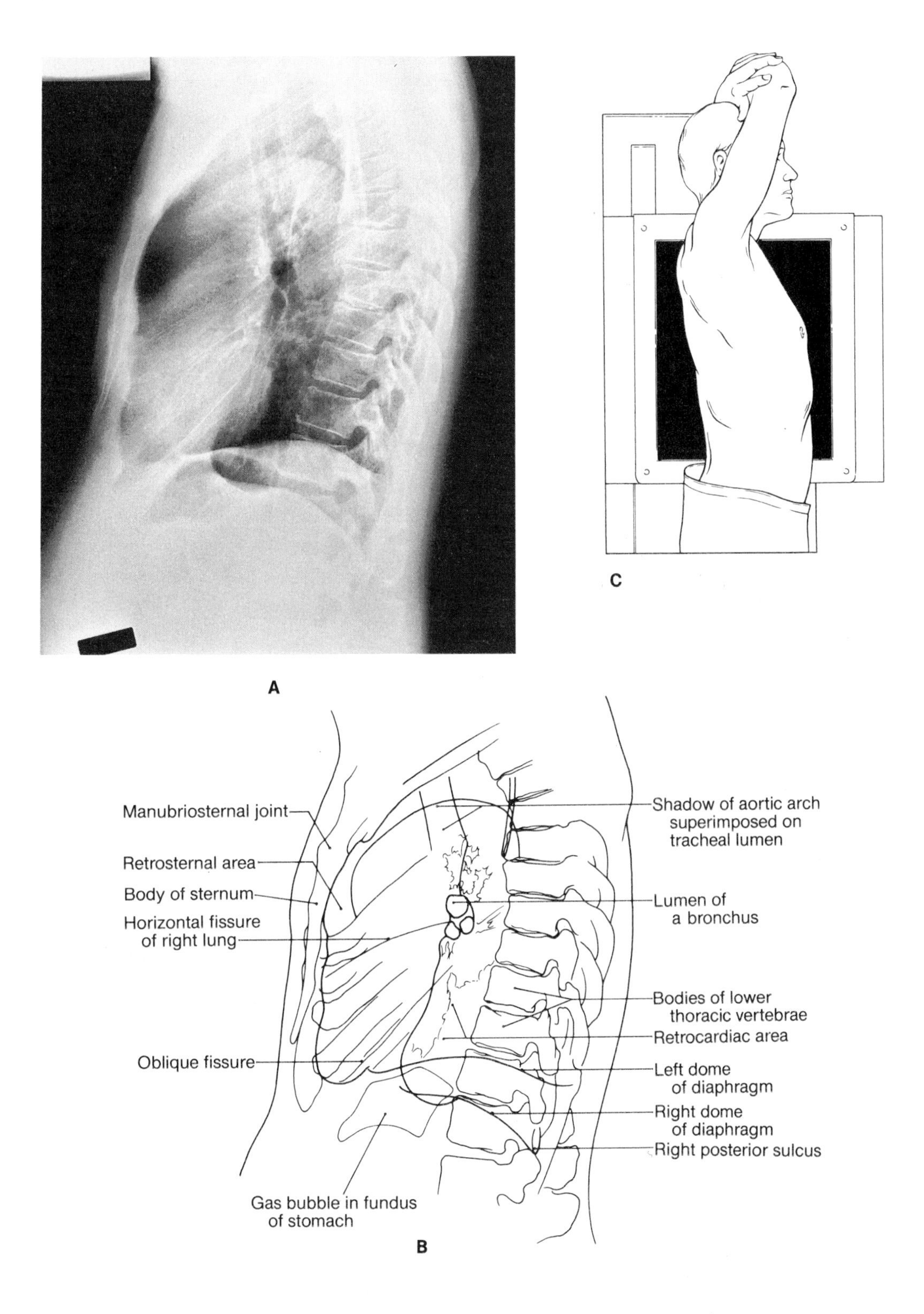

Figure 3-4. (*A*) Left lateral chest film of the same 54-year-old male as in Figure 3-1, (*B*) its schematic representation, and (C) the orientation of the patient's thorax relative to the x-ray beam and film cassette for the radiograph. (See section II B.)

(1) The T4–T5 intervertebral disk lies at the level of the manubriosternal joint (i.e., at the level of the sternal angle).
(2) The bodies of the thoracic vertebrae appear progressively more radiolucent inferiorly. This happens because
(a) The lateral chest film superimposes the radiodensities of the posterior parts of both lungs on the images of the bodies of the thoracic vertebrae.
(b) The radiolucency of the parenchyma of each lung appears to increase inferiorly as the chest widens.

c. The radiograph shows most of the **ribs** as they extend first posteriorly from their articulation with the vertebral column and then anteroinferiorly through the anterolateral chest wall.

d. The platelike body of each **scapula** casts a radiopaque profile superimposed upon the thoracic vertebrae.

3. Diaphragm and underlying abdominal viscera. The domes of the diaphragm and their underlying abdominal viscera cast nearly superimposed, domed water-density shadows at the bases of the lung fields.

a. The level of the left dome is generally but not always lower than that of the right dome.

b. The domes can be unambiguously distinguished if a radiolucent **gas bubble** in the **fundus of the stomach** underlies one but not the other dome: it is the **left dome** that caps the gas bubble. If the **inferior vena cava** can be observed extending from the diaphragmatic domes to the posterior border of the cardiac shadow, the **right dome** can be unambiguously identified from its effacement by the inferior vena cava.

4. Mediastinal viscera

a. The chambers of the **heart** cast a bulbous shadow overlying the anterosuperior margins of the domes of the diaphragm.
(1) The anterior wall of the **right ventricle** defines the lower half of the anterior border of the cardiac shadow.
(2) The posterior wall of the **left ventricle** defines the lower third of the posterior border of the cardiac shadow.
(3) The posterior wall of the **left atrium** defines the middle third of the posterior border of the cardiac shadow.

b. The three segments of the **thoracic aorta** cast a cane-shaped shadow in the radiograph.
(1) The shadow of the **ascending aorta** projects upward from the superior limit of the anterior border of the cardiac shadow.
(2) The shadow of the **aortic arch** arches over the cardiac shadow and into the radiolucent space anterior to the bodies of the third and fourth thoracic vertebrae.
(3) The shadow of the **descending thoracic aorta** parallels the curved stack of the bodies of the lower thoracic vertebrae.

c. The **tracheal lumen** appears as an almost vertical radiolucent band which ends immediately behind the superior limit of the posterior border of the cardiac shadow.
(1) The highest part of the aortic arch crosses the tracheal lumen in the superior mediastinum.
(2) The tracheal lumen is bordered posteriorly by a distinct water-density stripe; the stripe represents the posterior tracheal wall and collapsed esophagus together.

d. The **left pulmonary artery** casts an arched water-density band that crosses the lower part of the tracheal lumen; the **right pulmonary artery** casts an oblate water-density shadow anterior to the lower part of the tracheal lumen.

5. Lung markings

a. The radiolucent area bounded by the sternum anteriorly and the cardiac shadow and ascending aorta posteriorly is called the **retrosternal area**.
(1) The retrosternal area shows the superimposed radiolucencies of principally the anterior bronchopulmonary segments of the **upper lobes** of both lungs.
(2) The anteroinferior corner of the retrosternal area is called the **anterior costophrenic angle**. The sharply acute angle represents the superimposed projections of the anterior aspect of each lung's costodiaphragmatic margin into its costodiaphragmatic recess.

b. The radiolucent area directly posterior to the lower part of the cardiac shadow is called the **retrocardiac area**.
(1) The retrocardiac area shows the superimposed radiodensities of the basal bronchopulmonary segments of the **lower lobes** of both lungs.

(2) The posteroinferior corner of the retrocardiac area is called the **posterior costophrenic angle**, or **posterior sulcus**. The sharply acute angle represents the superimposed projections of the posterior aspect of each lung's costodiaphragmatic margin into its costodiaphragmatic recess.

c. The **oblique fissure** of each lung commonly casts a fine water-density line extending anteroinferiorly from the level of the body of the fourth or fifth thoracic vertebra to the location of the anteroinferior heart border. A fine horizontal line extending anteriorly from about the midregion of the right lung's oblique fissure represents the lung's **horizontal fissure**.

d. The radiodensities of the lungs' **hila** are superimposed in the region directly posterior to the upper part of the cardiac shadow. In this region of the superimposed hila, the walls of a few lobar or segmental **bronchi** frequently are sufficiently parallel to the path of the x-ray beam for each to cast a fine water-density circle around an air-density interior.

III. CT SCANS OF THE THORAX.

The **mediastinal viscera** and **blood vessels** exhibit fairly constant relationships in normal individuals. These relationships can be summarized by reference to six distinct levels within the superior mediastinum and upper part of the inferior mediastinum. The discussion of the relationships at each level begins with the most posterior structures and ends with the most anterior structures.

A. Relationships at the level of the origin of the three branches of the aortic arch (Figure 3-5). This level lies just inferior to the thoracic inlet; that is, just below the upper boundary of the superior mediastinum.

1. The **esophagus** appears in transverse section directly anterior to and slightly to the left of the body of a thoracic vertebra. A patent lumen is occasionally evident.

2. The **trachea** appears in transverse section directly anterior to and slightly to the right of the esophagus. The trachea generally exhibits an inverted U-shaped border anterolaterally and a linear border posteriorly.

3. The brachiocephalic artery, left common carotid artery, and left subclavian artery each appears in transverse section.
   a. The **brachiocephalic artery** lies anterior to and to the right of the trachea.
   b. The **left common carotid artery** lies anterior to and to the left of the trachea.
   c. The **left subclavian artery** lies to the left of the posterior border of the trachea.

4. The **right brachiocephalic vein** appears in transverse section, and lies to the right of the brachiocephalic artery. The **left brachiocephalic vein** appears in oblique section; as it extends to the right, it passes anterior to the left common carotid artery and brachiocephalic artery.

5. The **thymus** (if present) casts a triangular image directly anterior to the left brachiocephalic vein.

B. Relationships at the level of the aortic arch (Figure 3-6)

1. The **esophagus** and **trachea** each appear in transverse section; they show the same relationships relative to each other and to the vertebral column as they show at the level of the origin of the three branches of the aortic arch.

2. The upper end of the **azygos vein** appears in transverse section posterior to the trachea and to the right of the esophagus.

3. The longitudinally sectioned aortic arch casts a curved image which begins directly to the left of the right brachiocephalic vein, sweeps around the left anterolateral side of the trachea, and ends directly to the left of the esophagus.

4. The **left brachiocephalic vein** is obliquely sectioned at its union with the transversely sectioned **right brachiocephalic vein**.

C. Relationships at the level of the aortic-pulmonary window (Figure 3-7). The **aortic-pulmonary window** is the space in the superior mediastinum that extends from the bifurcation of the pulmonary trunk to the undersurface of the aortic arch.

1. As at the two higher levels (see sections III A and B), the transversely sectioned **esophagus** lies directly anterior to and to the left of the body of a thoracic vertebra.

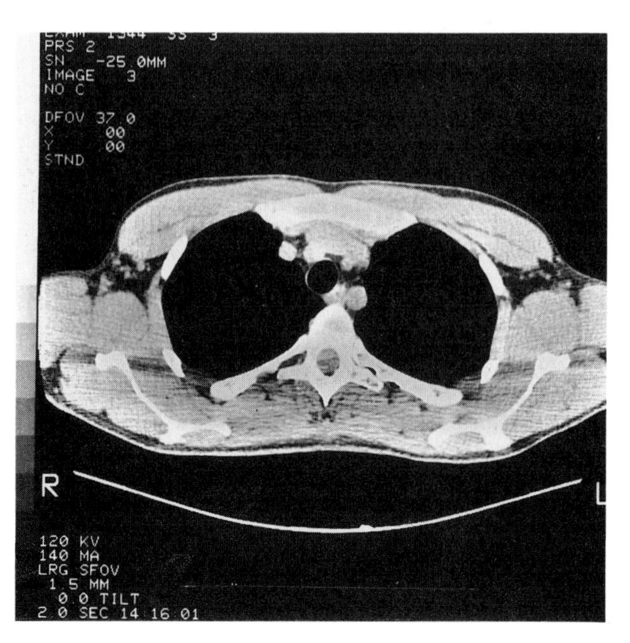

A

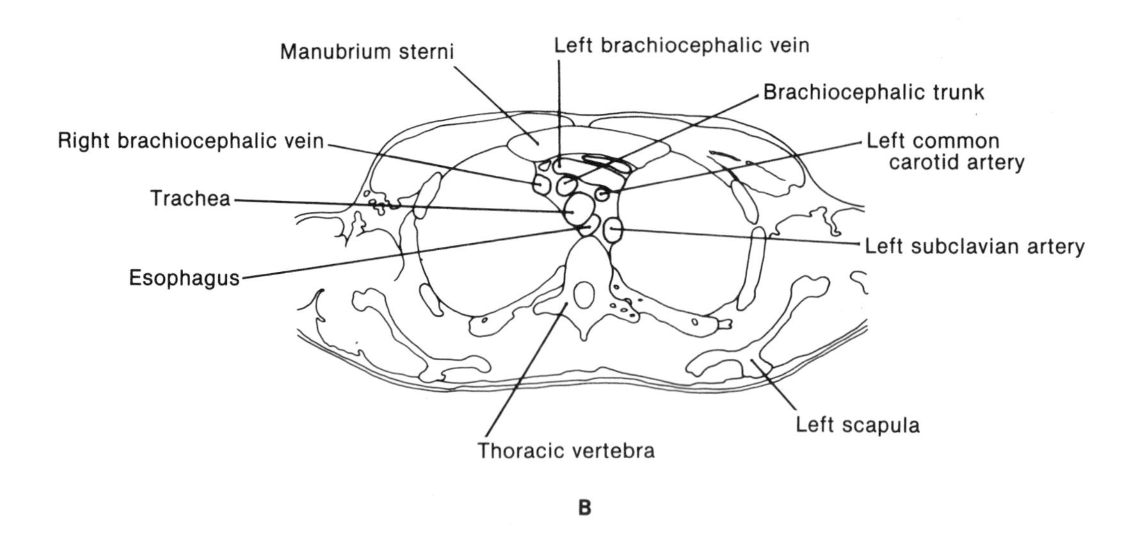

B

Figure 3-5. (*A*) CT scan at the level of the origin of the three branches of the aortic arch that demonstrates the mediastinal viscera, and (*B*) its schematic representation. (*C*) CT scan at the identical level that demonstrates segments of blood vessels of the lungs (lung window; i.e., a CT scan taken with equipment settings adjusted to show the lung tissues), and (*D*) its schematic representation. (*E*) Appearance and relationships of the major mediastinal viscera at this level. (See section III A.)

Figure 3-5. *continued*

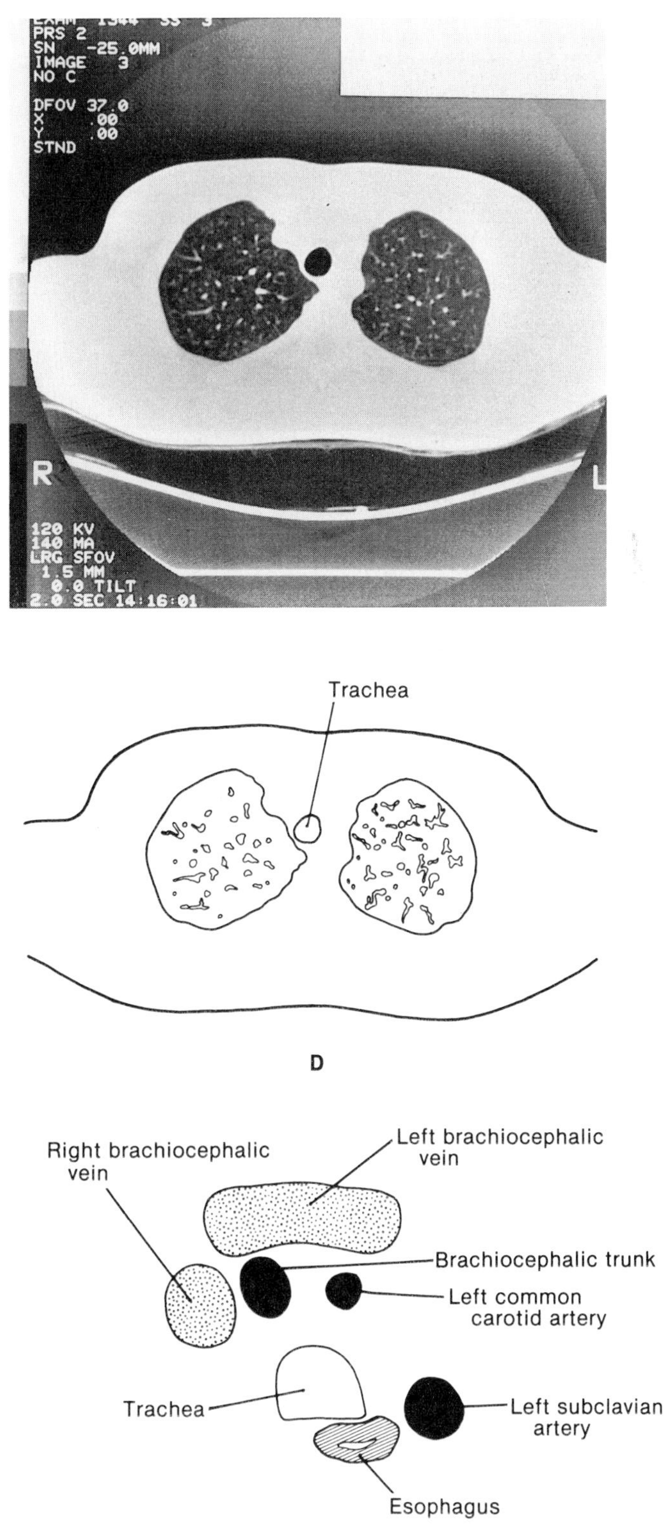

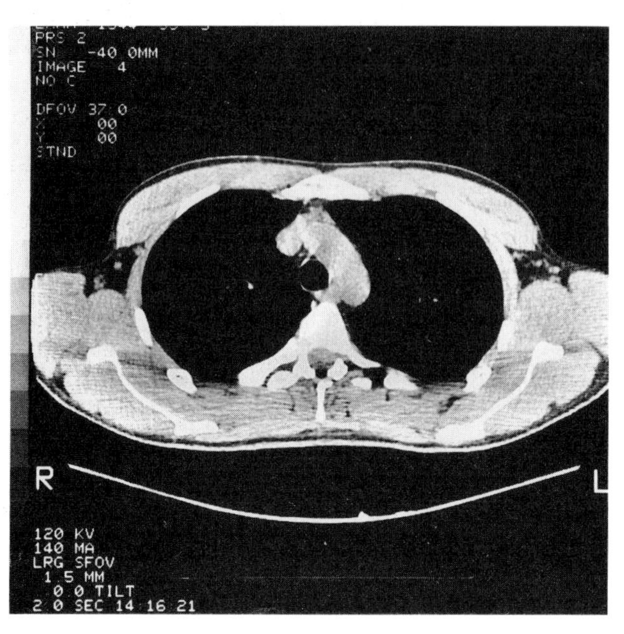

A

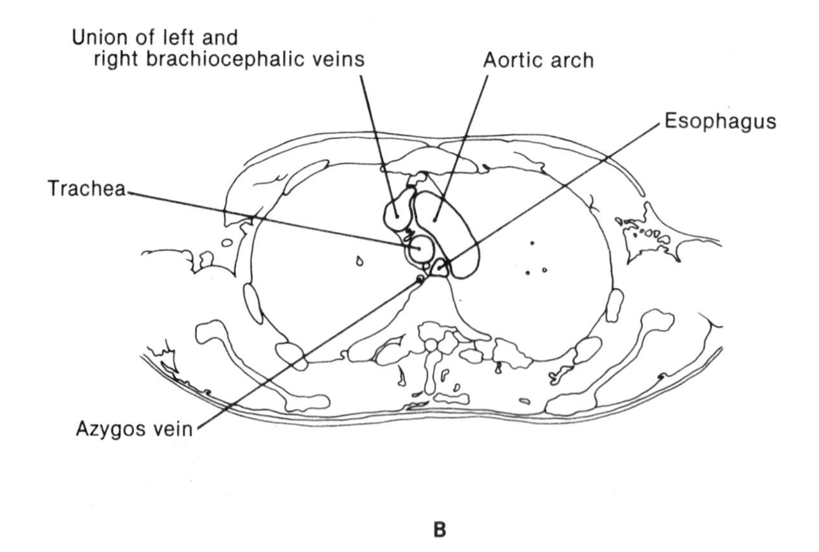

B

Figure 3-6. (*A*) CT scan at the level of the aortic arch that demonstrates the mediastinal viscera, and (*B*) its schematic representation. (*C*) CT scan at the identical level (lung window) that demonstrates segments of blood vessels of the lungs, and (*D*) its schematic representation. (*E*) Appearance and relationships of the major mediastinal viscera at this level. (See section III B.)

Figure 3-6. *continued*

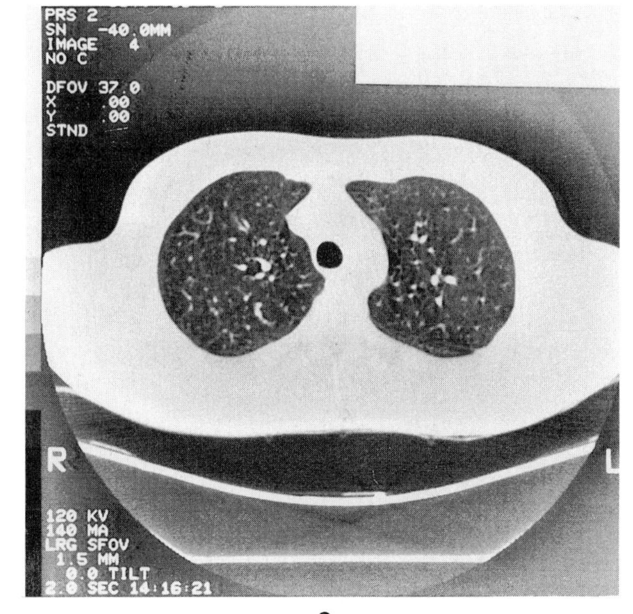

C

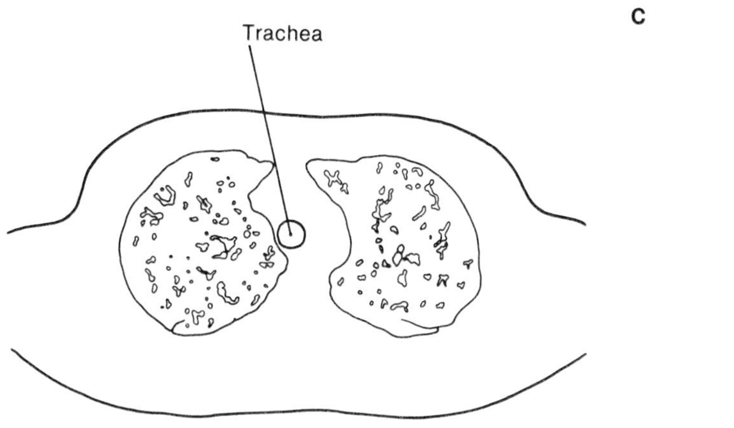

D

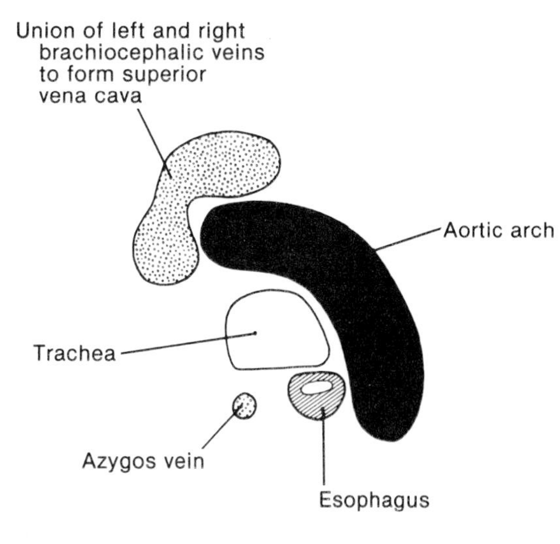

E

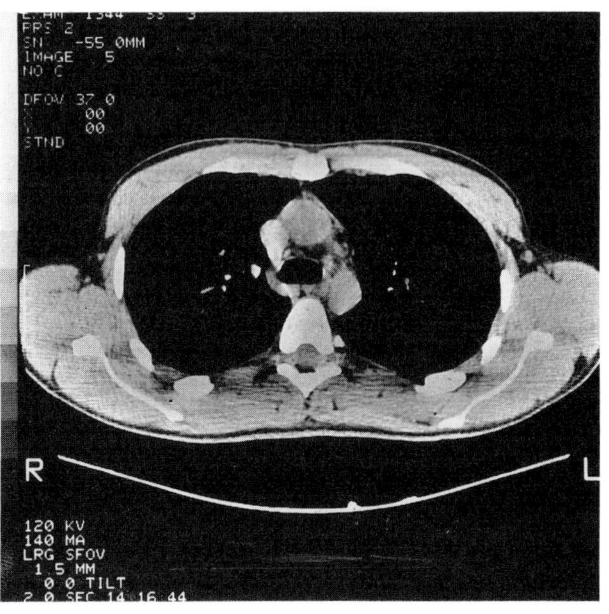

A

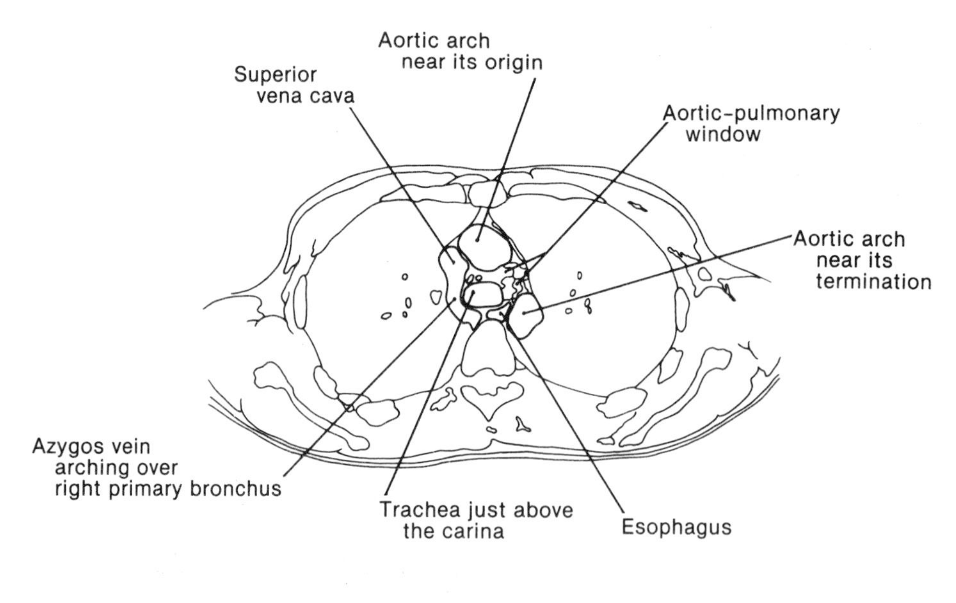

B

Figure 3-7. (*A*) CT scan at the level of the aortic–pulmonary window that demonstrates the mediastinal viscera, and (*B*) its schematic representation. (C) CT scan at the identical level (lung window) that demonstrates segments of blood vessels of the lungs and the oblique fissure of the left lung, and (*D*) its schematic representation. (E) Appearance and relationships of the major mediastinal viscera at this level. (See section III C.)

Figure 3-7. *continued*

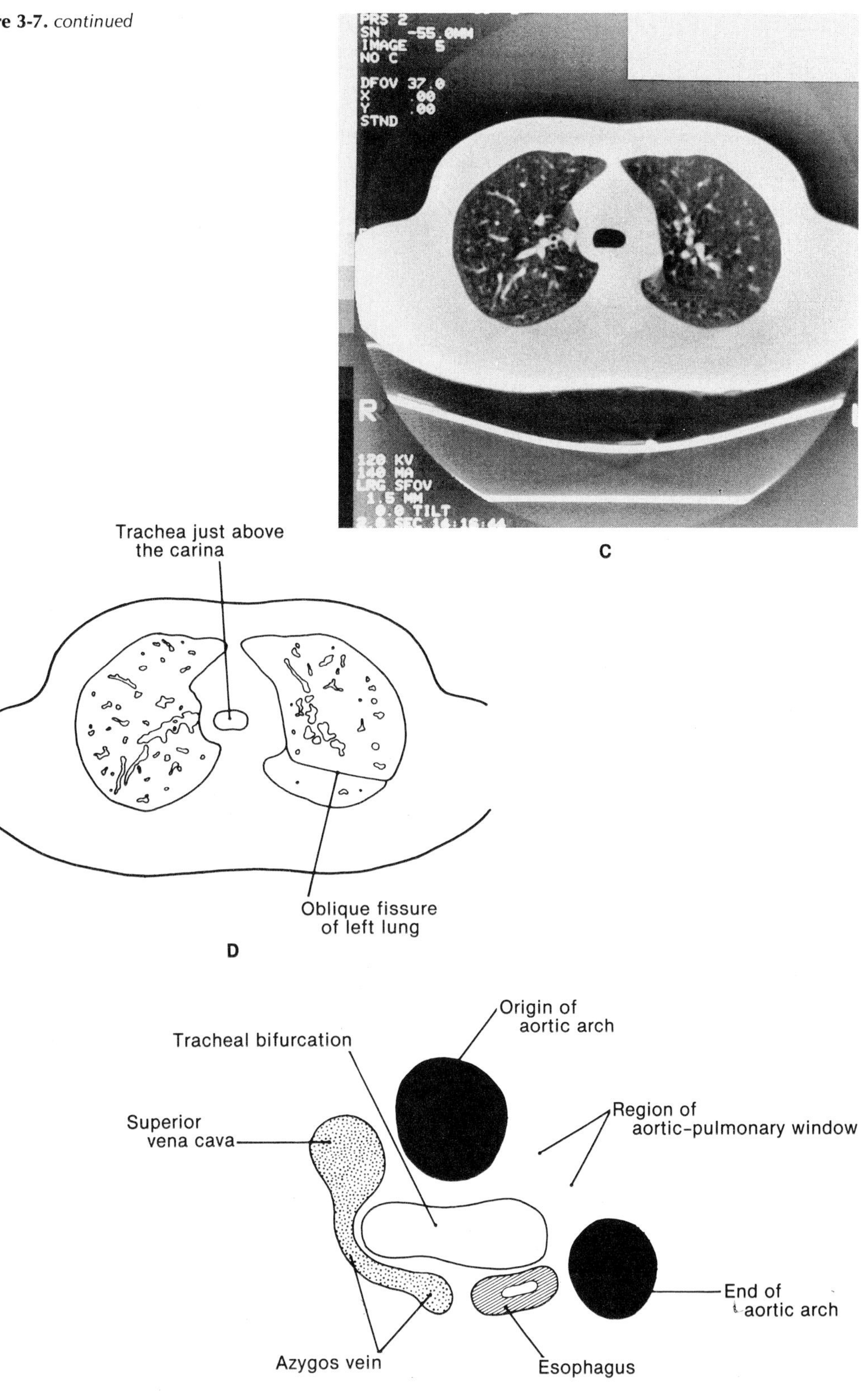

2. The **main stem bronchi** appear in oblique section just above or below the level of the carina.
3. The **azygos vein** appears in longitudinal section at the level where it arches over the right main stem bronchus and ends via union with the **superior vena cava** (which appears in transverse section).
4. The **origin of the aortic arch** lies transversely sectioned directly anterior to the origin of the main stem bronchi; the **end of the arch** lies transversly sectioned directly to the left of the esophagus.
5. The region in the scan between the origin and end of the aortic arch represents the **aortic–pulmonary window**.

D. Relationships at the level of the origin of the left pulmonary artery (Figure 3-8). This level lies in the upper part of the inferior mediastinum.

1. The **azygos vein**, **esophagus**, and **descending thoracic aorta** all appear in transverse section in the posterior mediastinum.
2. The **left main stem bronchus** appears in almost transverse section directly anterior to and between the esophagus and the descending thoracic aorta.
3. The scan is near or at the level at which the **right main stem bronchus** bifurcates into the right upper lobe bronchus and the intermediate bronchus. The **right upper lobe bronchus** is commonly called the **eparterial bronchus** because it is the only lobar bronchus in either lung to lie superior to its neighboring pulmonary artery.
4. The **pulmonary trunk** appears in transverse section anterior to and to the left of the left main stem bronchus. The **left pulmonary artery** appears in almost longitudinal section as it curves posterolaterally toward the hilum of the left lung.
5. The **ascending aorta** lies transversely sectioned anterior to and between the main stem bronchi.
6. The transversely sectioned **superior vena cava** lies anterior to the origin of the eparterial bronchus.

E. Relationships at the level of the origin of the right pulmonary artery (Figure 3-9)

1. As in the preceding level, the **azygos vein**, **esophagus**, and **descending thoracic aorta** all appear in transverse section in the posterior mediastinum.
2. The scan is near or at the level at which the **left main stem bronchus** bifurcates into the **left upper and left lower lobar bronchi**.
3. The **intermediate bronchus** of the right lung lies to the right of the bifurcation of the left main stem bronchus.
4. The **pulmonary trunk** appears in transverse section anterior to the bifurcation of the left main stem bronchus. The **right pulmonary artery** appears in almost longitudinal section as it passes posterior to the ascending aorta and superior vena cava and anterior to the intermediate bronchus in its route to the hilum of the right lung.

F. Relationships at the level of the roots of the ascending aorta and pulmonary trunk (Figure 3-10)

1. As in the preceding two levels, the **azygos vein**, **esophagus**, and **descending thoracic aorta** all appear in transverse section in the posterior mediastinum.
2. Lobar or segmental **bronchi** lie on either side of the oblate outline of the left atrium.
3. The **roots** of the **ascending aorta** and **pulmonary trunk** lie directly anterior to the left atrium. A portion of the **right ventricle** may be evident anterior to and between the roots of the ascending aorta and pulmonary trunk.
4. A crescent-shaped **right atrium** lies directly to the right of the root of the ascending aorta.

IV. COMMON ABNORMAL FINDINGS IN CHEST FILMS. Abnormal findings in chest films are generally not pathognomonic of a specific disease or pathologic process: in most instances, a number of diseases or processes can produce each type of abnormal finding.

A. **Bones and soft tissues of the chest wall**

1. **Blurring of the outline of a companion clavicular shadow in a PA chest film**
   a. **Bilateral blurring** may be due to **excessive fat deposition** in the superficial fascia of the supraclavicular fossa of both shoulders.
   b. **Unilateral blurring** may be produced by **enlarged supraclavicular lymph nodes.**

2. **Lytic or sclerotic lesions in the bodies or pedicles of the vertebrae.** Such lesions can be produced by **metastases** from primary tumors of the bronchi, breast, prostate, kidney, thyroid, and other sources, as well as by **primary bone lesions**.

3. **Lytic or sclerotic lesions in the ribs.** Such lesions can be produced by **metastases** from primary tumors of the bronchi, breast, prostate, kidney, thyroid, and other sources, as well as by **primary bone lesions**. Metastatic lytic lesions are most readily observed in the cortex of the superior rib border.

4. **Discontinuities of the cortical bone of the ribs. Rib fractures** present in this way. Most rib fractures result from the application of compression forces on the chest wall.

5. **Notches in the inferior borders of the posterior body segments of the upper ribs in a PA chest film.** Individuals suffering from congenital **aortic coarctation** may exhibit such notches.
   a. Congenital constriction of the aorta generally occurs at a site immediately distal to the origin of the left subclavian artery.
   b. The impediment to aortic blood flow imposed by the coarctation commonly results in a relatively high flow of blood from the internal thoracic arteries through the intercostal arteries to the descending thoracic aorta.
   c. The walls of the intercostal arteries develop dilatations because of the abnormally high blood flow, and the dilatations produce extrinsic pressure defects on the adjacent ribs. The notching is most prominent along the posterior body segments because it is along these segments that the intercostal arteries lie closest to the overlying costal groove.

B. **Diaphragmatic domes and underlying abdominal cavity**

1. **Flattening of the domes of the diaphragm. Asthma** and **emphysema** are common causes of flattening of the domes. Flattening is indicated if the vertical distance from the midpoint of a dome to the line extending between the vertices of the cardiophrenic and lateral costophrenic angles in a PA chest film is less than 1.5 cm.

2. **A subdiaphragmatic region with a radiographic density of air**
   a. The air-density region may be sandwiched between the undersurface of the right diaphragmatic dome and the superior surface of the liver or may lie directly beneath the left diaphragmatic dome. Either finding indicates a **pneumoperitoneum** (i.e., the presence of gas in the abdominal cavity). When a dome of the diaphragm overlies an intra-abdominal air bubble, the dome appears as a curved, 2- to 3-mm-thick water-density band.
   b. Abdominal free air may be normal after recent abdominal surgery, or abnormal following rupture of an abdominal hollow viscus.

C. **Mediastinal viscera**

1. **Enlargement or distortion of the cardiovascular shadow in a PA chest film.** An enlarged relative size of the cardiovascular shadow or a distortion of its left or right borders is commonly an indicator of a disease or process which has produced either **myocardial hypertrophy** or **chamber enlargement**.
   a. The **cardiothoracic ratio** is the greatest ratio of the transverse dimension of the cardiovascular shadow to the transverse dimension of the thoracic cavity. A cardiothoracic ratio greater than 0.5 is indicative of either generalized cardiomegaly or pericardial effusion. This measurement is valid only in a PA chest film taken at deep inspiration in an erect patient. Other considerations may further modify the clinical significance of a ratio greater than 0.5.
   b. **Enlargement of the left atrium** can alter the appearance of the PA chest film in several ways.
      (1) It can alter the appearance of the **cardiovascular shadow's borders** in one or both of two ways:
         (a) The part of the shadow's left border that is outlined by the auricle of the left atrium is normally an indentation between the outlines cast by the pulmonary trunk and the left ventricle. Left atrial enlargement can fill out this indentation and thus straighten the left border.

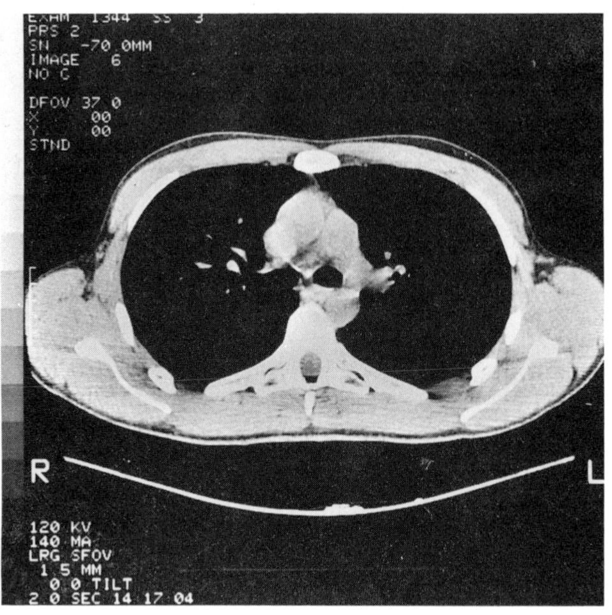

A

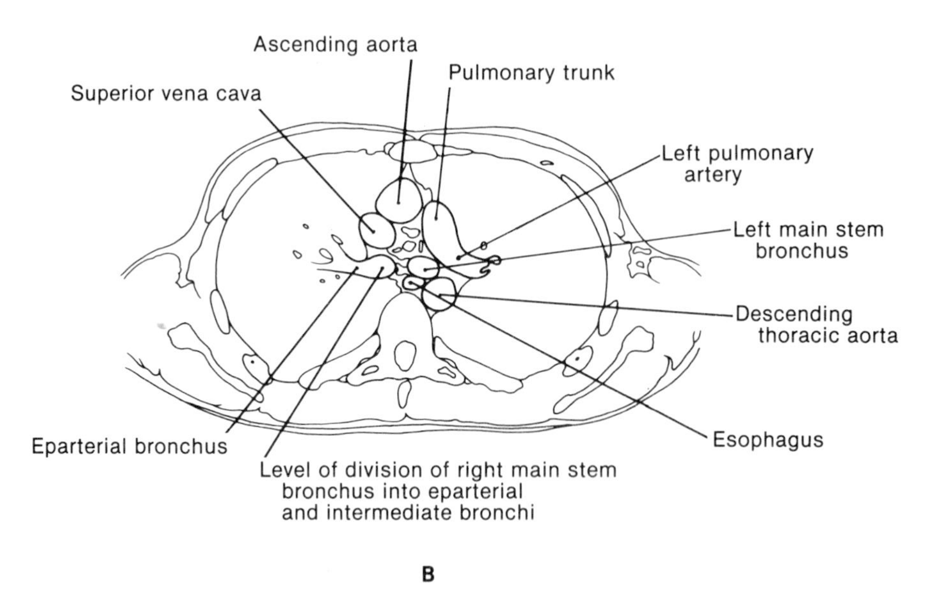

B

Figure 3-8. (*A*) CT scan at the level of the origin of the left pulmonary artery that demonstrates the mediastinal viscera, and (*B*) its schematic representation. (*C*) CT scan at the identical level (lung window) that demonstrates segments of bronchi and blood vessels of the lungs, and (*D*) its schematic representation. (*E*) Appearance and relationships of the major mediastinal viscera and pulmonary structures at this level. (See section III D.)

Figure 3-8. *continued*

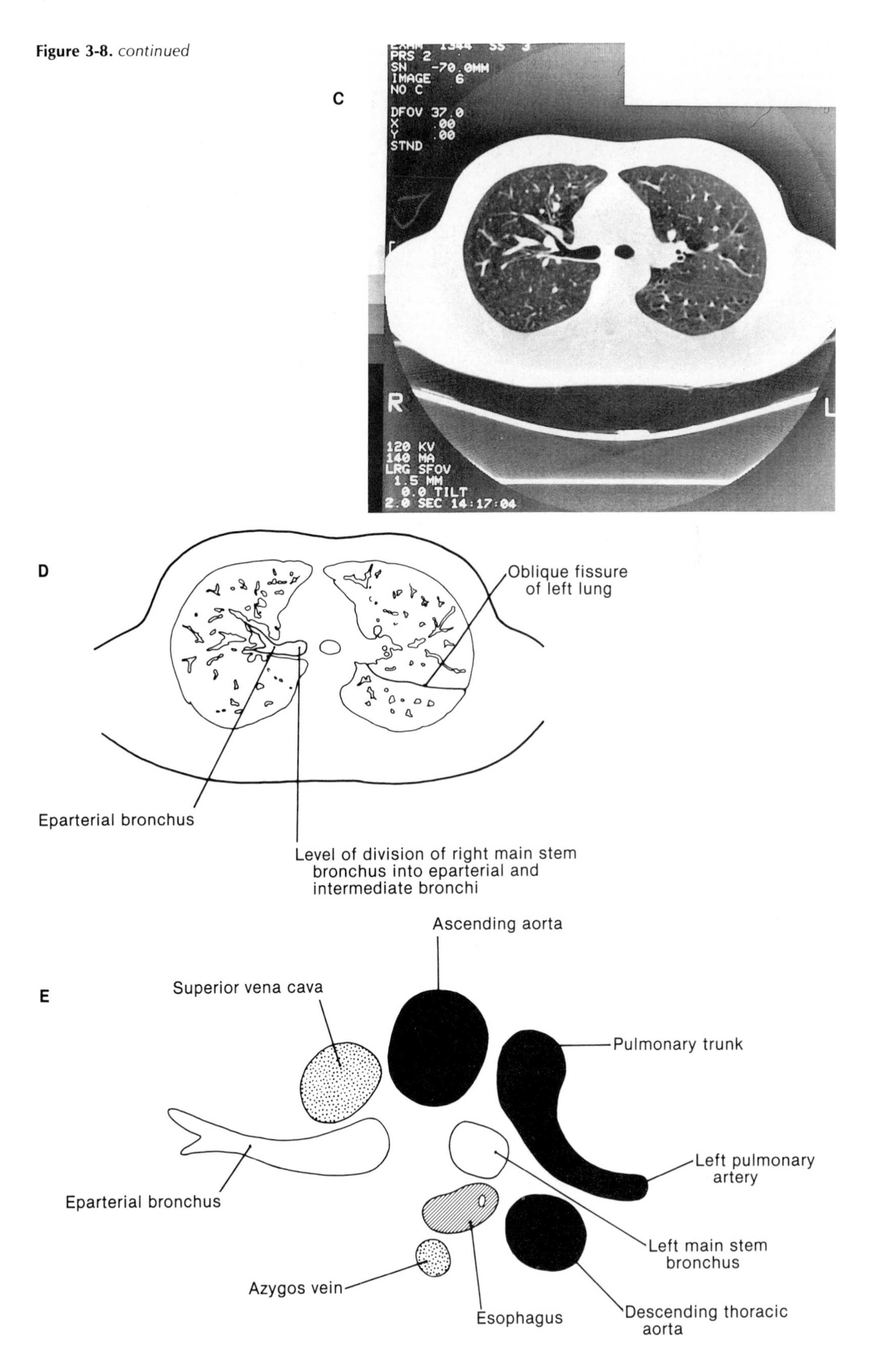

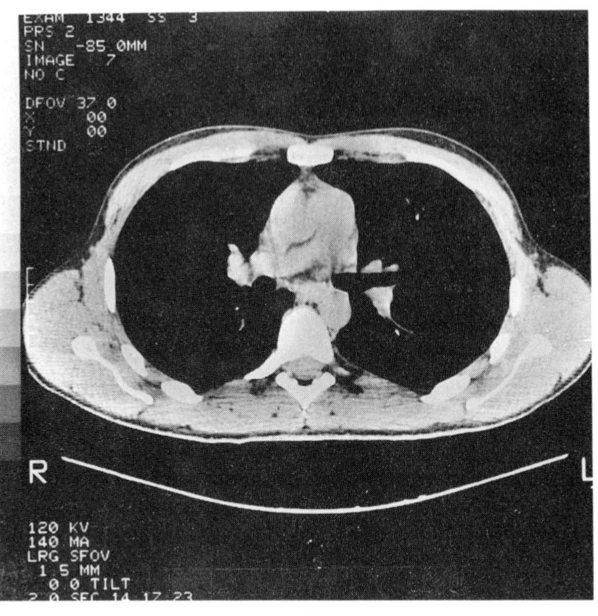

A

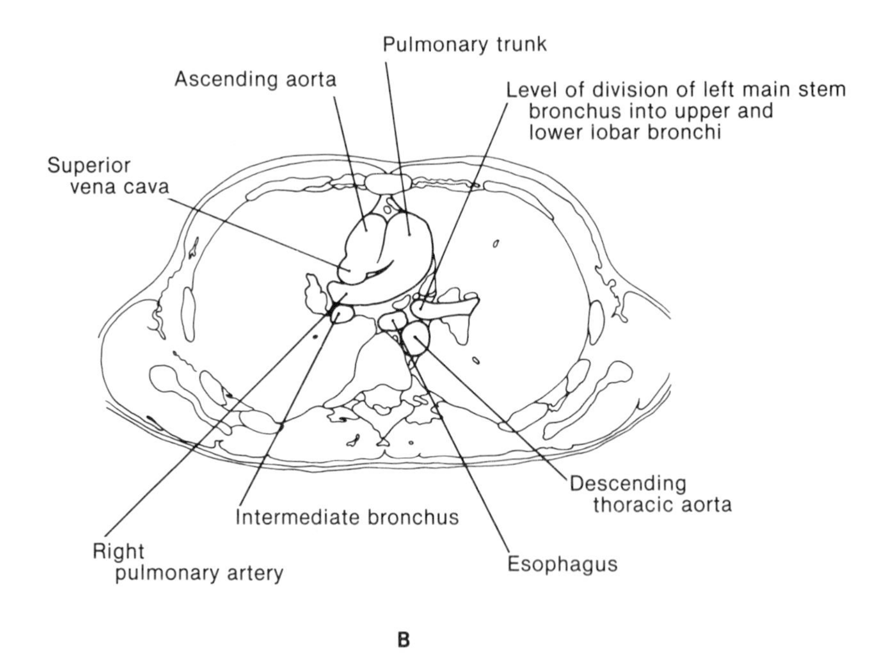

B

Figure 3-9. (*A*) CT scan at the level of the origin of the right pulmonary artery that demonstrates the mediastinal viscera, and (*B*) its schematic representation. (*C*) CT scan at the identical level (lung window) that demonstrates segments of bronchi and blood vessels of the lungs, and (*D*) its schematic representation. (*E*) Appearance and relationships of the major mediastinal viscera and pulmonary structures at this level. (See section III E.)

Figure 3-9. *continued*

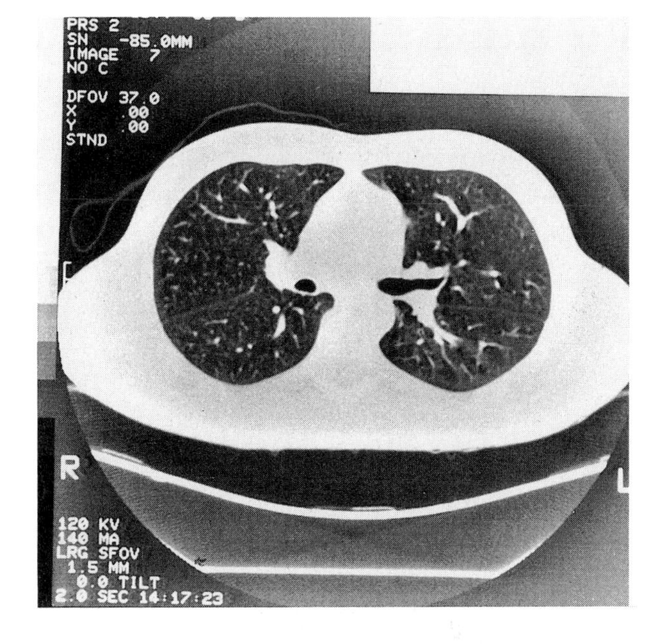

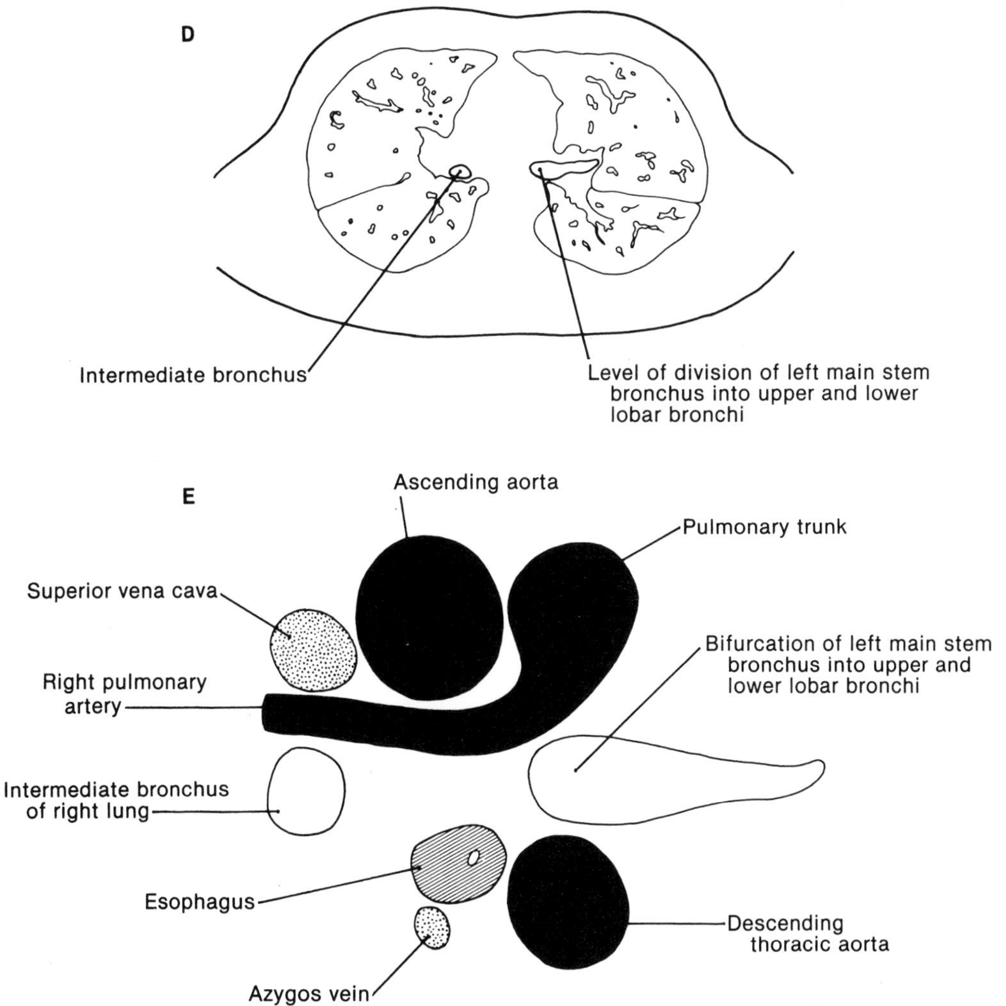

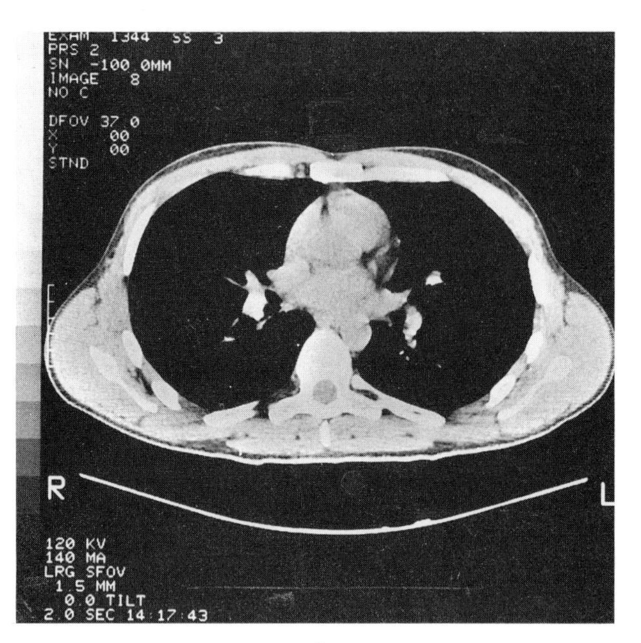

A

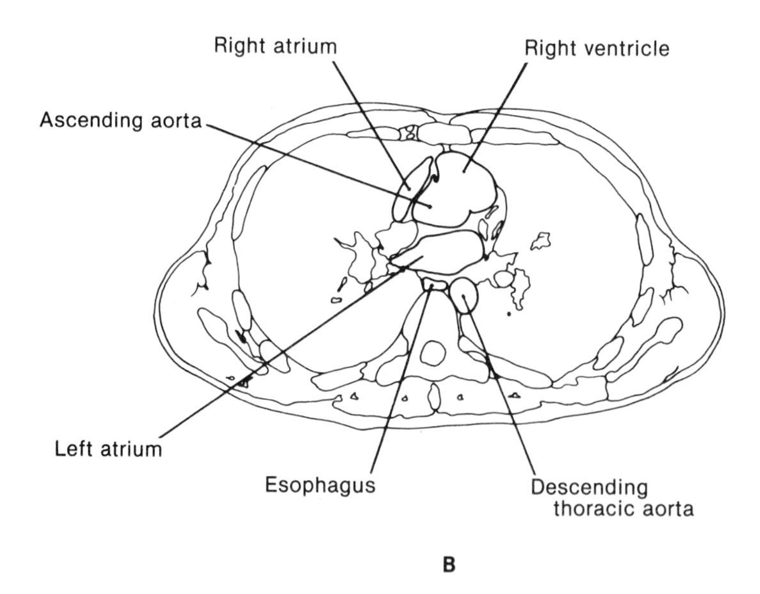

B

Figure 3-10. (*A*) CT scan at the level of the roots of the ascending aorta and pulmonary trunk that demonstrates the mediastinal viscera, and (*B*) its schematic representation. (*C*) CT scan at the identical level (lung window) that demonstrates segments of bronchi and blood vessels of the lungs, and (*D*) its schematic representation. (*E*) Appearance and relationships of the major mediastinal viscera and pulmonary structures at this level. (See section III F.)

Figure 3-10. *continued*

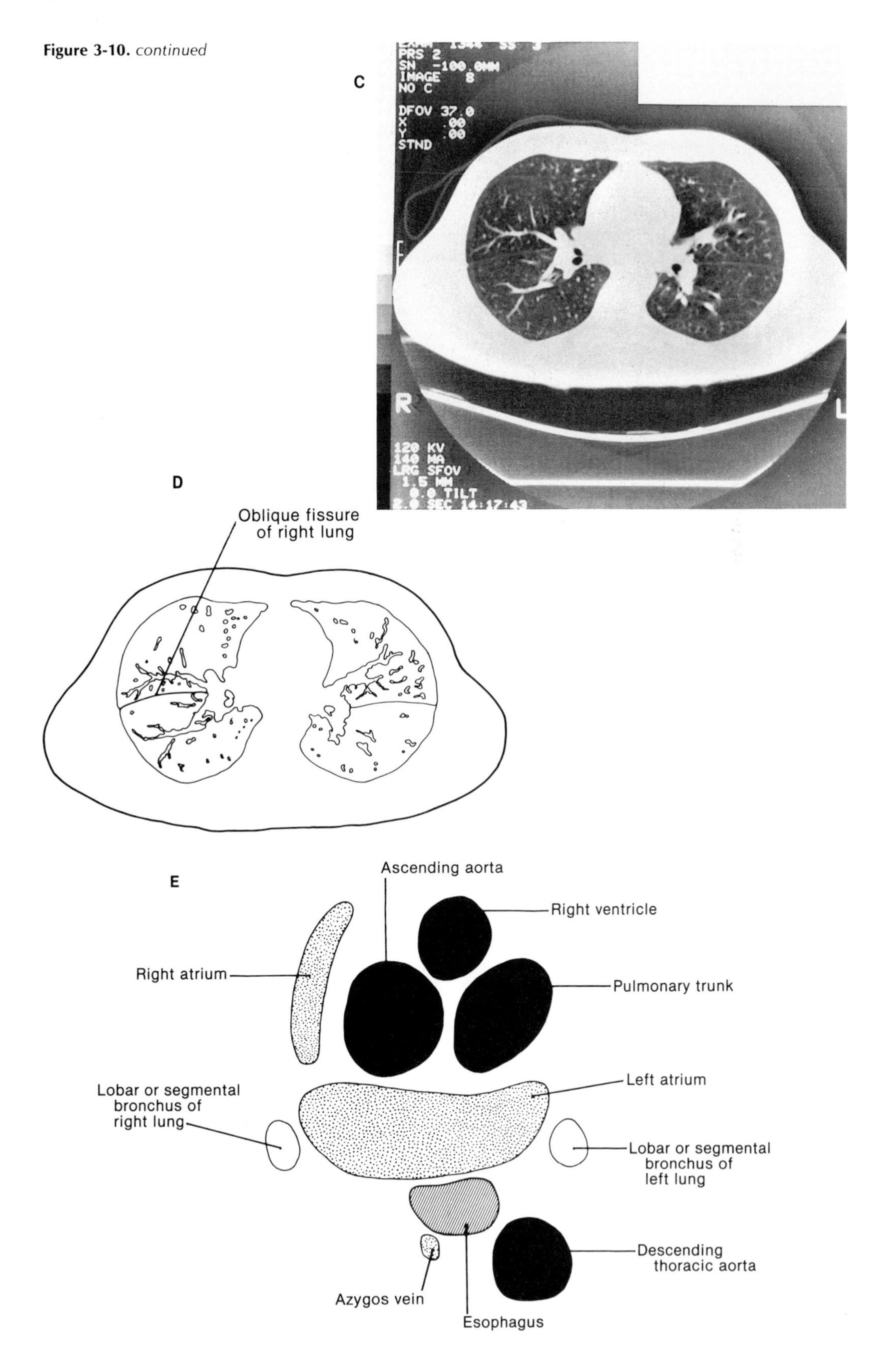

(b) Left atrial enlargement can distend the chamber's right border, bringing it closer to the heart's right border and thereby increasing the radiopacity of the lower right side of the cardiovascular shadow. This increase in radiopacity generally extends almost to the lower right border of the shadow, and thus produces a distinct radiopaque border immediately medial to that part of the shadow's right border outlined by the right atrium.

(2) An enlarged left atrium may elevate the left main stem bronchus.

c. **Enlargement of the right ventricle** can elevate the apex and straighten the cardiovascular shadow's left border.

d. **Enlargement of the left ventricle** can lower the apex and increase the outward lower bulging of the cardiovascular shadow's left border.

2. **Marked increase of the carinal angle in a PA chest film.** A marked widening of the angle between the main stem bronchi can be produced by
   a. **Enlargement of the left atrium**
   b. **Enlargement of the subcarinal lymph nodes**

3. **Widening and blurring of the lateral margin of the right tracheal stripe in a PA chest film.** Such a finding commonly indicates **enlarged tracheobronchial lymph nodes**.

4. **A water-density retrosternal or retrocardiac mass in a lateral chest film**
   a. The most common **retrosternal masses** are intrathoracic **goiters**, **teratomas**, **thymomas**, and **lymphoma**.
   b. The most common **retrocardiac masses** are neurogenic **tumors**, **hiatal hernias**, and **aneurysms** of the descending thoracic aorta.

5. **Generalized shift of mediastinal structures.** Such a shift may be indicative of a **tension pneumothorax** in the pleural cavity contralateral to the side of the shift. Shifts may also be due to **postsurgical or postinfectious volume loss** on the side to which the mediastinum shifts.

D. Lung fields

1. **Pulmonary nodules**
   a. **Radiographic definition.** The term **pulmonary nodule** refers to any radiopacity with a fairly well defined circular or elliptic border in a lung field.
   b. **Radiographic appearance**
      (1) **Limits of visibility.** Individual calcified pulmonary nodules are visible down to a size of approximately 1 mm. For solitary pulmonary nodules with a radiographic density of water, the lower limit of visibility is about 3 mm.
      (2) Individual nodules may exhibit nonuniform radiopacity because of cavitation or inhomogeneous calcification.
      (3) Small pulmonary nodules are most easily detected in the radiolucent interspaces of the lung fields.
   c. **Significance.** Nodules may represent **benign granulomas**, **primary malignant neoplasms**, or **metastatic deposits**.

2. **Consolidation**
   a. **Definition.** The term **consolidation** refers to any process in which the air in one or more acini of a lung is isovolumetrically replaced with fluid or, rarely, tissue. (The **acini** of a lung are its basic respiratory units; each acinus consists of a terminal bronchiole and the respiratory airways it serves: the respiratory bronchioles, alveolar ducts, alveolar sacs, and alveoli.)
   b. **General features of consolidated areas.** Areas of consolidation can vary in size from 5 mm (which is the smallest size of an acinus) to the entire lung field.
      (1) If a pathologic process produces multiple foci of consolidation, the foci commonly appear initially as ill-defined and irregularly shaped areas; this occurs because the accumulating fluid tends to disperse in a rather arbitrary fashion throughout the pulmonary parenchyma via the pores of Kohn and the canals of Lambert.
      (2) If the pathologic process continues unabated, the foci tend to coalesce into areas of homogeneous radiopacity; these areas acquire well-defined borders upon reaching pleural surfaces, such as those bordering the interlobar fissures.
   c. **Radiologic signs**
      (1) **Air bronchogram**
         (a) When the consolidation process in a lung region does not replace the air in the larger conducting bronchial passageways, the lumina of the air-filled bronchi appear in chest films as branching, radiolucent bands within the relatively radiopaque consolidated lung region. Such a finding is called an **air bronchogram**.

(b) An air bronchogram can only be produced by an intrapulmonary process, although this may be a process other than consolidation.

(2) Silhouette sign

(a) Any loss of the silhouettes of the mediastinal viscera that define the borders of the cardiovascular shadow along the medial margins of the lung fields in a PA chest film, or any loss of the silhouettes of the domes of the diaphragm along the inferior margins of the lung fields, is called the **silhouette sign**.

(b) Some of the bronchopulmonary segments in each lung directly face the mediastinal viscera or diaphragmatic domes; if these segments acquire a radiographic density equal to that of the mediastinal viscera or diaphragmatic domes, a silhouette sign is produced because part or all of the border between the radiopaque segments and the mediastinal viscera or diaphragmatic domes cannot be discerned.

(c) Consolidation is a process which commonly generates such an increase in the radiographic density of these segments.

(i) Consolidation of the **anterior segment** of the **right** lung's **upper lobe** may obscure the silhouettes of the superior vena cava, the ascending aorta, and the upper end of the right atrium along the right border of the cardiovascular shadow.

(ii) Consolidation of the **medial segment** of the **right** lung's **middle lobe** may obscure the silhouette of the right atrium along the right border of the cardiovascular shadow.

(iii) Consolidation of the **apical posterior segment** of the **left** lung's **upper lobe** may obscure the silhouette of the aortic knob.

(iv) Consolidation of the **anterior segment** of the **left** lung's **upper lobe** may obscure the silhouette of the upper part of the left ventricle along the left border of the cardiovascular shadow.

(v) Consolidation of **one or both** of the **left** lung's **lingular segments** may obscure the silhouette of most of the left ventricle along the left border of the cardiovascular shadow.

(vi) Consolidation of any of the **basal segments** of the **lower lobe** in **each lung** may obscure part of the silhouette of the underlying diaphragmatic dome.

(d) The silhouette sign can also be produced by processes other than consolidation of appropriate bronchopulmonary segments.

3. Linear radiopacities. Connective tissue septa thickened by disease or engorged lymphatics present as water-density lines less than 1 mm thick called **Kerley lines**. When present in the bases of the lung fields, Kerley lines characteristically present as horizontal, nonbranching lines that abut perpendicularly against the pleural border of the lung fields.

4. Shift of a lung fissure. A shift of an interlobar fissure commonly accompanies significant **atelectasis** of a lung lobe.

a. Shifts of the left lung's oblique fissure

(1) In atelectasis of the left lung's upper lobe, the oblique fissure shows an almost parallel shift anteriorly in the lateral chest film. Corresponding signs of **left upper lobe atelectasis** in the PA chest film commonly include:

(a) Increased radiopacity in the superior part of the left lung field (which may obscure the silhouette of the aortic knob)

(b) Decreased radiopacity in the inferior part of the left lung field (due to hyperinflation of the left lower lobe)

(c) Elevation of the left hilum

(d) Deviation of the trachea to the left

(2) In atelectasis of the left lung's lower lobe, the oblique fissure shows an almost parallel shift posteriorly in the lateral chest film. Corresponding signs of **left lower lobe atelectasis** in the PA chest film commonly include:

(a) Increased radiopacity in the inferior part of the left lung field

(b) Decreased radiopacity in the superior part of the left lung field

(c) Depression of the left hilum

b. Shifts of the right lung's horizontal and oblique fissures

(1) In atelectasis of the right lung's upper lobe, the horizontal fissure shows upward rotation about the hilum in both the lateral and PA chest films. Corresponding signs of **right upper lobe atelectasis** commonly include:

(a) Forward rotation about the hilum of the upper part of the lung's oblique fissure in the lateral chest film

(b) Increased radiopacity in the upper part of the right lung field in the PA chest film

(c) Decreased radiopacity in the lower part of the right lung field in the PA chest film

(d) Elevation of the right hilum
(e) Deviation of the trachea to the right in the PA chest film
(f) The **S sign of Golden** in the PA chest film if the hilar area of the upper lobe bears a **tumor mass**: The tumor mass prevents the hilar end of the horizontal fissure from rotating upward, and thus the horizontal fissure assumes the shape of the letter S in the PA chest film.

(2) In atelectasis of either the middle or the lower lobe of the right lung, its horizontal fissure shows downward rotation about the hilum in both the lateral and PA chest films.

(a) **Right middle lobe atelectasis** is indicated if the downward rotation of the horizontal fissure in the lateral chest film is associated with forward rotation about the hilum in the lower part of the lung's oblique fissure. Corresponding signs of right middle lobe atelectasis commonly include:

(i) A wedge of increased radiopacity between the downwardly rotated horizontal fissure and the forwardly rotated part of the oblique fissure in the lateral chest film. The apex of the wedge points toward the hilum unless there is a tumor mass in the hilar area of the middle lobe. A tumor mass in the hilar area prevents the hilar end of the horizontal fissure from rotating downward and the hilar end of the oblique fissure from rotating upward, thereby rendering a wedge whose apex points away from the hilum.
(ii) Obscurity of the silhouette of the right atrium along the right border of the cardiovascular shadow in the PA chest film.

(b) **Right lower lobe atelectasis** is indicated if the downward rotation of the horizontal fissure in the lateral chest film is associated with a posterior parallel shift of the lung's oblique fissure. Corresponding signs of right lower lobe atelectasis in the PA chest film commonly include:

(i) Increased radiopacity in the inferior part of the right lung field
(ii) Decreased radiopacity in the superior part of the right lung field
(iii) Depression of the right hilum

5. **Blunting of the costophrenic angles.** Blunting of the costophrenic angles is often an indication of **pleural effusion**.

a. If a person is in the erect position, nonencapsulated fluid in the pleural cavity will accumulate in the **costodiaphragmatic recess**. This recess rims the **subpulmonic pleural space** (the space sandwiched between the base of the lung and the underlying dome of the diaphragm).

(1) Pooling occurs first along the posterior margin of the recess (where the recess reaches its most inferior extent), and then progressively spreads to the lateral and anterior margins of the recess if the volume of the effusion increases even further.
(2) The posterior and anterior costophrenic angles are thus, respectively, the first and last costophrenic angles to show evidence of pooling of a nonencapsulated pleural effusion in the erect patient.

b. **Progressive pooling** at any of the costophrenic angles (posterior, lateral, or anterior) first diminishes the depth of the angle, then blunts the angle, and finally generates a fluid-filled recess bearing a curved meniscus.
c. Blunting of a lateral costophrenic angle in a PA chest film of an adult does not occur until 200 to 500 ml of fluid has accumulated in the subpulmonic pleural space.
d. Blunting may also represent **scarring of parietal pleura** resulting from old infections, trauma, or surgery.

6. **Loss of vascular markings in the apical area of a lung field.** This is an indication of a small **pneumothorax**. The area devoid of lung vascular markings will be medially bordered by a thin water-density line that represents the visceral pleura lining the retracted lung apex.

STUDY QUESTIONS

Directions: Each question below contains five suggested answers. Choose the **one best** response to each question.

1. All of the following structures participate in defining the right border of the cardiovascular shadow in a PA chest film EXCEPT the

(A) superior vena cava
(B) brachiocephalic artery
(C) right atrium
(D) right ventricle
(E) inferior vena cava

2. All of the following structures participate in defining the left border of the cardiovascular shadow in a PA chest film EXCEPT the

(A) left subclavian artery
(B) descending thoracic aorta
(C) left ventricle
(D) auricle of the left atrium
(E) pulmonary trunk

3. All of the following are correct statements regarding a CT scan of the thorax at a level above the aortic arch EXCEPT

(A) the right brachiocephalic vein appears in transverse section
(B) the left brachiocephalic vein appears in oblique section
(C) the thymus (if present) lies directly anterior to the left brachiocephalic vein
(D) the esophagus lies directly posterior to and slightly to the left of the trachea
(E) the left subclavian artery is the most anteriorly positioned of the branches of the aortic arch

4. All of the following are correct statements regarding a CT scan of the thorax at the level of the aortic–pulmonary window EXCEPT

(A) the origin and end of the aortic arch both appear in transverse section
(B) the pulmonary trunk lies directly between the origin and end of the aortic arch
(C) the superior vena cava lies directly to the right of the origin of the aortic arch
(D) the scan is approximately at the level of the carina
(E) the esophagus lies directly anterior to and slightly to the left of the vertebral column

5. All of the following are correct statements regarding CT scans at the origins of the left and right pulmonary arteries EXCEPT

(A) as the left pulmonary artery extends into the hilum of the left lung, it passes between the left main stem bronchus and the descending thoracic aorta
(B) as the right pulmonary artery extends into the hilum of the right lung, it passes between the superior vena cava and the intermediate bronchus of the right lung
(C) the CT scan showing the emanation of the left pulmonary artery from the pulmonary trunk lies at a level above that of the scan showing the emanation of the right pulmonary artery from the pulmonary trunk
(D) the CT scan showing the emanation of the left pulmonary artery from the pulmonary trunk lies at a level above that of the scan showing the division of the left main stem bronchus into its upper and lower lobar bronchi
(E) the CT scan showing the emanation of the right pulmonary artery from the pulmonary trunk lies at a level below that of the scan showing the division of the right main stem bronchus into its eparterial and intermediate bronchi

6. All of the following are correct statements regarding a CT scan of the thorax at the level of the roots of the ascending aorta and pulmonary trunk EXCEPT

(A) the azygos vein, esophagus, and descending thoracic aorta all appear in transverse section in the posterior mediastinum
(B) the root of the pulmonary trunk lies directly to the left of the root of the ascending aorta
(C) the right atrium lies directly to the right of the root of the ascending aorta
(D) the roots of the ascending aorta and pulmonary trunk lie directly anterior to the left atrium
(E) a portion of the left ventricle may be evident anterior to and between the roots of the ascending aorta and pulmonary trunk

7. Loss of the silhouettes of the superior vena cava and ascending aorta in a PA chest film can occur upon consolidation of which bronchopulmonary segment of the right lung?

(A) Apical segment of the upper lobe
(B) Anterior segment of the upper lobe
(C) Posterior segment of the upper lobe
(D) Lateral segment of the middle lobe
(E) Medial segment of the middle lobe

8. Loss of the silhouette of the right atrium in a PA chest film can occur upon consolidation of which bronchopulmonary segment of the right lung?

(A) Anterior segment of the upper lobe
(B) Medial segment of the middle lobe
(C) Apical segment of the lower lobe
(D) Anterior basal segment of the lower lobe
(E) Medial basal segment of the lower lobe

9. Which bronchopulmonary segment of the right lung's lower lobe does not directly face the underlying diaphragmatic dome?

(A) Apical
(B) Medial basal
(C) Posterior basal
(D) Lateral basal
(E) Anterior basal

10. Loss of the silhouette of the aortic knob in a PA chest film can occur upon consolidation of which bronchopulmonary segment of the left lung?

(A) Apical posterior segment of the upper lobe
(B) Superior lingular segment of the upper lobe
(C) Inferior lingular segment of the upper lobe
(D) Apical segment of the lower lobe
(E) Medial basal segment of the lower lobe

11. The sternal angle lies at the level of the intervertebral disk between the

(A) first and second thoracic vertebrae
(B) second and third thoracic vertebrae
(C) third and fourth thoracic vertebrae
(D) fourth and fifth thoracic vertebrae
(E) fifth and sixth thoracic vertebrae

12. All of the following structures pass through the esophageal opening of the diaphragm EXCEPT

(A) the anterior vagal trunk
(B) the posterior vagal trunk
(C) the branches of the left gastric artery
(D) the tributaries of the left gastric vein
(E) the azygos vein

13. All of the following are correct statements regarding the left coronary artery and its branches EXCEPT

(A) the left coronary artery emerges from the sinus of the left cusp of the aortic valve
(B) the circumflex and left anterior descending arteries are branches of the left coronary artery
(C) the nutrient artery for the SA node is a branch of the left coronary artery in about 10% of the population
(D) the posterior descending artery arises from the left coronary artery in about 10% of the population
(E) the most commonly occluded major coronary arterial vessel is a branch of the left coronary artery

14. All of the following structures are located in the posterior mediastinum EXCEPT

(A) the trachea
(B) the vagus nerves
(C) the esophagus
(D) the thoracic duct
(E) the phrenic nerves

15. All of the following are correct statements regarding the aortic arch EXCEPT

(A) the aortic arch lies in the superior mediastinum
(B) the aortic arch begins in front of the right pulmonary artery
(C) the aortic arch ends behind the left pulmonary artery
(D) the aortic arch restricts expansion of a segment of the esophagus during peristaltic transport of food boli
(E) the aortic–pulmonary window is traversed by the left and right recurrent laryngeal nerves

16. The mitral component of the first heart sound is best heard over the

(A) apex beat
(B) anterior end of the right fifth intercostal space
(C) anterior end of the left fifth intercostal space
(D) anterior end of the right second intercostal space
(E) anterior end of the left second intercostal space

Directions: Each question below contains four suggested answers of which **one or more** is correct. Choose the answer

A if **1, 2, and 3** are correct
B if **1 and 3** are correct
C if **2 and 4** are correct
D if **4** is correct
E if **1, 2, 3, and 4** are correct

17. Anatomic structures that normally contribute significantly to the radiopaque markings of the hila in the lung fields of a PA chest film include the

(1) pulmonary artery
(2) secondary bronchi
(3) pulmonary veins
(4) bronchopulmonary lymph nodes

18. Which of the following findings would negate the worthiness of a PA chest film?

(1) The clavicles do not have companion shadows
(2) The costal cartilages of the upper ribs are not visible
(3) Not all the ribs have companion shadows
(4) The bodies of the thoracic vertebrae are not discernible within the cardiovascular shadow

19. Which of the following findings would be distinctly abnormal with respect to the appearance of the trachea in PA chest films of adults?

(1) The radiopaque stripe representing the right tracheal wall measures 9 to 10 mm in width
(2) The radiopaque stripe representing the left tracheal wall is not observed
(3) The inferior angle between the main stem bronchi at the carina measures 100°
(4) The trachea deviates slightly to the right in the upper chest

20. PA and lateral chest films are taken of an adult in whom there is a nonencapsulated pleural effusion in the left lung. Which of the following statements would be correct regarding the order of appearance of pleural effusion in the costophrenic angles of chest films if the films are taken with the patient standing upright?

(1) The pleural effusion collects in the posterior costophrenic angle of a lateral chest film before it collects in the anterior costophrenic angle
(2) The pleural effusion collects in the left lateral costophrenic angle of a PA chest film before it collects in the anterior costophrenic angle of a lateral chest film
(3) The pleural effusion collects in the left lateral costophrenic angle of a PA chest film after it collects in the posterior costophrenic angle of a lateral chest film
(4) Evidence of pleural effusion in a PA chest film does not occur until a minimum of 25 ml of fluid has collected in the pleural cavity

21. Significant atelectasis of the left lung's upper lobe is commonly accompanied by which of the following findings?

(1) Anterior shift of the left lung's oblique fissure
(2) Increased radiopacity in the inferior part of the left lung field
(3) Elevation of the left hilum
(4) Deviation of the trachea to the right

SUMMARY OF DIRECTIONS

A	B	C	D	E
1, 2, 3 only	1, 3 only	2, 4 only	4 only	All are correct

22. A young child has a congenital aortic coarctation located immediately distal to the origin of the left subclavian artery. Correct statements regarding the development of notches in the ribs of the patient include which of the following?

(1) Rib notches do not develop in the first and second ribs
(2) The notches in the upper ribs are more prominent than those in the lower ribs
(3) The notches along the posterior body segment of a rib are more prominent than those along the anterior body segment
(4) The notches develop along the superior border of each affected rib

23. Correct statements regarding the general features of consolidated areas in lung fields include which of the following?

(1) The minimum dimension for an area of consolidation is 1 cm
(2) Foci of consolidation initially have a spherical shape
(3) Areas of consolidation generally do not acquire well-defined borders until they reach intersegmental connective tissue sheaths
(4) Consolidation of a lung region generally occurs without a net change in the volume of the region

24. The phrenic nerves provide which of the following types of innervation?

(1) Sensory innervation for the parietal pleura overlying the central tendon of the diaphragm
(2) Sensory innervation for the mediastinal pleura
(3) Sensory innervation for the parietal peritoneum underlying the central tendon of the diaphragm
(4) Motor innervation for the diaphragm

25. Correct statements regarding the cardiac shadow in a lateral chest film include which of the following?

(1) The shadow of the ascending aorta projects upward from the superior limit of the posterior border of the cardiac shadow
(2) The left ventricle defines the lower half of the shadow's anterior border
(3) The right ventricle defines the lower third of the shadow's posterior border
(4) The left atrium defines the middle third of the shadow's posterior border

26. The walls of the left or right atria contain which of the following parts of the heart's conducting system?

(1) SA node
(2) AV node
(3) Internodal tracts
(4) Purkinje fibers

27. Which of the following could be radiographic findings in a patient with an enlarged left atrium?

(1) An increase in the carinal angle in a PA chest film
(2) A straightened left border of the cardiovascular shadow in a PA chest film
(3) A distinct vertical radiopaque border immediately medial to the right border of the cardiovascular shadow in a PA chest film
(4) A posterior bulge of the middle third of the posterior border of the cardiac shadow in a lateral chest film

28. Significant atelectasis of the right lung's middle lobe is commonly accompanied by which of the following findings?

(1) Upward rotation about the hilum of the right lung's horizontal fissure
(2) Forward rotation about the hilum of the lower part of the right lung's oblique fissure
(3) Deviation of the trachea to the right
(4) Obscurity of the outline of the right atrium

Directions: Each question below contains four suggested answers. Choose the **one best** response to each question.

29. Fissures that are generally evident in both PA and lateral chest films include which of the following?

(A) The oblique fissure of the left lung
(B) The horizontal fissure of the right lung
(C) Both fissures
(D) Neither fissure

30. In a PA chest film, a retrosternal mediastinal mass with a radiographic density of water may obscure the silhouette of

(A) the right atrium
(B) the aortic knob
(C) both structures
(D) neither structure

31. In a PA chest film, a retrocardiac mediastinal mass with a radiographic density of water may obscure the outline of

(A) the descending thoracic aorta
(B) the apex of the heart
(C) both structures
(D) neither structure

32. Correct statements about the site of an aspirated object include which of the following?

(A) When a person standing or seated upright accidentally aspirates a small object into the trachea, the object will most likely pass into the left main stem bronchus
(B) When a supine person accidentally aspirates a small object into either lung, the object will most likely lodge in the lower lobe's posterior basal segment
(C) Both statements
(D) Neither statement

33. Correct statements about surface projections of the lungs include which of the following?

(A) The apex of each lung projects above the middle third of the clavicle
(B) Each lung's upper lobe is the lobe which casts the largest surface projection to the back of the chest
(C) Both statements
(D) Neither statement

34. Correct statements about the spinous processes of the thoracic vertebrae include which of the following?

(A) The spinous process of the first thoracic vertebra is the highest palpable spinous process in the vertebral column
(B) The tip of the spinous process of the third thoracic vertebra lies at the level of the body of the fourth thoracic vertebra
(C) Both statements
(D) Neither statement

35. The retrosternal area in a lateral chest film displays a lateral projection of

(A) the anterior segments of both lungs' upper lobes
(B) possibly the thymus in a child
(C) both structures
(D) neither structure

36. The retrocardiac area in a lateral chest film displays a lateral projection of

(A) the basal segments of both lungs' lower lobes
(B) the descending thoracic aorta
(C) both structures
(D) neither structure

37. PA chest films of neonates and young children differ from those of adults in which of the following ways?

(A) The anterior body segments of the ribs slope downward less markedly in PA chest films of neonates and children
(B) A solid mediastinal viscus may outline the cardiovascular shadow in PA chest films of neonates and children but does not outline the shadow in PA chest films of adults
(C) Both findings
(D) Neither finding

38. Correct statements about the visibility of pulmonary nodules includes which of the following?

(A) The lower limit of visibility of individual calcified pulmonary nodules is about 1 mm
(B) The lower limit of visibility of individual pulmonary nodules with a radiographic density of water is about 3 mm
(C) Both statements
(D) Neither statement

39. Horizontal, nonbranching water-density lines in the base of a lung field commonly represent

(A) thickened bronchial walls
(B) swollen lymphatics
(C) both disorders
(D) neither disorder

40. The costodiaphragmatic margin of each lung at midinspiration in quiet breathing lies at

(A) the level of the sixth rib anteriorly at the midclavicular line
(B) the level of the tenth rib laterally at the midaxillary line
(C) both rib levels
(D) neither rib level

ANSWERS AND EXPLANATIONS

1. The answer is D. [*I E 1 b, e; II A 3 a (1); Figure 3-3*] The great veins and arteries extending to and from the upper border of the heart on the right side of the body (namely, the right brachiocephalic vein, superior vena cava, ascending aorta, and brachiocephalic artery) define the upper part of the right border of the cardiovascular shadow in a PA chest film. The right atrium defines almost all of the lower part of the right border of the shadow. The union of the inferior vena cava with the floor of the right atrium casts a curvilinear outline at the base of the shadow's right border. The right ventricle forms most of the heart's sternocostal surface, and is not a component of the right border of the cardiovascular shadow.

2. The answer is B. [*I E 1 f; II A 3 a (2), d; Figure 3-3*] The left subclavian artery and left brachiocephalic vein outline the uppermost part of the cardiovascular shadow's left border in a PA chest film. The terminal part of the aortic arch and pulmonary trunk outline the next lowest part of the shadow's left border. The auricle of the left atrium and the left ventricle form the heart's left border, and thus outline the lower part of the shadow's left border. The left border of the descending thoracic aorta is visible within the cardiovascular shadow, but the descending thoracic aorta does not contribute to the left border of the cardiovascular shadow.

3. The answer is E. [*III A; Figure 3-5*] In a CT scan taken at a level above the aortic arch, the thymus (if present) is the most anterior mediastinal viscus. The left and right brachiocephalic veins are the next most posterior major structures within the superior mediastinum; the obliquely sectioned left brachiocephalic vein lies directly behind the thymus, and the transversely sectioned right brachiocephalic vein lies at the right edge of the superior mediastinum. The three branches of the aortic arch lie posterior to the brachiocephalic veins; the left subclavian artery is the most posteriorly positioned branch and the branch furthest to the left. The esophagus lies slightly to the left of center between the trachea and vertebral column.

4. The answer is B. [*III C; Figure 3-7*] In a CT scan at the level of the aortic–pulmonary window, the pulmonary trunk is not evident in the space between the origin and end of the aortic arch, as the aortic–pulmonary window lies immediately above the bifurcation of the pulmonary trunk into the left and right pulmonary arteries. The scan lies just above or below the carina; the scan commonly shows the azygos vein arching over the right main stem bronchus to unite with the superior vena cava. The position of the esophagus, directly anterior to and slightly to the left of the vertebral column, remains constant as the esophagus descends through the superior mediastinum and posterior mediastinum.

5. The answer is A. [*III D 2–4, E 2–4; Figures 3-8, 3-9*] Whereas the left pulmonary artery ascends as it extends from the pulmonary trunk to the left lung, the right pulmonary artery descends as it extends from the pulmonary trunk to the right lung. This difference is the anatomic basis for the fact that the CT scan showing the emanation of the left pulmonary artery from the pulmonary trunk lies at a level higher than that for the scan showing the emanation of the right pulmonary artery from the pulmonary trunk.

As the left pulmonary artery extends into the hilum of the left lung, the artery lies anterior to both the left main stem bronchus and the descending thoracic aorta and superior to the bifurcation of the left main stem bronchus into its upper and lower lobar bronchi. As the right pulmonary artery extends into the hilum of the right lung, the artery passes first between the superior vena cava and intermediate bronchus of the right lung and then beneath the right lung's eparterial bronchus.

6. The answer is E. [*III F; Figure 3-10*] The CT scan at the level of the roots of the ascending aorta and pulmonary trunk generally shows the uppermost parts of the chambers that form the heart's right border, base, and most of its sternocostal surface. The left ventricle is not visible. The uppermost part of the right ventricle may be evident anterior to and between the roots of the ascending aorta and pulmonary trunk; the right ventricle forms most of the heart's sternocostal surface. The scan shows the right atrium forming the heart's right border and the left atrium forming most of its base. The right atrium lies immediately to the right of the root of the ascending aorta. The left atrium lies posterior to the roots of the ascending aorta and pulmonary trunk and anterior to the viscera of the posterior mediastinum.

7. The answer is B. [*IV D 2 c (2) (c) (i); Table 3-1*] There are bronchopulmonary segments in each lung that directly face one or more of the mediastinal viscera that define the outline of the cardiovascular shadow in a PA chest film. Consolidation of these segments can obscure the outlines of these mediastinal viscera. The anterior bronchopulmonary segment of the right lung's upper lobe directly faces the superior vena cava and ascending aorta.

8. The answer is B. [*IV D 2 c (2) (c) (ii); Table 3-1*] The medial and lateral segments of the right lung's middle lobe each directly face the right atrium. Consolidation of either segment can obscure the outline of the right atrium in a PA chest film.

9. The answer is A. [*IV D 2 c (2) (c) (vi)*] The basal segments of each lung's lower lobe are the only segments that directly face the underlying diaphragmatic dome on each side. Accordingly, the basal segments are the only segments whose consolidation can potentially obscure the silhouette of the diaphragmatic dome in both PA and lateral chest films.

10. The answer is A. [*IV D 2 c (2) (c) (iii)*] The apical posterior segment of the left lung's upper lobe directly faces the aortic knob. Consolidation of the segment can obscure the outline of the aortic knob in a PA chest film.

11. The answer is D. [*II B 2 b (1)*] The sternal angle is the posterior angle between the manubrium and the body of the sternum at the manubriosternal joint. The sternal angle is easily palpated as a rather prominent transverse ridge in the midline of the anterior chest wall, at the level of the T4–T5 intervertebral disk. It marks the level in the thorax at which the mediastinum is divided into the superior mediastinum and inferior mediastinum. It also marks the union of the costal cartilages of the second ribs with the sternum; this relationship permits identification of the second ribs and all the lower ribs in the chest wall.

12. The answer is E. [*I B 2 b*] The esophageal opening of the diaphragm transmits the esophagus, anterior and posterior vagal trunks, esophageal branches of the left gastric artery, and esophageal tributaries of the left gastric vein. The left gastric vein is a tributary of the portal vein. The aortic opening of the diaphragm transmits the azygos vein.

13. The answer is C. [*I E 2 a (2) (b); b*] The left coronary artery emerges from the sinus of the left cusp of the aortic valve and extends for only a relatively short distance on the heart's surface before dividing into the left anterior descending and the circumflex arteries. The circumflex artery is the most commonly occluded major artery of the heart. The nutrient artery for the SA node is a branch of the right coronary artery in 55% of the population and a branch of the circumflex artery in the remainder of the population. The posterior descending artery is an extension of the right coronary artery in 90% of the population and an extension of the circumflex artery in the remainder of the population.

14. The answer is E. [*I G 1–5*] The phrenic nerves descend through first the superior mediastinum and then the middle mediastinum as they extend from the neck to the diaphragm. As they descend through the middle mediastinum, the phrenic nerves course alongside the pericardial sac and pass in front of the roots of the lungs. The lower end of the trachea lies behind the pericardial sac in the upper part of the posterior mediastinum. In the posterior mediastinum, the esophagus lies directly anterior to and slightly to the left of the vertebral column. The vagus nerves descend through the posterior mediastinum in close association with the esophagus. As the thoracic duct ascends through the posterior mediastinum, it lies, for the most part, directly behind the esophagus.

15. The answer is E. [*I F 1 b, G 2 b (1) (a)*] The aortic arch begins in front of the right pulmonary artery at the level of the sternal angle, arches over the pulmonary trunk bifurcation in the superior mediastinum, and ends behind the left pulmonary artery at the level of the sternal angle. It is the most superior structure to restrict expansion of the esophagus during peristaltic transport of food boli. The aortic–pulmonary window is traversed by the left but not the right recurrent laryngeal nerve.

16. The answer is A. [*I E 4 b (1) (a)*] The mitral and tricuspid components of the first heart sound are best heard, respectively, over the apex beat and over the anterior end of the left fifth intercostal space. The aortic and pulmonary components of the second heart sound are best heard, respectively, over the anterior ends of the right and left second intercostal spaces.

17. The answer is B (1, 3). [*II A 4 a (1), b, c*] The radiopaque markings of the hilum in each lung field primarily represent the shadows of the pulmonary artery and its lobar branches and the pulmonary veins and their immediate tributaries. The walls of most of the lobar and segmental bronchi are too obliquely oriented to cast distinct shadows. Normal lymph nodes are too small to cast shadows.

18. The answer is D (4). [*II A 1 b (2)*] An inability to discern the bodies of the thoracic vertebrae within the cardiovascular shadow negates the capacity to detect anterior or posterior mediastinal masses with a radiographic density of water. The absence of clavicular companion shadows bilaterally may be due to excessive fat deposition in the superficial fascia of the supraclavicular fossae. Costal cartilages are normally not visible and rib companion shadows are inconstantly visible in PA chest films.

19. The answer is B (1, 3). [*II A 3 c; IV C 2, 3*] The normal width of the right tracheal stripe in adults is 4 to 5 mm; a width of 9 to 10 mm commonly indicates enlarged tracheobronchial lymph nodes. A radiopaque stripe representing the left tracheal wall is only infrequently apparent. The inferior angle between the main stem bronchi normally measures 60° to 75°. Slight deviation of the lower third of the trachea to the right is a common, normal finding.

20. The answer is A (1, 2, 3). [*I C 1 c (2); II A 4 f; B 5 a (2), b (2); IV D 5 a, c*] A nonencapsulated pleural effusion pools in the costodiaphragmatic recess that rims the subpulmonic pleural space. Pooling occurs first along the posterior part of the recess since this is the most inferior part of the recess. The posterior costophrenic angle in a lateral chest film provides a cross-sectional view of the posterior part of the recess, and thus is the first of the costophrenic angles to show evidence of the pleural effusion. The left lateral costophrenic and anterior costophrenic angles are, respectively, the second and last costophrenic angles to show evidence of the pleural effusion; this is because the margin of the costodiaphragmatic recess ascends as it extends from its posterior end to its anterior end.

Evidence of pleural effusion in a lateral costophrenic angle on a PA chest film does not occur until 200 to 500 ml of fluid has collected in the subpulmonic pleural space.

21. The answer is B (1, 3). [*IV D 4 a (1)*] Significant atelectasis of a lung's lobe produces shifts of the fissures that border the lobe and compensatory hyperinflation of one or both of the other lobes of the lung. Marked atelectasis of the left lung's upper lobe produces an anterior shift of the lung's oblique fissure and hyperinflation of the lower lobe. The left hilum becomes elevated as a consequence of the upper lobe's diminished volume; the upper lobe's increased radiopacity may obscure the outline of the aortic knob in a PA chest film. The expanded volume and diminished radiopacity of the lower lobe produces an area of diminished radiopacity in the lower part of the left lung field in a PA chest film. The trachea is deviated toward the left side as a consequence of the average pressure in the left pleural cavity being less than that in the right pleural cavity.

22. The answer is A (1, 2, 3). [*I A 3 c (2); IV A 5*] The impediment to aortic blood flow imposed by congenital aortic coarctation results in a relatively high flow of blood from the internal thoracic arteries to those intercostal arteries which arise posteriorly from the descending thoracic aorta. Since the posterior intercostal arteries of the first and second intercostal spaces arise from the superior intercostal artery (a branch of the costocervical trunk of the subclavian artery), the intercostal arteries of the uppermost two intercostal spaces do not participate in the collateral blood flow, and thus rib notches do not develop in the first and second ribs. The intercostal arteries in the upper intercostal spaces bear a greater abnormally high flow of blood than the intercostal arteries in the lower intercostal spaces, and thus the notches in the higher ribs are more prominent than those in the lower ribs. The notches are most prominent along the posterior body segment of a rib because it is along these segments that the intercostal arteries lie closest to the overlying costal groove. The notches develop along the inferior border of each affected rib.

23. The answer is D (4). [*IV D 2 a, b*] Consolidation is any process in which the air in one or more acini is isovolumetrically replaced with fluid or tissue. The minimum dimension for an area of consolidation is that of an acinus (5 mm). Foci of consolidation initially have irregular shapes and poorly defined borders. Areas of consolidation acquire well-defined borders upon reaching pleural surfaces.

24. The answer is E (all). [*I B 1 a*] The phrenic nerves are commonly derived from spinal nerves C3, C4, and C5. Pathologic processes in the thorax (such as pleurisy or lower lobar pneumonia) which irritate the parietal pleura overlying the central tendon of the diaphragm may elicit referred pain to the point of the shoulder (which receives its cutaneous innervation from C3 and C4). Pathologic processes or traumatic injuries in the abdomen (such as cholecystitis or a ruptured spleen) which irritate the parietal peritoneum underlying the central tendon of the diaphragm can also elicit referred pain to the point of the shoulder. The phrenic nerves provide motor innervation for the diaphragm.

25. The answer is D (4). [*II B 4 a, b (1)*] In a lateral chest film, the anterior wall of the right ventricle outlines the lower half of the anterior border of the cardiac shadow. The posterior walls of the left ventricle and left atrium outline, respectively, the lower and middle thirds of the shadow's posterior border. The shadow of the ascending aorta projects upward from the superior limit of the anterior border of the cardiac shadow.

26. The answer is A (1, 2, 3). [*IE 3 a–c, e*] The SA node is a crescent-shaped cluster of specialized myocardial cells which extends from the superior vena caval opening in the right atrium into the upper end of the crista terminalis. The myocardial cells of the SA node generate the contraction signal which begins electrical activity in the heart during each cardiac cycle. The internodal tracts extend from the SA node through the walls of the right atrium, and terminate in the AV node. There is dispute concerning the specific location of the tracts. The tracts rapidly transmit the contraction signal from the SA node to the AV node. The AV node is an oval-shaped cluster of specialized myocardial cells located in the posteroinferior region of the interatrial septum, close to the orifice of the coronary sinus and the fibrous anulus of the tricuspid valve. At the appropriate moment during the cardiac cycle, the AV node relays the contraction signal to the AV bundle. The Purkinje fibers are dispersed throughout the ventricular musculature.

27. The answer is E (all). [*II B 4 a (3); IV C 1 b (1), 2 a*] The left atrium forms most of the base of the heart. Since its posterior wall defines the middle third of the posterior border of the cardiac shadow in a lateral chest film, left atrial enlargement produces a posterior bulge in this part of the cardiac shadow's posterior border. The left atrium's auricle is the only part of the chamber to directly define a part of the silhouette (specifically, the middle part of the left border) of the cardiovascular shadow in a PA chest film. Enlargement of the left atrium can straighten the left border of the silhouette by filling out the indentation between the outlines of the pulmonary trunk and the left ventricle. Left atrial enlargement can laterally displace the right border of the left atrium and thus increase the radiopacity of the lower part of the shadow's right side. This increase in radiopacity produces a distinct radiopaque border immediately medial to that part of the shadow's right border outlined by the right atrium. The left atrium lies anteroinferior to the tracheal bifurcation. Left atrial enlargement can distend the chamber posterosuperiorly, and thus widen the carinal angle.

28. The answer is C (2, 4). [*IV D 4 b (2) (a)*] Marked atelectasis of the right lung's middle lobe produces a downward rotation about the hilum of the lung's horizontal fissure in both lateral and PA chest films, accompanied by a forward rotation of the lower part of the oblique fissure. The increased radiopacity of the middle lobe commonly obscures the outline of the right atrium in a PA chest film. Tracheal deviation does not generally occur because there is not a significant change in the average pressure of the right pleural cavity following collapse of the comparatively small middle lobe.

29. The answer is B. [*II A 4 h, B 5 c*] Whereas the horizontal fissure of the right lung is generally evident in both PA and lateral chest films, the oblique fissures of the lungs are evident in the lateral chest film only. The pleural surfaces that are apposed across a fissure together cast a water-density line in a chest film if the near-planar pleural surfaces are almost parallel to the path of the x-rays in the x-ray beam. The oblique fissures of the lungs are not evident in the PA chest film because they are oriented obliquely to the path of the x-rays.

30. The answer is A. [*IV D 2 c (2)*] The silhouette sign in chest films may be produced when any mass with a radiographic density of water directly faces the mediastinal viscera or the diaphragmatic domes. Although consolidation of appropriate bronchopulmonary segments commonly produces it, the silhouette sign can also result from other pathologic processes. A retrosternal mediastinal mass can directly face the anterior aspect of the right side of the pericardial sac, and thus obscure the outline of the right atrium in a PA chest film. A retrosternal mediastinal mass cannot, however, directly face the end of the aortic arch, as the end of the aortic arch is located at the boundary between the superior mediastinum and posterior mediastinum. Accordingly, a retrosternal mediastinal mass cannot obscure the aortic knob in a PA chest film.

31. The answer is A. [*IV D 2 c (2)*] A retrocardiac mediastinal mass with a radiographic density of water can produce the silhouette sign in chest films if the mass directly faces a part of the descending thoracic aorta, and thus obscures the outline of the descending thoracic aorta within either the cardiovascular shadow of a PA chest film or the retrocardiac area of a lateral chest film. A retrocardiac mediastinal mass cannot, however, directly face the apex of the heart, and thus cannot obscure its outline in a PA chest film.

32. The answer is D. [*I C 2 c, G 1 b*] When a person standing or seated upright accidentally aspirates a small object into the trachea, the object will most likely pass into the right main stem bronchus because this is more vertical and larger than the left main stem bronchus. When a supine person accidentally aspirates a small object into either lung, the object will most likely lodge in the lower lobe's apical segment, because this segment has the segmental bronchus that arises most directly and posteriorly from the main stem bronchus.

33. The answer is D. [*I C 1 a, b; II A 4 e*] The apex of each lung field projects above the medial third of the clavicle. The apex of the lung and the parietal pleura facing it are thus always in jeopardy when a penetrating wound is suffered above the medial third of the clavicle. If the parietal pleura is penetrated, air may enter the pleural cavity (producing a pneumothorax) or blood may enter the pleural cavity (producing a hemothorax). These considerations explain why a pneumothorax or hemothorax is always a risk when the subclavian vein is accessed along that part of its course which lies above and behind the medial third of the clavicle.

Because of the relatively low surface projection of each lung's oblique fissure to the front of the chest wall, each lung's upper lobe is the lobe which casts the largest surface projection to the front of the chest. Because of the relatively high surface projection of each lung's oblique fissure to the back of the chest wall, each lung's lower lobe is the lobe which casts the largest surface projection to the back of the chest.

34. The answer is B. [*I A 1 a*] The spinous process of the seventh cervical vertebra is the highest palpable spinous process in the vertebral column; the spinous processes of the second through sixth cervical vertebrae are difficult to palpate because of the overlying ligamentum nuchae. The tip of the spinous process of each thoracic vertebra rests at about the level of the body of the vertebra immediately below.

35. The answer is C. [*I G 6; II B 5 a (1)*] The retrosternal area in a lateral chest film shows the superimposed radiodensities of principally the anterior bronchopulmonary segments of both lungs' upper lobes. The relatively prominent thymus in a child may extend inferiorly as far as the anterior mediastinum.

36. The answer is C. [*II B 4 b (3), 5 b (1)*] The retrocardiac area in a lateral chest film superimposes the radiodensities of the basal segments of both lungs' lower lobes upon the radiodensities of the posterior mediastinal viscera. The descending thoracic aorta, the esophagus, and the lower end of the trachea are the most prominent posterior mediastinal viscera in the lateral chest film.

37. The answer is C. [*I G 6; II A 1 c (2), 3 b*] The anterior body segments of the ribs slope downward less markedly in PA chest films of neonates and children than in PA chest films of adults because the ribs lie almost horizontally in a neonate's or young child's chest wall. The marked oblique lie of the ribs in an adult's chest wall is diminished during inspiration; these rib movements significantly contribute to inspiration in adults because the movements account for most of the increases in the anteroposterior and transverse dimensions of the chest wall during inspiration. By contrast, the slight oblique lie of the ribs in a neonate's or young child's chest wall precludes rib movements from significantly contributing to inspiration. A neonate's or young child's breathing is therefore essentially just diaphragmatic breathing.

The thymus is a relatively prominent mediastinal viscus in neonates and young children. Its outline in PA chest films of neonates and young children may define the upper parts of the left and right borders of the cardiovascular shadow. The thymus degenerates by late adolescence, and is not seen in PA chest films of adults.

38. The answer is C. [*IV D 1 b (1)*] A calcified pulmonary nodule smaller than 1 mm, or a water-density nodule smaller than 3 mm, is generally not visible radiographically. Small pulmonary nodules are most easily detected in the radiolucent interspaces of the lung fields. Evaluation of solitary pulmonary nodules is significantly aided if chest films taken during the last 2 years can be compared. A pulmonary nodule which has not increased in size during the last 2 years is not a primary malignancy.

39. The answer is B. [*IV D 3*] Horizontal, nonbranching water-density lines in the base of a lung field (Kerley lines) commonly represent engorged lymphatics or interlobular connective tissue septa thickened by disease; the lines abut perpendicularly against the pleural border of the lung fields. Thickened bronchial walls present as small radiopaque circles when viewed in cross section and as branching pairs of parallel lines when viewed en face.

40. The answer is A. [*I C 1 c (1)*] The lower margin of each lung at midinspiration in quiet breathing lies at the level of the sixth rib anteriorly at the midclavicular line, the eighth rib laterally at the midaxillary line, and the tenth rib posteriorly at the lateral border of the vertebral column. There is a potential recess two rib spaces high in each pleural cavity between the costodiaphragmatic margins of the lung and the pleural cavity at midinspiration in quiet breathing.

4
Abdomen

I. ANATOMY OF THE ABDOMEN, PELVIS, AND PERINEUM

A. Abdominopelvic walls

1. Anterolateral abdominal wall

a. Muscles

(1) The chief muscles of the anterolateral abdominal wall are **external oblique**, **internal oblique**, **transversus abdominis**, and **rectus abdominis.**

(a) Actions. All the muscles can flex the lumbar part of the vertebral column and aid in respiration, micturition, defecation, and parturition; their muscle tone decreases during inspiration and increases during expiration, micturition, defecation, and parturition.

(b) Innervation. External oblique, internal oblique, and transversus abdominis are each innervated by the anterior rami of spinal nerves T7 through T12 and L1. Rectus abdominis is innervated by the anterior rami of T7 through T12.

(2) Rectus sheath. The aponeurotic tendons of external oblique, internal oblique, and transversus abdominis form the rectus sheath on each side. The lateral margin of each sheath is called its **linea semilunaris**. The medial margins of the left and right sheaths are united along a fibrous midline raphe, called the **linea alba**.

(3) Inguinal canal

(a) The inguinal canal is the passageway in the anterolateral abdominal wall via which the spermatic cord in the male and the round ligament of the uterus in the female traverse the abdominal wall.

(i) The lower free borders of internal oblique and transversus abdominis form the canal's roof.

(ii) External oblique's aponeurosis forms most of the canal's anterior wall.

(iii) The inguinal ligament forms the canal's floor.

(iv) Transversalis fascia forms most of the canal's posterior wall.

(b) The canal begins deeply at the deep inguinal ring, and ends superficially at the superficial inguinal ring.

b. Neurovascular elements

(1) The anterior rami of spinal nerves T7 through T12 and L1 provide the **sensory supply** of the anterolateral abdominal wall's skin and peritoneal lining.

(a) T7 innervates the skin over the xiphoid process.

(b) T10 innervates the skin around the umbilicus.

(c) L1 innervates the skin immediately above the pubic crests.

(2) The chief **arteries** of the anterolateral abdominal wall are the lumbar branches of the abdominal aorta and the superior and inferior epigastric arteries.

(3) The **paraumbilical region** is a region of **portal–systemic anastomoses** between tributaries of the **lumbar veins** and tributaries of the **paraumbilical veins**. The lumbar and paraumbilical veins are, respectively, tributaries of the inferior vena cava and the portal vein.

2. Scrotum. The scrotum in the male (and the **labia majora** in the female) forms as an outpouching of the anterolateral abdominal wall.

a. A sac of five **tissue layers** envelops the contents of the scrotum on each side. Proceeding from the most superficial to the deepest, these layers are the

(1) Skin

(2) Superficial fascia with its dartos muscle

(3) External spermatic fascia (which is derived from the external oblique muscle)

(4) Cremasteric fascia (which is derived from the internal oblique muscle). The **cremaster muscle** in the cremasteric fascia is innervated by the genital branch of the genitofemoral nerve; the cremaster muscle can elevate the testis in the scrotum, and thus aids in regulating the temperature of the testis by controlling the proximity of the testis to the trunk of the body.
(5) Internal spermatic fascia (which is derived from the transversalis fascia)

b. The **contents of the scrotum** include the testis, epididymis, and vas deferens.

3. Posterior abdominal wall

a. Muscles

(1) **Quadratus lumborum** aids in inspiration and can laterally flex the lumbar part of the vertebral column. It is innervated by T12 and L1 through L3 (or L4).
(2) **Psoas major and iliacus** act together as the most powerful flexor of the thigh at the hip joint. Psoas major is innervated by L1 through L4; iliacus is innervated by the femoral nerve.

b. Lumbar plexus. The lumbar plexus arises from the anterior rami of L1, L2, L3, and part of L4. The major **branches** of the lumbar plexus and their **segmental derivation** are as follows:

(1) Iliohypogastric nerve (L1)
(2) Ilioinguinal nerve (L1)
(3) Genitofemoral nerve (L1 and L2)
(4) Lateral cutaneous nerve of the thigh (L2 and L3)
(5) Femoral nerve (L2, L3, and L4)
(6) Obturator nerve (L2, L3, and L4)

4. Pelvic walls

a. Skeletal framework. The skeletal framework of the pelvic basin is the **bony pelvis.**

(1) The **superior opening** of the pelvis is called the **pelvic inlet**. The border of the pelvic inlet is called the **pelvic brim** (pelvic rim), and it is formed
   (a) Anteriorly by the **pubic crests** of the innominate bones
   (b) Laterally by the **iliopectineal lines** of the innominate bones
   (c) Posteriorly by the **sacral promontory** (i.e., the anterosuperior edge of the body of the first sacral vertebra)
(2) The **inferior opening** of the pelvis is called the **pelvic outlet**, and it is bordered
   (a) Anteriorly by the **pubic arch**
   (b) Laterally by the **ischial tuberosities**
   (c) Posteriorly by the **sacrotuberous ligaments** and the **coccyx**

b. Muscles

(1) **Levator ani.** The paired levator ani muscles form most of the floor of the pelvis; their muscle tone increases during forced expiration. Levator ani is innervated by fibers which arise from the pudendal nerve and from S4.
(2) **Coccygeus.** The paired coccygeus muscles form the most posterior part of the pelvic floor. Coccygeus is innervated by fibers which arise from S4 and S5.
(3) **Obturator internus** lines the lateral pelvic wall. It is innervated by the nerve to obturator internus.
(4) **Piriformis** lines the posterior pelvic wall. It is innervated by fibers derived from S1 and S2.

c. Sacral plexus. The sacral plexus arises from the lumbosacral trunk (which is derived from the anterior rami of L4 and L5), the anterior rami of S1, S2, and S3, and part of the anterior ramus of S4. The major **branches** of the sacral plexus and their **segmental derivation** are as follows:

(1) Superior gluteal nerve (L4, L5, and S1)
(2) Inferior gluteal nerve (L5, S1, and S2)
(3) Nerve to quadratus femoris (L4, L5, and S1)
(4) Nerve to obturator internus (L5, S1, and S2)
(5) Posterior cutaneous nerve of the thigh (S1, S2, and S3)
(6) Sciatic nerve (L4, L5, S1, S2, and S3)
(7) Pudendal nerve (S2, S3, and S4)

B. Divisions of the abdominopelvic cavity

1. Quadrants of the abdominopelvic cavity. The intersection of the median sagittal plane with the horizontal plane which passes through the umbilicus divides the cavity into its four quadrants:

a. Right upper quadrant
b. Left upper quadrant
c. Left lower quadrant
d. Right lower quadrant

2. **Regions of the abdominopelvic cavity**
   a. **Boundaries separating the regions**
      (1) The **subcostal plane** is a horizontal plane which passes anteriorly through the lowest points of the costal margins.
      (2) The **transtubercular plane** is a horizontal plane which passes through the iliac tubercles of the innominate bones.
      (3) The **midclavicular planes** are the vertical planes which bisect the clavicles.
   b. The midclavicular planes divide the parts of the abdominopelvic cavity above the subcostal plane, between the subcostal and transtubercular planes, and below the transtubercular plane into three regions each.
      (1) The three **regions above the subcostal plane** are
         (a) The right hypochondriac region
         (b) The epigastric region
         (c) The left hypochondriac region
      (2) The three **regions between the subcostal and transtubercular planes** are
         (a) The right lumbar region
         (b) The paraumbilical region
         (c) The left lumbar region
      (3) The three **regions below the transtubercular plane** are
         (a) The right iliac fossa (right inguinal region)
         (b) The hypogastric region
         (c) The left iliac fossa (left inguinal region)

C. **Anatomic features and relations of the viscera supplied by the celiac artery** (*NOTE:* This section and the following sections are organized by blood supply as an aid in learning this important information. In general, the lymphatic drainage from an abdominal organ flows in directions opposite to that of its blood supply.)

1. **Lower third of the esophagus**
   a. The lower third of the esophagus is supplied by the left gastric artery.
   b. The boundary between the middle and lower thirds of the esophagus is a region of **portal-systemic anastomoses** between tributaries of the **azygos system of veins** and tributaries of the **left gastric vein**. The azygos system of veins and the left gastric vein are, respectively, tributaries of the superior vena cava and the portal vein.

2. **Stomach**
   a. The stomach openings at the esophageal and duodenal junctures are called, respectively, the **cardiac** and **pyloric openings**.
   b. The stomach has a small upper curved border and a large lower curved border which are called, respectively, its **lesser** and **greater curvatures**. The lesser curvature is indented along its lower margin by a sharply defined notch called the **incisura angularis**.
   c. **Parts.** The stomach is descriptively divisible into three parts:
      (1) The **fundus** is the part which lies above the cardiac opening. The fundus generally occupies a posterosuperior location within the left hypochondriac region.
      (2) The **body** is the part that extends from the level of the cardiac opening to the incisura angularis. The body of the stomach is quite mobile and variable in shape. The most anterior part of the stomach, it can extend from the epigastric and left hypochondriac regions above to the hypogastric and left inguinal regions below.
      (3) The **gastric antrum** extends from the incisura angularis to the pyloric opening. The thickened wall musculature at the pyloric opening is called the **pylorus**, or **pyloric sphincter**. The pylorus sometimes lies at the level of the body of the first lumbar vertebra in a supine patient.
   d. **Ligaments.** The stomach is an intraperitoneal organ with two extensive peritoneal ligaments extending from it.
      (1) The **lesser omentum** extends mainly from the porta hepatis of the liver to the lesser curvature of the stomach and the superior border of the proximal half of the first part of the duodenum (the duodenal bulb). The lesser omentum transmits
         (a) The portal vein to the porta hepatis
         (b) The hepatic artery proper to the porta hepatis

(c) The common bile duct toward the duodenum

(2) The **greater omentum** extends from the greater curvature of the stomach and the inferior border of the proximal half of the first part of the duodenum to the root of the transverse mesocolon, the diaphragm, and, laterally, the spleen.

e. The stomach and its omenta divide the peritoneal cavity into its **greater** and **lesser sacs.**

(1) The lesser sac lies behind the lesser omentum and the stomach and between the anterior and posterior folds of the greater omentum.

(2) The **epiploic foramen** is the only **opening** between the lesser and greater sacs of the peritoneal cavity. The epiploic foramen is bordered

(a) Superiorly by the caudate process of the liver's caudate lobe

(b) Anteriorly by the right free edge of the lesser omentum

(c) Inferiorly by the proximal half of the first part of the duodenum

(d) Posteriorly by the inferior vena cava

f. Blood supply

(1) The **short gastric arteries** supply the fundus of the stomach.

(2) The **left gastric artery** supplies the stomach regions bordering the upper part of its lesser curvature.

(3) The **right gastric artery** supplies the stomach regions bordering the lower part of its lesser curvature.

(4) The **left gastroepiploic artery** supplies the stomach regions bordering the upper part of its greater curvature.

(5) The **right gastroepiploic artery** supplies the stomach regions bordering the lower part of its greater curvature.

3. Duodenum

a. As the duodenum extends from the pyloric opening of the stomach to the duodenojejunal flexure, it traces a C-shaped course around the head of the pancreas.

b. Parts. The duodenum is descriptively divisible into four parts:

(1) **First part**

(a) The first part arches over the head of the pancreas.

(b) The common bile duct and gastroduodenal artery pass behind the first part of the duodenum.

(2) **Second part**

(a) The second part descends along the right margin of the head of the pancreas.

(b) The common bile duct and main pancreatic duct unite in the posteromedial wall of the second part and open into the duodenal lumen at the site of the **major duodenal papilla.**

(3) **Third part.** The third part arches under the head of the pancreas.

(4) **Fourth part**

(a) The fourth part ascends along the lower margin of the neck and adjoining body region of the pancreas.

(b) The superior mesenteric artery and vein pass anterior to the border between the third and fourth parts of the duodenum.

c. The duodenum is the most fixed segment of the small intestine, as all of the duodenum is secondarily retroperitoneal except for the proximal half of the first part, which is intraperitoneal. (A **secondarily retroperitoneal organ** is an organ that was initially intraperitoneal during fetal development but became retroperitoneal by the time of birth.)

d. Blood supply. The **superior pancreaticoduodenal artery** is the branch of the celiac arterial tree which supplies the duodenum.

4. Pancreas

a. Parts. The pancreas is descriptively divisible into four parts:

(1) **Head.** The head of the pancreas is partially encircled by the first, second, and third parts of the duodenum.

(2) **Neck**

(a) The neck of the pancreas lies at the level of the body of the first lumbar vertebra.

(b) The **portal vein** is formed behind the neck of the pancreas by the union of the splenic and superior mesenteric veins. Its tributaries drain the gastrointestinal tract from the lower third of the esophagus to the upper half of the anal canal, and the spleen, the pancreas, and the gallbladder.

(c) The **celiac trunk** and **superior mesenteric artery** arise from the abdominal aorta directly above and behind the neck of the pancreas, respectively.

(3) **Body**
  (a) As the **splenic artery** extends from the celiac trunk to the lienorenal ligament, it exhibits a serpentine course immediately above the body and tail of the pancreas.
  (b) As the **splenic vein** extends from the lienorenal ligament to its union with the superior mesenteric vein, it follows a course immediately posterior to the tail and body of the pancreas. The **inferior mesenteric vein** commonly joins the splenic vein along the latter's course behind the body of the pancreas.

(4) **Tail.** The tail of the pancreas faces the hilum of the spleen.

b. All of the pancreas is secondarily retroperitoneal except for its tail, which lies within the lienorenal ligament.

c. **Blood supply.** The **splenic** and **superior pancreaticoduodenal arteries** are the branches of the celiac arterial tree which supply the pancreas.

5. Spleen

a. The long axis of the spleen parallels the downward course of the posterolateral body segment of the left tenth rib; the spleen lies under the cover of the left ninth, tenth, and eleventh ribs.

b. The spleen's anteroinferior border is firm and notched, and cannot be palpated at or near the left costal margin in an adult if the spleen is not enlarged.

c. **Ligaments.** The spleen is an intraperitoneal organ with two peritoneal ligaments extending from it.
  (1) The **lienorenal ligament** directs the hilum of the spleen to face the anterior surface of the left kidney and the tail of the pancreas.
  (2) The **gastrosplenic ligament** is part of the greater omentum; it directs the hilum of the spleen to face the fundus of the stomach.

d. **Blood supply.** The **splenic artery** supplies the spleen.

6. Liver

a. The anterior intersection of the right fifth rib with the midclavicular plane marks the level of the highest point of the liver in the right hypochondriac region on full expiration.

b. The porta hepatis of the liver's visceral surface lies approximately at the level of the celiac trunk.

c. The anteroinferior border of the liver is generally palpable along the right costal margin on full inspiration.

d. **Ligaments.** Most of the liver's exterior is covered with peritoneum. The margin of the liver's bare area is closely associated with five peritoneal ligaments that extend from the liver to the anterolateral abdominal wall and diaphragm; namely:
  (1) The falciform ligament
  (2) The left and right coronary ligaments
  (3) The left and right triangular ligaments

e. **Lobes.** The falciform ligament's margin of attachment to the liver's anterior surface demarcates the border between the liver's **left and right lobes**. Grooves and fissures on the liver's visceral surface further subdivide the right lobe into its **quadrate and caudate lobes**.

f. **Blood supply.** The hepatic artery proper and portal vein supply the liver.
  (1) The **left hepatic artery** and **left branch of the portal vein** supply the liver's left lobe, quadrate lobe, and all of the caudate lobe except for its caudate process.
  (2) The **right hepatic artery** and **right branch of the portal vein** supply the remainder of the liver.

g. **Hepatic ducts**
  (1) The **left hepatic duct** collects bile from the liver's left lobe, quadrate lobe, and all of the caudate lobe except for its caudate process.
  (2) The **right hepatic duct** collects bile from the remainder of the liver.
  (3) The left and right hepatic ducts unite at the porta hepatis to form the **common hepatic duct.**

7. Gallbladder

a. **Parts.** The expanded blind end of the gallbladder is called its **fundus**, the tapered open end its **neck**, and the intervening region its **body**.

b. The fundus projects below the liver's anteroinferior margin, generally at about the level of the tip of the ninth costal cartilage.

c. The anterior surfaces of the body and neck of the gallbladder generally lie directly against the lower part of the liver's visceral surface, leaving only the fundus and the posteroinferior surfaces of the body and neck covered with peritoneum.

d. **Ducts.** The **cystic duct** extends from the neck of the gallbladder to unite with the common hepatic duct to form the **common bile duct**.

e. **Blood supply.** The **cystic artery** supplies the gallbladder and its cystic duct.

D. Anatomic features and relations of the viscera supplied by the superior mesenteric artery

1. **Duodenum.** The inferior pancreaticoduodenal artery is the branch of the superior mesenteric artery which supplies the duodenum.

2. **Pancreas.** The inferior pancreaticoduodenal artery is the branch of the superior mesenteric artery which supplies the pancreas.

3. **Jejunum and ileum**

   a. The jejunum and ileum are the intraperitoneal, highly coiled segments of the small intestine. The **jejunum** comprises roughly the proximal two-fifths and the **ileum** the distal three-fifths of the **small intestine**, which extends from the duodenojejunal flexure (at the **ligament of Treitz**) to the ileocecal junction.

   b. An extensive peritoneal ligament called the **mesentery of the small intestine** attaches the jejunum and ileum to the posterior abdominal wall along a margin called the **root of the mesentery of the small intestine**.

   c. **Qualitative differences between the jejunum and ileum**

      (1) The walls of the proximal jejunal loops are thicker than the walls of the distal ileal loops because the plicae circulares of the jejunal mucosa are thicker and more numerous than those of the ileal mucosa.

      (2) The vascularity in the jejunal wall is denser than that in the ileal wall.

      (3) The aggregates of lymphoid tissue called **Peyer's patches** are less numerous in the jejunum than in the ileum.

      (4) The number of arterial tiers in the mesentery to the proximal jejunum is less than that in the mesentery to the distal ileum.

      (5) The vasa recta in the mesentery to the proximal jejunum are longer than those in the mesentery to the distal ileum.

      (6) The mesentery to the jejunum bears less fat than the mesentery to the ileum.

   d. **Blood supply.** The jejunum and ileum are supplied by jejunal and ileal branches of the superior mesenteric artery.

4. **Vermiform appendix**

   a. The vermiform appendix forms a blind appendage at the lower end of the cecum.

   b. The vermiform appendix is intraperitoneal, and is suspended from the mesentery of the small intestine via a peritoneal ligament called the **mesoappendix**.

   c. The vermiform appendix is not fixed in position. It most commonly lies either behind the cecum or draped over the pelvic brim.

   d. The **appendicular artery** (which is a branch of the ileocolic artery) supplies the vermiform appendix.

5. **Cecum**

   a. The cecum lies fixed against the posterior abdominal wall in the right inguinal region. Although it is intraperitoneal, it is not suspended from the posterior abdominal wall via a peritoneal ligament.

   b. The **ileocecal valve** guards the opening of the ileum into the cecum; the ileocecal valve is not always competent.

   c. The anterior and posterior **cecal arteries** (which are branches of the ileocolic artery) supply the cecum.

6. **Ascending colon**

   a. The ascending colon is the large bowel segment that ascends from the level of the ileocolic junction to the hepatic (right colic) flexure. It is secondarily retroperitoneal.

   b. The **right colic artery** and ascending branch of the **ileocolic artery** supply the ascending colon.

7. **Transverse colon**

   a. The transverse colon is the large bowel segment that extends from the hepatic flexure to the splenic (left colic) flexure.

   b. The transverse colon is intraperitoneal, and is suspended from the posterior abdominal wall by a peritoneal ligament called the **transverse mesocolon**.

   c. The **middle colic artery** supplies the proximal two-thirds of the transverse colon.

E. Anatomic features and relations of the viscera supplied by the inferior mesenteric artery

1. **Distal third of the transverse colon.** The **left colic artery** supplies the distal third of the transverse colon.

2. **Descending colon**
   a. The descending colon is the large bowel segment that descends from the splenic flexure to the left inguinal region. It is secondarily retroperitoneal.
   b. The **left colic artery** supplies the descending colon.

3. **Sigmoid colon**
   a. The sigmoid colon extends from the descending colon to the rectum. It is intraperitoneal, and lies suspended from the posterior abdominal and pelvic walls by a fan-shaped peritoneal ligament called the **sigmoid mesocolon**.
   b. The **sigmoid branches** of the inferior mesenteric artery supply the sigmoid colon.

4. **Rectum and anal canal**
   a. The rectum and anal canal are the terminal segments of the digestive tract; the rectum lies in the pelvic cavity, and the anal canal traverses the perineum.
   b. The **superior rectal artery** (which is the terminal continuation of the inferior mesenteric artery) supplies the rectum and the upper half of the anal canal; it is almost the sole arterial supply of the mucosal lining of these digestive tract segments.

F. Anatomic features and relations of the viscera supplied by direct branches of the abdominal aorta or the renal arteries

1. **Adrenal glands**
   a. The retroperitoneal adrenal gland on each side lies atop the superior pole of the kidney.
   b. A branch of the inferior phrenic artery (the **superior adrenal artery**), a branch of the abdominal aorta (the **middle adrenal artery**), and a branch of the renal artery (the **inferior adrenal artery**) supply each gland.
   c. The left adrenal vein drains into the left renal vein, and the right adrenal vein drains into the inferior vena cava.

2. **Kidneys and ureters**
   a. The retroperitoneal **kidneys** are nestled within the paravertebral gutters in the upper quadrants.
      (1) Each kidney lies anterior to the costovertebral angle near the midline of the back; its superior pole extends above the posterior body segment of the twelfth rib. The right kidney lies slightly lower than its left counterpart.
      (2) Whereas the right kidney is in direct contact anteriorly with the duodenum and hepatic flexure, the left kidney is in direct contact anteriorly with the pancreas and splenic flexure.
   b. The retroperitoneal **ureters** emerge from the hila of the kidneys, descend in front of the psoas major muscles, cross the pelvic brim anterior to the bifurcations of the common iliac arteries, and finally travel alongside the lateral pelvic walls before piercing the upper lateral corners of the posterior surface of the urinary bladder.
   c. **Blood supply**
      (1) The renal arteries supply the kidneys.
      (2) Branches of the renal arteries and the abdominal aorta supply the ureters.

3. **Uterus, uterine tubes, and ovaries**
   a. The **uterus** is a hollow, pear-shaped organ which is descriptively divided into a cervix and a body.
      (1) The **cervix** protrudes through the uppermost anterior wall of the vagina; the cervix thus has an upper, supravaginal part and a lower, intravaginal part.
      (2) The **body** comprises the upper two-thirds of the viscus.
         (a) The **fundus** of the uterus is that region which lies above the points where the uterine tubes enter into the uterus.
         (b) The **round ligament of the uterus** extends from the body of the uterus on each side to gain entrance into the inguinal canal via the deep inguinal ring.
   b. When the bladder is empty, it is common for the uterus to be both anteverted and anteflexed.
   c. Each **uterine tube** is divided for descriptive purposes into four segments:
      (1) The **uterine**, or **intramural**, **segment** traverses the wall of the uterus.

(2) The next most lateral part is the narrowest segment, and thus is called the **isthmus**.

(3) The isthmus is continuous laterally with the widest and longest segment, the **ampulla**.

(4) The most lateral segment is funnel-shaped, and thus is called the **infundibulum**.

d. Each **ovary** lies suspended from the broad ligament of the uterus and embraced by the **fimbriae** (i.e., the finger-like processes) at the end of the uterine tube.

e. Blood supply and venous drainage

(1) The **ovarian artery** on each side supplies the ovary, uterine tube, and fundus of the uterus.

(2) Whereas the **left ovarian vein** drains into the left renal vein, the **right ovarian vein** drains into the inferior vena cava.

4. Testis

a. The **testicular artery** supplies the testis and epididymis.

b. The **testicular vein** on each side arises from the pampiniform plexus of veins in the spermatic cord. Whereas the left testicular vein drains into the left renal vein, the right testicular vein drains into the inferior vena cava.

G. Anatomic features and relations of the viscera supplied by the internal iliac artery

1. Rectum and anal canal

a. The paired **middle rectal arteries** supply mainly the muscularis externa layers of the rectum and anal canal. The paired **inferior rectal arteries** supply the lower half of the anal canal.

b. The border between the upper and lower halves of the anal canal is a region of **portal–systemic anastomoses** between tributaries of the **superior rectal vein** and tributaries of the paired **inferior rectal veins**. The superior rectal vein and the inferior rectal veins are, respectively, tributaries of the portal vein and the inferior vena cava.

2. Bladder

a. The inferolateral surfaces of the bladder rest upon the floor of the pelvis. In an adult, the superior surface is the only surface covered with peritoneum. In a male, the **prostate** surrounds the neck of the bladder.

b. In both sexes, the **superior vesical artery** supplies the upper part of the bladder. In the male, the **inferior vesical artery** supplies the lower part of the bladder, the prostate, and the seminal vesicles. In the female, the **vaginal artery** provides the major arterial supply to the lower part of the bladder.

3. Uterus. The **uterine artery** supplies the cervix of the uterus and that part of the body of the uterus below the entry sites of the uterine tubes.

4. Erectile tissues of the external genitalia

a. In both sexes, the erectile tissues of the external genitalia reside in the superficial perineal space of the perineum.

b. In both sexes, the **internal pudendal artery** supplies the erectile tissues of the external genitalia.

II. ABDOMINAL RADIOGRAPH

A. General features

1. The abdominal radiograph, or **abdominal plain film**, is a composite of the images cast by the lower thoracic vertebrae, lower ribs, lumbar vertebrae, sacrum, coccyx, upper parts of the innominate bones, soft tissues of the abdominal wall, and major viscera of the abdomen and pelvis (Figure 4-1).

2. The radiograph may be taken with the patient standing upright, lying supine (Figure 4-1C), or lying on the left or right side; such radiographs are named, respectively, **AP erect**, **AP supine**, and **left and right lateral decubitus** abdominal plain films.

B. Bony structures

1. Lower thoracic vertebrae and lower ribs. The radiograph shows the two or three lowest thoracic vertebrae, the entirety of the eleventh and twelfth ribs, and portions of the next one or two higher ribs.

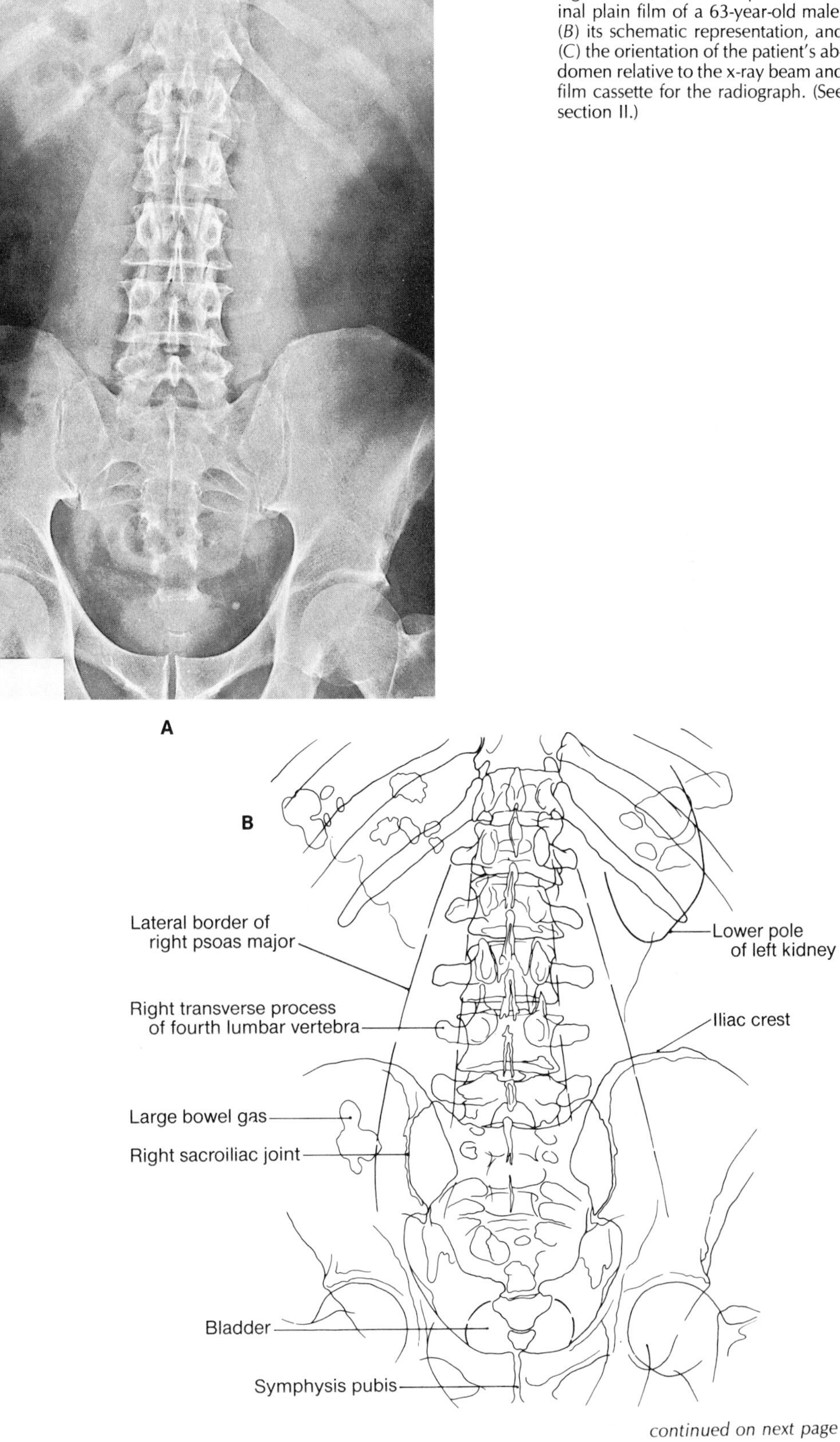

Figure 4-1. (*A*) An AP supine abdominal plain film of a 63-year-old male, (*B*) its schematic representation, and (C) the orientation of the patient's abdomen relative to the x-ray beam and film cassette for the radiograph. (See section II.)

continued on next page

Figure 4-1. *continued*

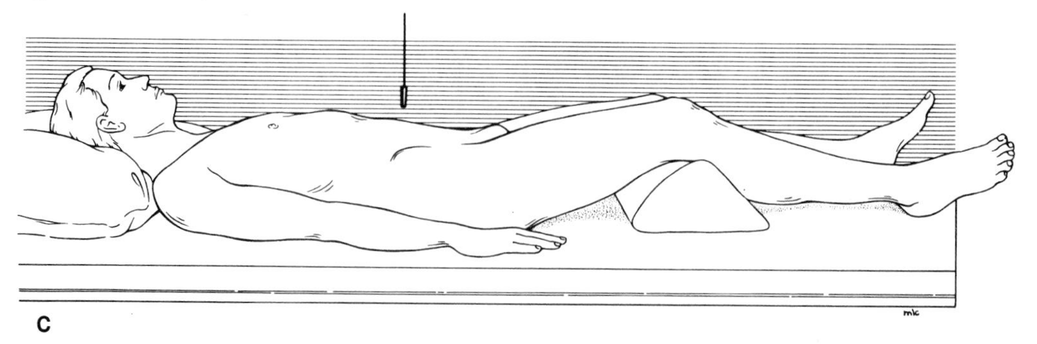

C

2. **Lumbar vertebrae.** The radiograph displays all five lumbar vertebrae (Figure 4-2).
   a. The **body** of each lumbar vertebra casts a rectangular outline whose sides are concave; that is, curved inward toward the midline.
   b. The elliptic outlines superimposed upon the lateral aspects of each vertebral body represent the vertebra's **pedicles.**
   c. The teardrop-shaped outline projecting below the lower border of each vertebral body in the midline represents the vertebra's **spinous process.**
   d. The **transverse processes** of each vertebra extend laterally beyond the sides of the vertebral body.
   e. Superior and inferior projections of the vertebral arch, called the **superior and inferior articular processes,** combine with the laminae to cast a butterfly-shaped outline that extends superiorly above the upper border of the vertebral body and inferiorly below the lower border of the vertebral body.
3. **Sacrum, coccyx, and innominate bones**
   a. The radiograph provides an anteroposterior projection of the sacrum, the coccyx, the upper parts of the innominate bones, and part or all of the femoral heads.
   b. Since the plane of the **pelvic inlet** lies roughly perpendicular to the path of the x-rays that pass through the pelvis, the radiograph projects a reasonably accurate shape of the pelvic inlet.

C. Soft tissues of the abdominal wall

1. **Flank region of the anterolateral abdominal wall.** The flank region of the anterolateral abdominal wall commonly exhibits a trilaminar composition in which the superficial and deep layers have a fat density (that is, the radiographic density of fat) and the intermediate layer has a water density (that is, the radiographic density of water).
   a. The **superficial layer** represents subcutaneous fat; its thickness is variable.
   b. The **intermediate layer** represents the cross-sectional shadow collectively cast by the external oblique, internal oblique, and transversus abdominis muscles in the flank region of the abdominal wall.
   c. The **deep layer,** which is called the **flank stripe,** represents the layer of **properitoneal fat,** the extraperitoneal fat sandwiched between the transversalis fascia and the peritoneum. (The superficial and deep borders of the flank stripe demarcate, respectively, the locations of the transversalis fascia and peritoneum.)
2. **Posterior abdominal wall**
   a. The lumbar vertebrae are flanked on each side by the water-density shadow cast by the **psoas major** muscle.
   b. The lateral border of each psoas major is sharply defined by a fat-density line which represents the cross-sectional appearance of the fat-laden fascial layer that envelops the muscle. It is important to note, however, that the right psoas major is not outlined by a fat line in many normal adults and children.

D. Abdominopelvic viscera

1. **Liver.** The liver casts a large water-density shadow in the right upper quadrant.
   a. The liver's **posteroinferior border** may sometimes be directly outlined by a fat-density

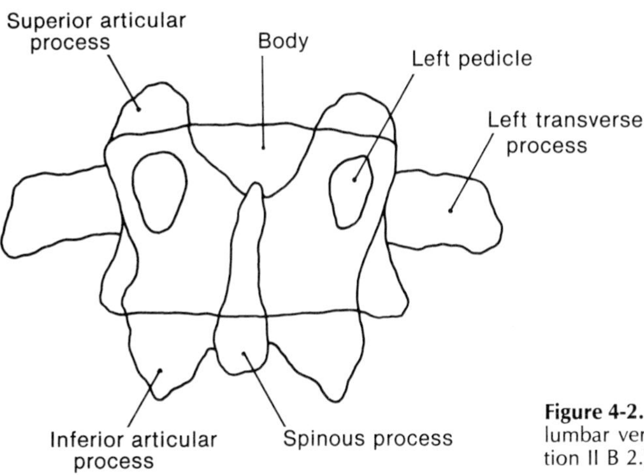

Figure 4-2. A schematic drawing of the appearance of a lumbar vertebra in an abdominal plain film. (See section II B 2.)

line. The fat line represents the extraperitoneal fat layer of the posterior abdominal wall into which the sharp posteroinferior border of the liver is embedded.

b. The **hepatic**, or **right colic**, **flexure** is in contact with the anteroinferior part of the liver's visceral surface. Intraluminal gas in the hepatic flexure may thus indirectly indicate this part of the liver's visceral surface.

2. Kidneys

a. The **lower halves of the kidneys** are commonly outlined by fat. The fat-density line that defines each kidney's margin represents the envelope of perirenal fat that surrounds the kidney.

b. The **hila** of the right and left kidneys closely approximate or overlap, respectively, the tip of the right transverse process of the second lumbar vertebra and the tip of the left transverse process of the first lumbar vertebra.

c. Mental reconstruction of the **upper halves of the kidneys** shows that, with the patient supine,

(1) The right kidney shadow is superimposed upon the twelfth rib

(2) The left kidney shadow is superimposed upon the eleventh and twelfth ribs

3. Spleen

a. The inferior pole and the lower diaphragmatic surface of the spleen are indirectly indicated by the extraperitoneal fat layer in many normal adults.

b. The upper visceral surface of the spleen may be indirectly indicated by gas in the fundus of the stomach.

c. The lower visceral surface of the spleen may be indirectly indicated by gas in the splenic flexure.

4. Stomach. The fundus of the stomach is frequently indicated in AP erect abdominal radiographs by the presence of a gas bubble. In such instances, the fundus of the stomach is observed to underlie the left dome of the diaphragm.

5. Small bowel

a. Individual segments of the small intestine may be identified in an **AP erect film** by either a small gas bubble or an **air–fluid line** (a linear boundary between an air-density area and a water-density area).

b. The amount and distribution of gas and the number and length of air–fluid lines in the small bowel are extremely variable. Most of the gas in the small bowel represents swallowed air.

6. Large bowel

a. Large bowel segments are generally identified easily if filled with gas. This is because the air-density areas representing the intraluminal gas are outlined by the distinctive sacculated, or haustrated, intraluminal border of the water-density shadows cast by the walls of the large bowel.

b. An AP erect film may also show a few air–fluid lines in the large bowel of a normal individual. As with gas in the small bowel, most of the gas in the large bowel represents swallowed air.

7. **Bladder and fundus of the uterus**
   a. The **bladder** in a normal **male** casts an ovoid water-density shadow in the suprapubic region of the radiograph.
   b. The superior border of the **bladder** in a normal **female** is outlined by a fat line and is broadly indented by the **fundus of the uterus** if the uterus is anteverted and anteflexed; the fundus of the uterus may cast an ovoid water-density shadow above the bladder shadow. The fat line between the superior wall of the bladder and the anterior wall of the fundus of the uterus represents the apposed fat layers of the extraperitoneal fat covering these walls.

III. CT SCANS OF THE ABDOMEN.

Some of the abdominal viscera and blood vessels exhibit fairly constant relationships among normal individuals. These relationships can be summarized by reference to the general appearance of CT scans at four broad abdominal levels.

A. CT scans between the levels of the central tendon and the esophageal opening of the diaphragm (Figure 4-3) portray the following structures:

1. **The descending thoracic aorta** and the **azygos vein** in the retrocrural space
   a. **Boundaries of the retrocrural space**
      (1) On each side of the vertebral column, a sinuous stripe extends anteriorly from the costovertebral region to a point directly anterior to or to the side of the descending thoracic aorta. These paired stripes represent the **left and right crura of the diaphragm**.
      (2) The retrocrural space is bounded anterolaterally by the paired crura of the diaphragm and posteriorly by the vertebral column. It represents the most inferior compartment of the inferior mediastinum.
   b. The **descending thoracic aorta** appears in transverse section in the retrocrural space anterior to and to the left of the vertebral column.
   c. The **azygos vein** appears in transverse section in the retrocrural space anterior to and to the right of the vertebral column.
2. **The inferior vena cava.** The vein appears in cross section in the upper abdomen, juxtaposed to the visceral surface of the liver and lying anterior to and to the right of the right crus.
3. **The liver** at the level of the union of the hepatic veins with the inferior vena cava. (The **hepatic veins** are better visualized if the abdominal vasculature bears contrast material.) The liver's image fills the entire right side of the abdominal cavity and anteriorly projects into the left side.
4. **The stomach** at or above its cardiac opening
   a. If the **cardiac opening** is imaged, it lies directly anterior to the descending thoracic aorta, and is continuous to the left with the stomach at the level of the boundary between the fundus and body of the stomach.
   b. The radiographic density of the luminal **contents of the stomach** (and small intestine) can be increased by the oral administration of a barium sulfate suspension before the scans are taken.
5. **The superior half of the spleen.** The organ displays a semilunar-shaped image whose convex diaphragmatic surface lies adjacent to obliquely sectioned posterior rib segments on the left side.
6. **The posterior parts of the costodiaphragmatic margins of the lungs**
   a. The radiolucent space directly posterior to the spleen represents the **costodiaphragmatic margin of the left lung** in the posterior part of the left costodiaphragmatic recess.
   b. The radiolucent space directly posterior to the liver represents the **costodiaphragmatic margin of the right lung** in the posterior part of the right costodiaphragmatic recess.

B. CT scans between the levels of the esophageal opening of the diaphragm and the superior pole of the left kidney (Figure 4-4) portray the following structures:

1. **The aorta and azygos vein** at or near their passage through the aortic opening of the diaphragm. The appearance of and the relationships among the **aorta**, **azygos vein**, **crura of the diaphragm**, and **vertebral column** are identical to those seen between the levels of the central tendon and the esophageal opening of the diaphragm (see section III A 1).

2. **The inferior vena cava.** The vein appears in transverse section immediately to the left of the liver's visceral surface, immediately anterior to the right adrenal gland, and to the right of the anterior end of the right diaphragmatic crus.
3. **The paired adrenal glands.** These cast relatively small triangular or stellate-shaped images lateral to the anterior parts of the diaphragmatic crura. The lower scans image the superior pole of the **left kidney** lying posterolateral to the left adrenal gland.

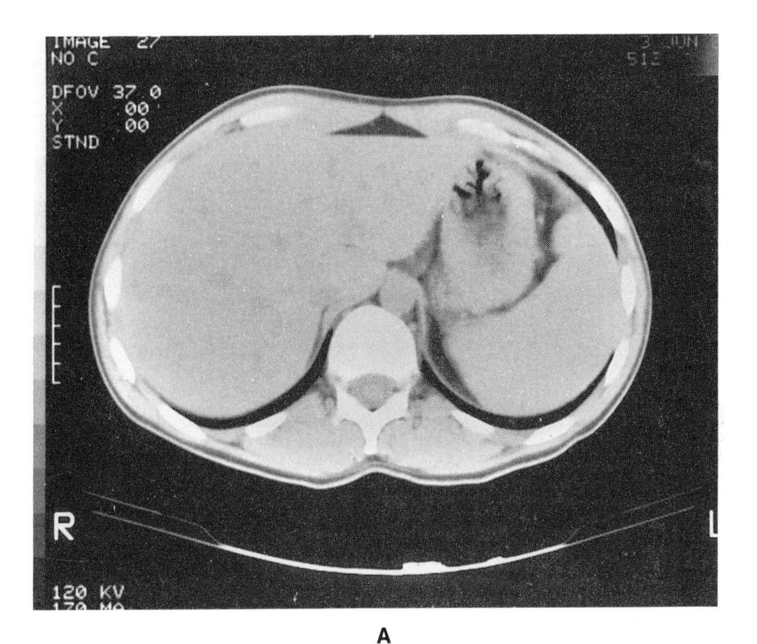

A

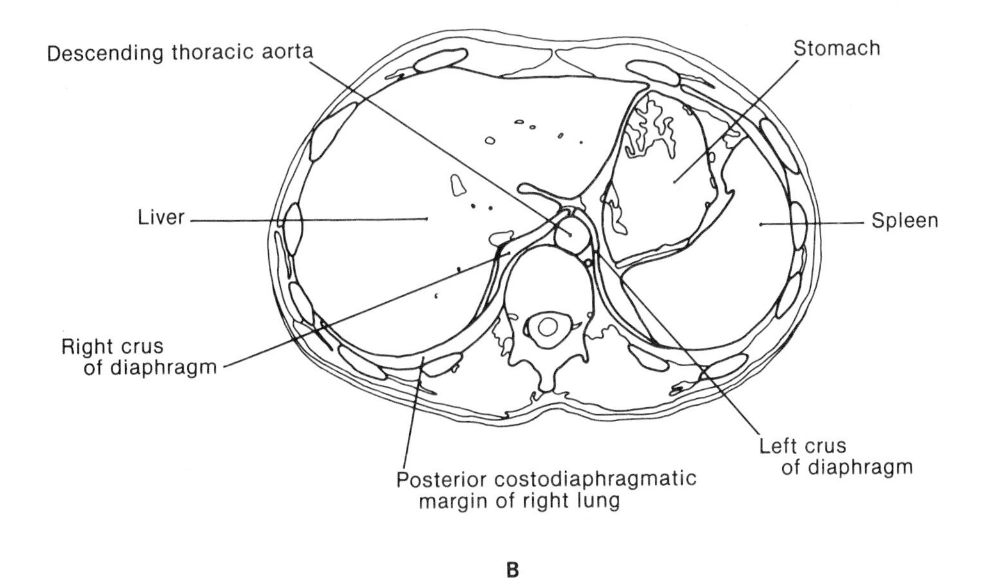

B

Figure 4-3. (*A*) CT scan between the levels of the central tendon and the esophageal opening of the diaphragm and (*B*) its schematic representation. (See section III A.)

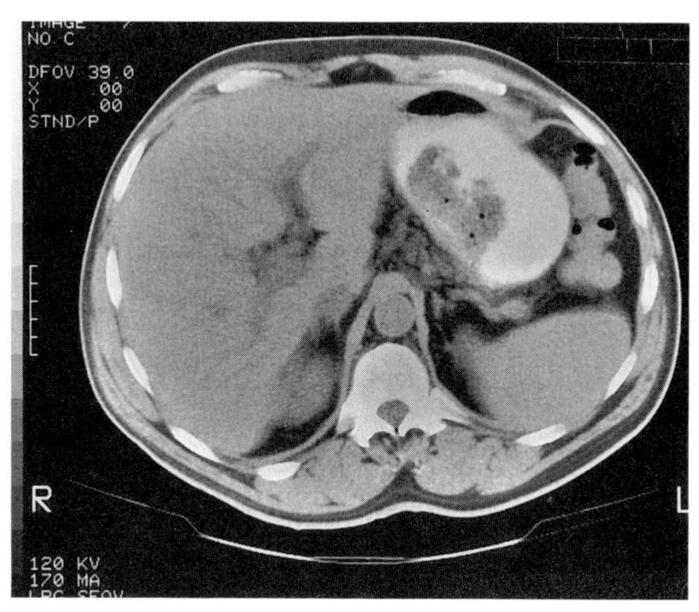

A

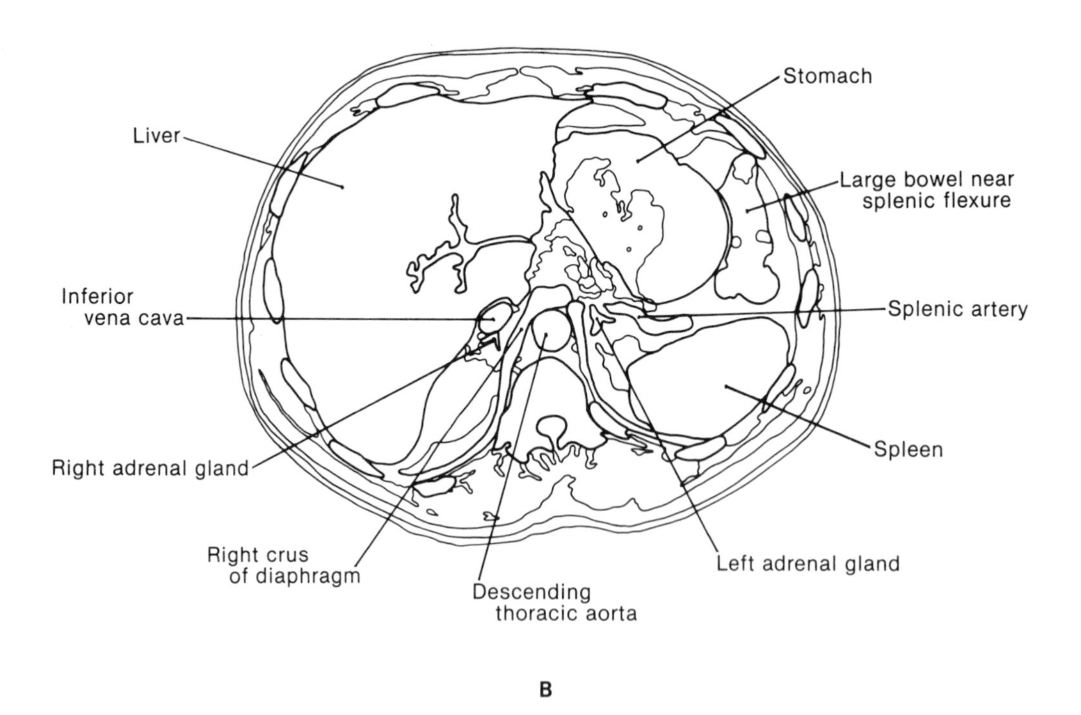

B

Figure 4-4. (*A*) CT scan between the levels of the esophageal opening of the diaphragm and the superior pole of the left kidney and (*B*) its schematic representation. (See section III B.)

4. **The celiac trunk or splenic artery**
   a. If the **celiac trunk** is imaged, it appears as a stout process projecting anteriorly from the abdominal aorta.
   b. If the **splenic artery** is imaged, it appears as a serpentine stripe in the left side of the abdominal cavity extending posterolaterally toward the general direction of the spleen.
5. **The inferior half of the spleen.** The appearance and relationships of the inferior half of the spleen are similar to those seen with the superior half of the spleen (see section III A 5).
6. **The tail of the pancreas**—this may or may not be portrayed. If the tail of the pancreas is imaged, it casts an irregularly shaped and poorly defined image close to the visceral surface of the spleen.
7. **The splenic flexure**, commonly imaged as an irregularly shaped radiolucent space with a fine, incomplete water-density border. It lies closely adjacent to the obliquely sectioned anterior rib body segments on the left side.
8. **The body of the stomach.** This casts an irregularly shaped image medial to the splenic flexure.
9. **The liver** at or near the porta hepatis. The liver's visceral surface may bear a cleft into which the ligamentum teres extends.

C. **CT scans between the levels of the superior and inferior poles of the kidneys** (Figure 4-5) portray the following structures:

1. **The abdominal aorta** at or near one of the following branches: the superior mesenteric artery, the left renal artery, or the right renal artery
2. **The inferior vena cava** at or near its union with the left or right renal vein
3. **The kidneys** lying in the paravertebral gutters. Individual scans may image a kidney's renal pelvis, ureter, renal artery, or renal vein.
4. **The head, neck, and body of the pancreas** and the large vessels posterior to the gland. The head, neck, and body of the pancreas collectively cast a poorly defined oblong image that extends across the breadth of the midregion of the abdominal cavity.
   a. The **splenic vein** may be imaged posterior to the body and neck of the pancreas. The right end of this image commonly represents the union of the splenic vein with the superior mesenteric vein to form the **portal vein**.
   b. The **superior mesenteric artery and vein** may be imaged posterior to the neck of the pancreas. The two vessels appear in transverse section; the larger vessel on the **right** represents the **vein**, and the smaller vessel on the **left** represents the **artery**.
5. One or more of the following segments of the **upper gastrointestinal tract:** the **body of the stomach**, **gastric antrum**, **pylorus**, or **duodenum**
   a. Scans that image the **gastric antrum and pylorus** show these segments lying anterior to the head of the pancreas.
   b. Scans that image the **second part of the duodenum** show this segment lying directly to the right of the head of the pancreas.
   c. Scans that image the **third and fourth parts of the duodenum** show these segments lying posterior to the superior mesenteric artery and vein.
6. The lower part of the **liver's right lobe**. Some scans may image an ovoid-shaped **gallbladder** juxtaposed to the visceral surface of the right lobe.
7. One or more of the following segments of the **large intestine**: the distal part of the **ascending colon**, the **hepatic flexure**, one or more parts of the **transverse colon**, or the proximal part of the **descending colon**. The scans also image segments of the **jejunum** and **ileum**.
8. The following **muscles and related structures**: the rectus abdominis, the linea alba, parts of the rectus sheaths, and the external oblique, internal oblique, and transversus abdominis muscles. The scans also image the psoas major muscles lying directly lateral to the vertebral column.

D. **CT scans at or near the bifurcation of the abdominal aorta into the left and right common iliac arteries** (Figure 4-6) portray the following structures:

1. The **inferior vena cava** at or near its origin from the union of the left and right common iliac veins

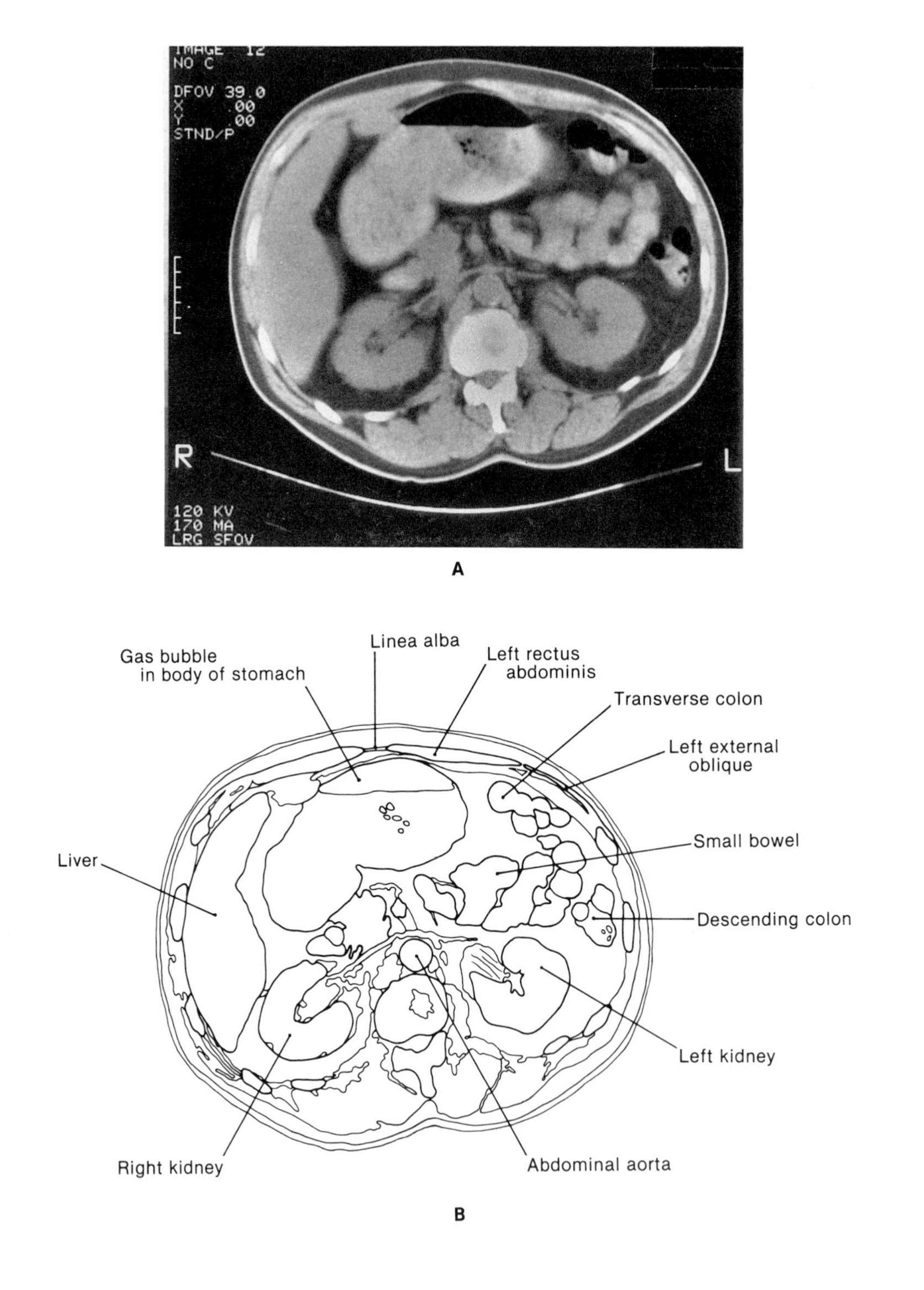

Figure 4-5. (*A*) CT scan between the levels of the superior and inferior poles of the kidneys and (*B*) its schematic representation. (See section III C.)

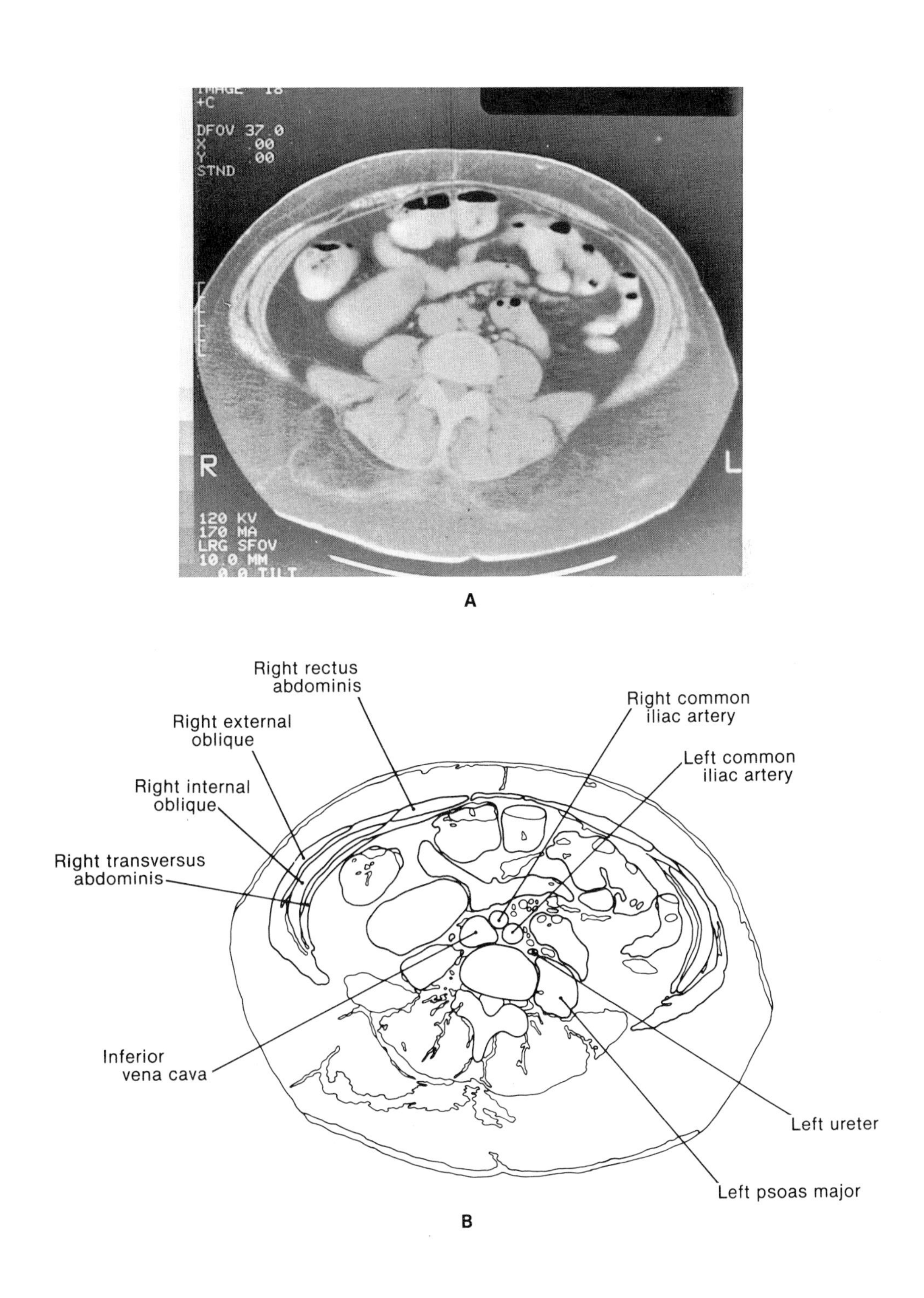

Figure 4-6. (*A*) CT scan below the bifurcation of the abdominal aorta into the left and right common iliac arteries and (*B*) its schematic representation. (See section III D.)

2. The **ureters**, each lying directly against the anterior surface of psoas major
3. One or more of the following segments of the **large intestine:** the **cecum**, proximal part of the **ascending colon**, or distal part of the **descending colon**. The scans also image segments of the **jejunum** and **ileum**.
4. The following **muscles and related structures**: the rectus abdominis, the linea alba, parts of the rectus sheaths, and the external oblique, internal oblique, and transversus abdominis muscles. The scans also image the psoas major muscles lying directly lateral to the vertebral column. A scan may also image the iliacus muscles lying directly anterior to the iliac fossae of the bony pelvis.

IV. COMMON ABNORMAL FINDINGS IN ABDOMINAL PLAIN FILMS. As is the case with chest films, abnormal findings in abdominal plain films are generally not pathognomonic of a specific disease or pathologic process: in most instances, a number of diseases or processes can produce each type of abnormal finding.

A. Loss of definition of fat lines

1. **Pathophysiology**
   a. Abdominal fat layers normally appear as fat lines when the abdominal plain film provides a transverse sectional view of the fat layer and the fat layer is bordered on one or both of its planar surfaces by tissues with a radiographic density of water.
   b. Fat lines suffer a loss of definition when the fat layer becomes edematous and thus acquires a radiographic density of water.
2. **Loss of definition of the flank stripes.** Inflammation of the extraperitoneal fat layer in the flank regions of the anterolateral abdominal wall can partially or completely obliterate the flank stripes.
3. **Loss of definition of the psoas fat line.** Inflammation of the fascial sheath about the psoas major can partially or completely obliterate the psoas fat line.

B. Evidence of bowel distension

1. **General features of large or small bowel distension**
   a. Mechanical obstruction or functional obstruction (cessation of peristaltic activity) along any bowel segment invariably leads to upstream distension of the bowel.
   b. Generally, the bowel upstream from the site of obstruction becomes distended with both gas and fluid.
      (1) The supine abdominal plain film under such conditions generally shows bowel loops distended by gas only.
      (2) The erect and lateral decubitus films show bowel loops bearing a number of air–fluid lines.

2. **General features of small bowel distension**
   a. Distended, gas-filled loops of small bowel are frequently traversed by thin, closely spaced, uninterrupted water-density lines; these lines represent the **submucosal circular folds** of the small intestine (called the **plicae circulares** by anatomists and the **valvulae conniventes** by clinicians).
      (1) The water-density folds are apparent because they are bordered by gas.
      (2) The circular folds are generally narrowed by small bowel distension; however, inflammation and edema of the small bowel may thicken them.
   b. Distended loops of small bowel show the following additional features:
      (1) They are frequently located centrally within the abdominal plain film.
      (2) Their radius of curvature is relatively small.
      (3) They seldom have a diameter greater than 5 cm.
      (4) They rarely contain solid fecal material.
   c. Mechanical obstruction generally produces the first radiographic signs of small bowel distension within several hours if the obstruction is complete.
   d. Localized inflammatory processes frequently produce **paralytic ileus** (i.e., peristaltic paralysis) along one or more of the small bowel segments which come into contact with the inflamed tissues. The one or two loops of distended small bowel generated under such circumstances are called **sentinel loops**, since they mark the site of localized inflammation.

3. General features of large bowel distension

a. Distended, gas-filled loops of large bowel are commonly traversed by thick, incomplete water-density bands spaced widely apart from each other; these bands represent the **crescentic submucosal (haustral) folds** that demarcate the border between adjacent haustra.

b. Distended loops of large bowel show the following additional features:

(1) They are frequently located peripherally within the abdominal plain film.

(2) Their radius of curvature is relatively large (approximating the breadth of the abdominal cavity itself).

(3) They generally have a diameter greater than 5 cm.

(4) They commonly contain solid fecal material.

c. Mechanical obstruction of the large bowel distal to the cecum leads to one of three characteristic **patterns of bowel distension**; the competency of the ileocecal valve determines the pattern that is manifested.

(1) Most commonly, the **ileocecal valve is competent and closed**.

(a) The closed ileocecal valve serves as a site of mechanical obstruction that leads to small bowel distension.

(b) The gas and fluid that accumulate in the large intestine upstream from the site of obstruction can lead to marked distension of the cecum (because the competency of the ileocecal valve prevents retrograde movement of gas and fluid from the cecum to the ileum), and thus place the cecum at risk of perforation.

(2) In the second pattern, the **ileocecal valve is competent and functional**; in other words, the valve permits only downstream movement of gas and fluid.

(a) Large bowl distension occurs from the ileocecal valve to the site of obstruction, but there is no small bowel distension.

(b) As is the case with a competent but closed ileocecal valve, this pattern can lead to marked distension of the cecum and thus place it at risk of perforation.

(3) In the third pattern, the **ileocecal valve is incompetent**. The incompetency of the ileocecal valve provides for progressive distension of both large and small bowel upstream from the site of obstruction, and thus moderates the extent to which the cecum can be distended.

C. Evidence of a pneumoperitoneum. Free gas in the abdominal cavity requires a period of 10 minutes to rise and collect in the most superior part of the cavity. A small pneumoperitoneum may thus not be evident in an abdominal radiograph unless the patient is requested to stand erect or lie horizontally for at least 10 minutes before the radiograph is taken.

1. The left lateral decubitus abdominal plain film and the erect PA chest film provide the most sensitive radiographic indications of a pneumoperitoneum; each radiograph permits detection of even a few milliliters of free abdominal gas.

a. The free gas in a **left lateral decubitus abdominal plain film** is observed between the liver and the right flank of the anterolateral abdominal wall.

b. The free gas in an **erect PA chest film** is observed beneath one or both diaphragmatic domes.

2. A **supine abdominal plain film** provides evidence of a pneumoperitoneum in relatively few cases.

a. The free gas may be observed in the right upper quadrant, outlining the liver. The gas typically collects in the subhepatic space or the hepatorenal recess.

b. The free gas may collect around a bowel segment, and thus outline the exterior of the segment.

c. The gas may collect on both sides of the falciform ligament; in such instances, the ligament appears as a fine vertical line of water density near the midline, outlined on both sides by regions of air density.

D. Evidence of fluid within the abdominal cavity

1. Large amounts of fluid in the **abdominopelvic cavity** cast a water-density haze that pervades the entire cavity.

2. Fluid in the left and right **lateral paracolic gutters** displaces the ascending and descending colon medially from the flank stripes.

E. Evidence of abnormal calcification

1. Only a fraction of all **gallstones** have enough calcium to cast a distinct image in an abdominal radiograph. They frequently show a laminated construction and a faceted surface.
2. **Phleboliths**, or **venous calcifications**, are normally encountered in the pelvic veins of an adult. Phleboliths frequently have a water-density center.
3. Approximately one-half of all **renal and ureteral stones** have enough calcium to cast a distinct image in an abdominal radiograph.
4. **Arterial calcification** occurs most commonly in the abdominal aorta and the iliac arteries. The walls of calcified arteries exhibit a line of calcific density that outlines their luminal border.

F. Lytic or sclerotic lesions of the bones. Such lesions can be produced by metastases from primary tumors, such as those of the bronchi, breast, prostate, kidney, or thyroid, or may represent primary bone tumors.

STUDY QUESTIONS

Directions: Each question below contains five suggested answers. Choose the **one best** response to each question.

1. All of the following structures are normally seen in CT scans that show the abdomen between the levels of the central tendon of the diaphragm and the esophageal opening of the diaphragm EXCEPT

(A) the azygos vein
(B) the fundus of the stomach
(C) the adrenal glands
(D) the crura of the diaphragm
(E) the posterior parts of the lungs' costodiaphragmatic margins

2. All of the following structures are normally seen in CT scans that show the abdomen between the levels of the esophageal opening of the diaphragm and the superior pole of the left kidney EXCEPT

(A) the splenic artery
(B) the body of the stomach
(C) the third and fourth parts of the duodenum
(D) the adrenal glands
(E) the liver at or near the porta hepatis

3. All of the following structures are normally imaged in CT scans that show the abdomen between the levels of the superior and inferior poles of the kidneys EXCEPT

(A) the origin of the superior mesenteric artery
(B) the body of the stomach
(C) the splenic vein
(D) the pylorus
(E) the tail of the pancreas

4. Which of the following parts of the stomach and duodenum has the most anterior lie in the abdominal cavity?

(A) Body of the stomach
(B) Fundus of the stomach
(C) Pylorus
(D) First part of the duodenum
(E) Second part of the duodenum

5. All of the following viscera border the lesser sac of the peritoneal cavity EXCEPT

(A) the spleen
(B) the stomach
(C) the pancreas
(D) the fundus of the gallbladder
(E) the caudate lobe of the liver

6. All of the following are correct statements regarding the qualitative differences between the jejunum and ileum EXCEPT

(A) the walls of the proximal jejunal coils are thicker than the walls of the distal ileal coils
(B) the vascularity in the jejunal wall is less dense than that in the ileal wall
(C) the mesentery to the jejunum bears less fat than the mesentery to the ileum
(D) Peyer's patches are less numerous in the jejunum than in the ileum
(E) the vasa recta in the mesentery to the proximal jejunum are longer than those in the mesentery to the distal ileum

7. All of the following are correct statements regarding the boundaries of the inguinal canal EXCEPT

(A) the inguinal ligament forms the canal's floor
(B) transversus abdominis forms most of the canal's posterior wall
(C) the lower free border of internal oblique forms part of the canal's roof
(D) external oblique's aponeurosis forms most of the canal's anterior wall
(E) the canal extends between the deep and superficial inguinal rings

8. Each of the following arteries is a branch of the celiac arterial tree EXCEPT

(A) the right gastric artery
(B) the left gastroepiploic artery
(C) the inferior pancreaticoduodenal artery
(D) the cystic artery
(E) an esophageal artery to the lower third of the esophagus

9. All of the following are correct statements regarding the segmental composition of nerves derived from the lumbar plexus EXCEPT

(A) the ilioinguinal nerve is derived from L2
(B) the iliohypogastric nerve is derived from L1
(C) the genitofemoral nerve is derived from L1 and L2
(D) the lateral cutaneous nerve of the thigh is derived from L2 and L3
(E) the obturator nerve is derived from L2, L3, and L4

10. All of the following viscera are supplied by a branch derived from the internal iliac artery EXCEPT

(A) the rectum
(B) the testis
(C) the urinary bladder
(D) the cervix of the uterus
(E) the anal canal

Directions: Each question below contains four suggested answers of which **one or more** is correct. Choose the answer

A if **1, 2, and 3** are correct
B if **1 and 3** are correct
C if **2 and 4** are correct
D if **4** is correct
E if **1, 2, 3, and 4** are correct

11. True statements about common general radiographic features of small bowel distension include which of the following?

(1) Supine films generally show small bowel loops distended only by gas
(2) Distended loops of small bowel are frequently located peripherally within the films
(3) Distended, gas-filled loops of small bowel are frequently traversed by thin, uninterrupted lines of water density
(4) Distended loops of small bowel frequently have a diameter greater than 5 cm

12. Secondarily retroperitoneal viscera include which of the following?

(1) Body of the pancreas
(2) Ascending colon
(3) Second part of the duodenum
(4) Descending colon

13. Structures that are transmitted by the lesser omentum either to or from the porta hepatis include which of the following?

(1) Hepatic artery proper
(2) Portal vein
(3) Common bile duct
(4) Inferior vena cava

14. In which of the following abdominopelvic cavity regions can the stomach be partially located?

(1) Left hypochondriac region
(2) Epigastric region
(3) Paraumbilical region
(4) Hypogastric region

15. Correct statements regarding the renal arteries and veins include which of the following?

(1) On each side, a branch of the renal artery supplies the ureter
(2) On the right side, the gonadal vein drains into the right renal vein
(3) On each side, a branch of the renal artery supplies the adrenal gland
(4) On the right side, the adrenal vein drains into the right renal vein

16. Muscles that increase in muscle tone during active, or forced, expiration include

(1) external oblique
(2) rectus abdominis
(3) internal oblique
(4) levator ani

17. Regions that are drained by tributaries of both the portal vein and the inferior or superior vena cava include which of the following?

(1) The border region between the middle and lower thirds of the esophagus
(2) the paraumbilical region of the anterolateral abdominal wall
(3) the border region between the upper and lower halves of the anal canal
(4) the border region between the second and third parts of the duodenum

Directions: Each question below contains four suggested answers. Choose the **one best** response to each question.

18. True statements regarding fat-density lines in an AP abdominal plain film include which of the following?

(A) The fat-density flank stripe of the anterolateral abdominal wall represents the wall's layer of subcutaneous fat
(B) The lateral border of the right psoas major muscle is not outlined by a fat line in many normal adults
(C) Both statements
(D) Neither statement

19. True statements regarding the images of abdominopelvic viscera in an AP abdominal plain film include which of the following?

(A) The liver's anteroinferior border may be directly outlined by fat
(B) The upper halves of the kidneys are superimposed upon the twelfth rib shadows
(C) Both statements
(D) Neither statement

20. True statements regarding the appearance of gas in the small bowel on an AP abdominal plain film include which of the following?

(A) Much of the gas in the small bowel represents swallowed air
(B) Most of the gas in the small bowel is generally located in the ileum
(C) Both statements
(D) Neither statement

21. An ileocecal valve in what state could lead to small bowel distension when the large bowel is obstructed distal to the cecum?

(A) Competent but closed
(B) Incompetent
(C) Either state
(D) Neither state

22. Which of the following radiographs will consistently provide evidence of a small pneumoperitoneum?

(A) An erect PA chest film
(B) An AP supine abdominal plain film
(C) Both kinds
(D) Neither kind

23. The kidneys, ureters, and urinary bladder can be rendered radiopaque by intravenous injection of a radiopaque substance that is excreted by the kidneys; radiographs taken under such conditions are called intravenous urograms. Which of the following statements would be correct regarding normal intravenous urograms in which most of the lengths of the ureters are filled with radiopaque medium?

(A) The uppermost segment of the left ureter overlies the tip of the left transverse process of the first lumbar vertebra
(B) The segments of the ureters between the levels of the third and the fifth lumbar vertebrae overlie the psoas major shadows
(C) Both statements
(D) Neither statement

24. True statements regarding the innervation of the anterolateral abdominal wall include which of the following?

(A) The skin overlying the tip of the xiphoid process is innervated by T5
(B) The skin in the midline immediately above the symphysis pubis is innervated by L2
(C) Both statements
(D) Neither statement

25. True statements regarding the palpation of a normal adult's liver and spleen at full inspiration include which of the following?

(A) It is generally possible to palpate the antero-inferior edge of the liver at or near the right costal margin
(B) It is generally possible to palpate the antero-inferior edge of the spleen at or near the left costal margin.
(C) Both statements
(D) Neither statement

ANSWERS AND EXPLANATIONS

1. The answer is C. [*III A 1 a (1), c, 4, 6; Figure 4-3*] The adrenal glands lie below the level of the esophageal opening of the diaphragm. CT scans between the levels of the central tendon and the esophageal opening of the diaphragm would include views of the cardiac opening of the stomach, the superior half of the spleen, the posterior part of the costodiaphragmatic recess of the pleural cavity on each side, and the upper levels of the retrocrural space. Scans of the retrocrural space show the descending thoracic aorta and azygos vein bounded anterolaterally by the diaphragmatic crura. The scans image the fundus of the stomach because it lies above the level of the cardiac opening of the stomach. The scans show the posterior parts of the lungs' costodiaphragmatic margins because the patient maintains full inspiration as the CT scans are taken (at full inspiration, the costodiaphragmatic margins of the lungs extend inferiorly almost completely into the costodiaphragmatic recesses of the pleural cavities).

2. The answer is C. [*III B 3, 4, 8, 9; Figure 4-4*] The third and fourth parts of the duodenum lie below the level of the superior pole of the left kidney. CT scans between the levels of the esophageal opening of the diaphragm and the superior pole of the left kidney would include views of the adrenal glands, the inferior half of the spleen, the celiac trunk or splenic artery, the splenic flexure, the body of the stomach, the liver at or near the porta hepatis, and the lower levels of the retrocrural space. If the splenic artery is imaged, it appears as a serpentine stripe extending posterolaterally toward the spleen. The body of the stomach has its superior limit at the level of the cardiac opening of the stomach, and it lies medial to the splenic flexure. The triangular or stellate-shaped images of the adrenal glands lie lateral to the anterior parts of the diaphragmatic crura. The liver is imaged at or near the porta hepatis because the porta hepatis lies at the level of the celiac trunk.

3. The answer is E. [*III C 1, 4 a, 5; Figure 4-5*] The tail of the pancreas would not be imaged since it projects toward the hilum of the spleen, whose inferior pole normally lies above the superior poles of the kidneys. CT scans between the levels of the superior and inferior poles of the kidneys would include views of the origin of the superior mesenteric artery from the abdominal aorta; the hila of the kidneys; the head, neck, and body of the pancreas; the body of the stomach; the gastric antrum, pylorus, and duodenum; the lower part of the liver's right lobe; parts of the large intestine from the distal part of the ascending colon to the proximal part of the descending colon; and the upper parts of the muscles of the anterolateral abdominal wall. The scans also image the splenic vein because the vein's middle and terminal parts lie behind the body and the neck of the pancreas, respectively.

4. The answer is A. [*I C 2 c, 3 c*] The body of the stomach extends anteriorly to the deep surface of the anterolateral abdominal wall. At the proximal end of the stomach, the fundus projects posterosuperiorly beneath the left dome of the diaphragm. The pylorus and proximal half of the first part of the duodenum lie near the posterior limit of the abdominal cavity in the midline since the distal half of the first part and the entirety of the remaining parts of the duodenum are retroperitoneal. In radiographic studies, knowing these relationships helps in differentially coating the mucosal lining of the upper gastrointestinal tract with a barium sulfate suspension. For example, an AP supine abdominal radiograph of a patient whose stomach interior is partially filled with a barium sulfate suspension will show the fundus of the stomach and the pylorus partly or completely filled with the radiopaque suspension but most of the body of the stomach only thinly coated with the suspension; the thin coat covering the mucosal lining of the body of the stomach provides evaluation of its topography.

5. The answer is D. [*I C 2 d, e*] The fundus of the gallbladder lies in the greater sac lateral to the epiploic foramen. The spleen and its lienorenal and gastrosplenic ligaments form the upper part of the left border of the lesser sac. The lesser omentum, stomach, and anterior fold of the greater omentum form the anterior wall of the lesser sac. The caudate lobe of the liver projects into the upper right part of the lesser sac. The pancreas lies retroperitoneally embedded against a part of the posterior abdominal wall region that forms the posterior wall of the lesser sac.

6. The answer is B. [*I D 3 c*] The density of blood vessels in the jejunal wall is greater than that in the ileal wall. Since the plicae circulares of the jejunal mucosa are thicker and more numerous than those of the ileal mucosa, the walls of the proximal jejunal coils are thicker than the walls of the distal ileal coils. The fat in the mesentery of the small intestine progressively increases from the duodenojejunal flexure to the ileocolic junction. The aggregates of lymphoid tissue called Peyer's patches are less numerous in the jejunum than in the ileum. The vasa recta in the mesentery to the proximal jejunum are longer than those in the mesentery to the distal ileum since the number of arterial tiers in the mesentery progressively increases from the duodenojejunal flexure to the ileocolic junction.

7. The answer is B. [*I A 1 a (3)*] Transversalis fascia forms most of the posterior wall of the inguinal canal; parts of the aponeuroses of internal oblique and transversus abdominis reinforce the part of the posterior wall that underlies the superficial inguinal ring. The deep and superficial inguinal rings mark, respectively, the lateral and medial ends of the inguinal canal. External oblique's aponeurosis forms most of the anterior wall of the inguinal canal; part of internal oblique strengthens the part of the anterior wall that overlies the deep inguinal ring. The inguinal ligament forms the floor of the inguinal canal, and the lower free borders of internal oblique and transversus abdominis form the roof of the inguinal canal.

The inguinal canal is a common site of herniation. In an indirect inguinal hernia, the contents protrude into the inguinal canal by passing through the deep inguinal ring (which lies lateral to the inferior epigastric artery). The neck of the sac of an indirect inguinal hernia thus always lies lateral to the inferior epigastric artery. In a direct inguinal hernia, the contents protrude into the inguinal canal through a distension of its posterior wall. The neck of the sac of a direct inguinal hernia always lies medial to the inferior epigastric artery and within the inguinal triangle. (The inguinal triangle is the area within the abdominal wall bounded by the inferior epigastric artery laterally, the lateral edge of rectus abdominis medially, and the inguinal ligament inferiorly.)

8. The answer is C. [*I C 1 a, 2 f (3), (4), 7 e; D 1*] The inferior pancreaticoduodenal artery is a direct branch of the superior mesenteric artery. The left gastric, splenic, and common hepatic arteries are direct branches of the celiac trunk. The esophageal arteries to the lower third of the esophagus are branches of the left gastric artery. The splenic artery gives rise to splenic branches, the left gastroepiploic artery, and the short gastric arteries. The common hepatic artery gives rise to the right gastric artery, the gastroduodenal artery, and the hepatic artery proper. The hepatic artery proper bifurcates into the left and right hepatic arteries, and the cystic artery arises from the right hepatic artery. The gastroduodenal artery bifurcates into the right gastroepiploic and superior pancreaticoduodenal arteries.

9. The answer is A. [*I A 3 b*] The iliohypogastric and ilioinguinal nerves are both derived from L1; each provides sensory innervation to the lower part of the anterolateral abdominal wall and motor innervation for external oblique, internal oblique, and transversus abdominis.

The genitofemoral nerve has two major branches: the femoral branch provides sensory innervation to the skin of the upper medial side of the thigh, and the genital branch provides sensory innervation to the skin of the mons pubis and labia majora in a female and to the skin of the scrotum in a male. In a male, the genital branch also innervates the cremaster muscle in the cremasteric fascia of the spermatic cord; the cremaster muscle acts to raise the testis in the scrotum. In a male, the femoral and genital branches of the genitofemoral nerve mediate a spinal cord reflex called the cremaster reflex, in which sudden stimulation of the upper medial surface of the thigh (such as that produced by a quick stroke of a fingernail) elicits a reflexive elevation of the ipsilateral testis.

The lateral cutaneous nerve of the thigh provides sensory innervation to the upper part of the lateral side of the thigh. The obturator nerve provides sensory innervation to the upper medial side of the thigh and motor innervation for the muscles of the medial compartment of the thigh (namely, gracilis, pectineus, adductor longus, adductor brevis, the adductor portion of adductor magnus, and obturator externus).

10. The answer is B. [*I F 4; G 1 a, 2 b, 3*] The testis is supplied by the testicular artery, which is a branch of the abdominal aorta. The cervix and the body of the uterus below the fundus are supplied by the uterine artery, which is a branch of the internal iliac artery. The rectum and anal canal are supplied by the superior rectal artery, which is the direct continuation of the inferior mesenteric artery, and by the middle rectal artery, which is a branch of the internal iliac artery. The anal canal is also supplied by the inferior rectal artery, which is a branch derived from the internal iliac artery. The upper part of the urinary bladder is supplied by the superior vesical artery, which is a branch of the internal iliac artery. The lower part of the urinary bladder is supplied by the inferior vesical artery in the male and the vaginal artery in the female; each of these arteries is a branch of the internal iliac artery.

11. The answer is B (1, 3). [*IV B 1 b (1), 2 a, b (1), (3)*] Although both gas and fluid typically accumulate in the small bowel upstream from a site of obstruction, a supine film generally shows small bowel loops distended by only gas since the film does not provide a cross-sectional view of the air–fluid interface in the loops. The thin, uninterrupted lines of water density represent the stretched plicae circulares. The distended loops are generally centrally located within the abdomen, and only infrequently have a diameter greater than 5 cm.

12. The answer is E (all). [*I C 3 c, 4 b; D 6 a; E 2 a*] All of the pancreas except for its tail is secondarily retroperitoneal. All of the duodenum except for the proximal half of its first part is secondarily retroperitoneal. The ascending colon and descending colon are the secondarily retroperitoneal segments of the large intestine.

13. The answer is A (1, 2, 3). [*I C 2 d (1)*] In the lesser omentum near its free right border, the portal vein and the hepatic artery proper are transmitted to the porta hepatis, and the common bile duct is transmitted from the porta hepatis. The portal vein lies posterior to and between the common bile duct and the hepatic artery proper, with the bile duct lying to the right of the artery. The inferior vena cava forms the posterior border of the epiploic foramen.

14. The answer is E (all). [*I B 2; C 2 c*] The stomach is the most mobile segment of the gastrointestinal tract. Its fundus is generally located in the left hypochondriac region, and its pylorus is generally located in the epigastric region. The body of the stomach can descend into the lower part of the abdominal cavity and even into the pelvic cavity, and thus can be partially located in the paraumbilical and hypogastric regions.

15. The answer is B (1, 3). [*I F 1 b, c, 2 c (2), 3 e (2), 4 b*] The ureters are mainly supplied by branches of the renal artery and abdominal aorta. The adrenal glands are each supplied by three arteries: a superior adrenal artery from the inferior phrenic artery, a middle adrenal artery from the abdominal aorta, and an inferior adrenal artery from the renal artery. On the right side, the adrenal and gonadal veins drain into the inferior vena cava; on the left side, the adrenal and gonadal veins drain into the left renal vein.

16. The answer is E (all). [*I A 1 a (1) (a), 4 b (1)*] During forced expiration, the muscles of the anterolateral abdominal wall and pelvic floor contract to increase pressure within the abdominopelvic cavity, and thus provide an impetus to force the relaxed diaphragm upward. External oblique, internal oblique, transversus abdominis, rectus abdominis, and pyramidalis are the muscles of the anterolateral abdominal wall. Levator ani and coccygeus form the muscular floor of the pelvis.

17. The answer is A (1, 2, 3). [*I A 1 b (3); C 1 b; G 1 b*] The middle third of the esophagus is drained by tributaries of the azygos vein (and thus the superior vena cava); the lower third of the esophagus is drained by tributaries of the left gastric vein, which drains into the portal vein. The paraumbilical region of the anterolateral abdominal wall is drained by the lumbar veins (which drain into the inferior vena cava) and the paraumbilical veins (which drain into the portal vein). The upper half of the anal canal is drained by the superior rectal vein (which drains into the portal vein via the inferior mesenteric and splenic veins), and the lower half of the anal canal is drained by the inferior rectal veins (which drain into the inferior vena cava via the internal pudendal, internal iliac, and common iliac veins). The duodenum is drained exclusively by tributaries of the portal vein.

18. The answer is B. [*II C 1 c, 2 b*] The flank region of the anterolateral abdominal wall casts a tripartite shadow. The superficial layer of fat density represents subcutaneous fat. The intermediate layer of water density represents the shadow collectively cast by the muscles in the flank region of the abdominal wall. The deep layer of fat density is called the flank stripe, and it represents the layer of extraperitoneal fat sandwiched between the transversalis fascia superficially and the peritoneum deeply. The lateral border of the right psoas major is not outlined by a fat line in many normal adults and children.

19. The answer is B. [*II D 1 a, 2 c*] The liver's posteroinferior border may be outlined by a fat-density line; the organ's anteroinferior border may on occasion be indirectly indicated by intraluminal gas in the hepatic flexure. The superior poles of both kidneys overlie the posterior body segments of the twelfth ribs; the left kidney is also superimposed on the eleventh rib.

20. The answer is A. [*II D 5*] Under normal conditions, gas in the small bowel represents both swallowed air and gas generated in the upper gastrointestinal tract. In normal individuals, most of the gas in the small bowel represents swallowed air. The distribution of gas within the small bowel is extremely variable.

21. The answer is C. [*IV B 3 c*] Obstruction of the large bowel distal to the cecum leads to one of three characteristic patterns of bowel distension. In the most common situation, the ileocecal valve is competent but closed, and small bowel distension follows because the closed valve represents a site of mechanical obstruction for the small bowel. Small bowel distension also occurs if the ileocecal valve is incompetent, as the incompetency of the valve permits the progressive retrograde accumulation of gas and fluid in both the large and small bowel upstream from the site of obstruction. Small bowel distension does not occur, however, if the ileocecal valve is competent and functional, since the valve permits downstream but not upstream movement of gas and fluid in the small bowel. A competent ileocecal valve, independently of whether it is functional or closed, does not permit upstream movement of gas and fluid from the cecum into the small intestine, and thus subjects the cecum to marked distension and the attendant risk of perforation.

22. The answer is A. [*IV C 1 2*] The erect PA chest film and left lateral decubitus abdominal film are the radiographs that provide the most sensitive indications of a pneumoperitoneum; each radiograph permits detection of even a few milliliters of free abdominal gas. The patient should be left in position for a minimum period of 10 minutes before either radiograph is taken, in order to permit the free abdominal gas to collect in the most superior part of the abdominopelvic cavity. A supine abdominal plain film may show free abdominal air if it collects in the subhepatic space, the hepatorenal space, around a bowel segment, or on both sides of the falciform ligament.

23. The answer is C. [*I F 2 b; II D 2 b*] The ureters transport urine from the major calyces of the kidneys to the urinary bladder; peristaltic contractions provide the impetus for the transport. Under normal conditions, intravenous urograms will show (during a period following intravenous injection of a radiopaque substance) the ureter almost entirely filled with radiopaque urine. The uppermost segment, or pelvis, of each ureter can be seen to curve inferiorly from the major calyces and narrow into the segment that overlies the psoas major shadows. More inferiorly, each ureter can be seen to cross the pelvic brim near the sacroiliac joint (which is the point on each side where the common iliac artery bifurcates into the external and internal iliac arteries) and empty into the urinary bladder (which is also filled with radiopaque urine).

24. The answer is D. [*I A 1 b (1)*] The anterior rami of spinal nerves T7 through T12 and L1 provide sensory innervation to the skin and peritoneal lining of the anterolateral abdominal wall. The dermatome of T7 includes the skin overlying the xiphoid process, that of T10 includes the skin of the paraumbilical region, and that of L1 includes the skin immediately above the pubic crests and symphysis pubis.

25. The answer is A. [*I C 5 b, 6 c*] Palpation of the abdomen (as the patient maintains deep inspiration) generally finds the anteroinferior border of the liver at or near the right costal margin. In a normal adult at deep inspiration, it is almost never possible to palpate the distinctively notched anteroinferior border of the spleen at or near the left costal margin. Palpation of the anteroinferior splenic border at or near the left costal margin may be normal in an infant, but is almost always indicative of splenomegaly in an adult.

5
Head and Neck

I. CRANIUM

A. Anatomy of the cranium

1. **Calvaria.** The calvaria is the domelike upper portion of the cranium.
   a. **Bones.** The calvaria of an adult consists of the upper parts of four bones:
      (1) The unpaired **frontal bone** anteriorly
      (2) The paired **parietal bones** on the sides
      (3) The unpaired **occipital bone** posteriorly
   b. **Articulations.** Between the bones of the calvaria in an adult are fibrous joints called **sutures**.
      (1) The **sagittal suture** is the midline suture between the paired parietal bones.
      (2) The **coronal suture** is the suture between the frontal bone and the paired parietal bones; the point of union between the coronal and sagittal sutures is called the **bregma**.
      (3) The **lambdoid suture** is the suture between the occipital bone and the paired parietal bones; the point of union between the lambdoid and sagittal sutures is called the **lambda**.
2. **Floor of the cranial cavity (base of the skull)**
   a. **Anterior cranial fossa**
      (1) **Components.** The anterior floor of the cranial cavity is formed by
         (a) The orbital plates of the **frontal bone**
         (b) The cribriform plate and crista galli of the **ethmoid bone**
         (c) The lesser wings and anterior part of the body of the **sphenoid bone**
      (2) **Relationships**
         (a) The anterior cranial fossa lodges the **frontal lobes** of the cerebral hemispheres.
         (b) It overlies the following structures:
            (i) Nasal cavities
            (ii) Frontal sinuses
            (iii) Ethmoid air cells
            (iv) Orbital cavities
      (3) **Openings and transmitted structures.** The perforations in the cribriform plate of the ethmoid bone transmit the afferent fibers of the **olfactory nerves** [first cranial nerve (CN I)] from the nasal cavities to the cranial cavity.
   b. **Middle cranial fossa**
      (1) **Components.** The middle floor of the cranial cavity is formed by
         (a) The greater wings and body of the **sphenoid bone**
         (b) The petrous and squamous parts of the **temporal bones**
      (2) **Relationships**
         (a) The middle cranial fossa lodges the following structures:
            (i) Pituitary gland
            (ii) Temporal lobes of the cerebral hemispheres
         (b) It overlies the following structures:
            (i) Sphenoid sinuses
            (ii) Infratemporal fossa on each side
            (iii) Inner ear on each side
            (iv) Middle ear and associated mastoid air cells on each side

(3) **Openings and transmitted structures**
- (a) The **optic canal** transmits the **optic nerve** (CN II) and **ophthalmic artery** between the cranial and orbital cavities.
- (b) The **superior orbital fissure** transmits the following structures between the cranial and orbital cavities:
  - (i) Oculomotor nerve (CN III)
  - (ii) Trochlear nerve (CN IV)
  - (iii) Ophthalmic division of the trigeminal nerve (CN V)
  - (iv) Abducent nerve (CN VI)
  - (v) Superior ophthalmic vein
- (c) The **foramen rotundum** transmits the **maxillary division** of the trigeminal nerve (CN V) from the cranial cavity to the pterygopalatine fossa.
- (d) The **foramen ovale** transmits the **mandibular division** of the trigeminal nerve (CN V) from the cranial cavity to the infratemporal fossa.
- (e) The **foramen spinosum** transmits the **middle meningeal artery** from the infratemporal fossa to the cranial cavity.

c. **Posterior cranial fossa**

(1) **Components.** The posterior floor of the cranial cavity is formed by
- (a) The petrous part of the **temporal bones**
- (b) The **occipital bone**

(2) **Relationships.** The posterior cranial fossa lodges the following structures:
- (a) Cerebellar hemispheres
- (b) Pons
- (c) Medulla oblongata

(3) **Openings and transmitted structures**
- (a) The **internal acoustic meatus** transmits
  - (i) The **facial nerve** (CN VII) between the cranial cavity and the facial canal
  - (ii) The **vestibulocochlear nerve** (CN VIII) from the inner ear to the cranial cavity
- (b) The **jugular foramen** transmits the **glossopharyngeal nerve** (CN IX), the **vagus nerve** (CN X), and the cranial and spinal parts of the **accessory nerve** (CN XI) from the cranial cavity to the neck; the jugular foramen is also the site at which the **internal jugular vein** begins as a continuation of the sigmoid sinus.
- (c) The **hypoglossal canal** transmits the **hypoglossal nerve** (CN XII) from the cranial cavity to the neck.
- (d) The **foramen magnum** transmits the **medulla oblongata**, the spinal part of the **accessory nerve**, and the **vertebral artery** between the cranial cavity and the cervical region.

3. **Circle of Willis**

a. **Description.** The **internal carotid** and **vertebral arteries** provide the blood supply to the brain. The vertebral arteries join on the ventral surface of the brainstem to form the **basilar artery**, and branches of the basilar artery combine with branches of the **internal carotid arteries** to form an **anastomotic arterial circle** at the base of the brain called the **circle of Willis**.

b. **Components.** The arteries that contribute to the circle are
- (1) The **anterior cerebral arteries**, which are branches of the internal carotid arteries
- (2) An **anterior communicating branch** between the left and right anterior cerebral arteries
- (3) The **posterior communicating branches** between the anterior and posterior cerebral arteries
- (4) The **posterior cerebral arteries**, which are branches of the basilar artery

4. **Dural venous sinuses**

a. **Cavernous sinuses**

(1) **Course.** The cavernous sinuses lie on either side of the hypophyseal fossa.

(2) **Transmitted structures**
- (a) The **interior** of the cavernous sinus is traversed by segments of
  - (i) The internal carotid artery
  - (ii) The abducent nerve
- (b) The **lateral wall** of the cavernous sinus transmits segments of
  - (i) The oculomotor nerve
  - (ii) The ophthalmic division of the trigeminal nerve
  - (iii) The maxillary division of the trigeminal nerve
  - (iv) The trochlear nerve

(3) **Relationships.** The cavernous sinus communicates directly with the following structures:
- (a) Superior ophthalmic vein
- (b) Greater petrosal sinus
- (c) Lesser petrosal sinus

b. Superior and inferior sagittal sinuses

(1) **Course.** The superior and inferior sagittal sinuses extend along the superior and inferior margins, respectively, of the falx cerebri.

(2) **Relationships.** The posterior ends of the superior and inferior sagittal sinuses are connected by the straight sinus.

c. Transverse sinuses. The transverse sinuses extend along the posterior margin of the tentorium cerebelli.

d. Confluence of sinuses (confluens sinuum). The confluence of sinuses is formed by the union of the posterior end of the superior sagittal sinus with the straight sinus, the occipital sinus, and the posterior ends of one or both transverse sinuses.

e. Sigmoid sinuses

(1) **Course.** Each sigmoid sinus exhibits an S-shaped course as it extends from the anterior end of the transverse sinus to the jugular foramen.

(2) **Relationships.** The greater and lesser petrosal sinuses unite with the sigmoid sinus at its superior and inferior ends, respectively.

5. Ventricular system of the brain

a. Components. Four ventricles comprise the cerebroventricular system.

(1) The left and right **lateral ventricles** are inferomedially located in the cerebral hemispheres. Each lateral ventricle consists of a **body** and three **horns**.
- (a) The **anterior horn** extends into the frontal lobe.
- (b) The **posterior horn** extends into the occipital lobe.
- (c) The **temporal horn** extends into the temporal lobe.

(2) The **third ventricle** lies inferior to and between the bodies of the lateral ventricles.

(3) The **fourth ventricle** lies in the midline between the pons and the cerebellum.

b. Intercommunications

(1) The lateral ventricles communicate with the third ventricle via the **interventricular foramen**.

(2) The third ventricle communicates with the fourth ventricle via the **cerebral aqueduct**.

(3) The fourth ventricle communicates inferiorly with the **central canal of the spinal cord**.

c. The **choroid plexuses** that line the margins of the ventricles produce **cerebrospinal fluid (CSF)**.

B. Major features of CT scans of the cranium

1. General considerations

a. The CT scans of the cranium displayed in Figures 5-2 through 5-6 are angled 15° relative to the orbitomeatal plane (Figure 5-1); this angulation is commonly employed because it provides superior visualization of the brainstem and cerebellum.

b. A radiopaque substance was administered intravenously before taking these CT scans in order to increase the radiopacity of the vascular structures of the cranium that lie outside the blood–brain barrier; such structures include the dural venous sinuses, basilar artery, cerebral arteries, and choroid plexus.

2. CT scans which image the cranium above the level of the lateral ventricles (Figure 5-2)

a. The **falx cerebri** appears as a dense sagittal line separating the paired cerebral hemispheres. The thickened anterior and posterior ends of the line represent cross-sectional views of the anterior and posterior parts of the **superior sagittal sinus**.

b. The central **white matter** of the **cerebral hemispheres** is less radiopaque and thus darker than the peripheral **gray matter**. The **sulci** (or **grooves**) and **gyri** (or **folds**) of the cerebral hemispheres are apparent because the **cerebrospinal fluid** (of the subarachnoid space) is also less radiopaque and thus darker than the peripheral gray matter.

c. The bones of the **calvaria** and the soft tissues of the **scalp** form the radiopaque border around the cranial cavity.

3. CT scans which image the cranium at the level of the bodies of the lateral ventricles (Figure 5-3)

a. The CSF-filled interiors of the bodies of the **lateral ventricles** appear as dark curved bands, separated by the **corpus callosum**. The radiopaque posterior margin of each lateral ventricle represents the **choroid plexus**.

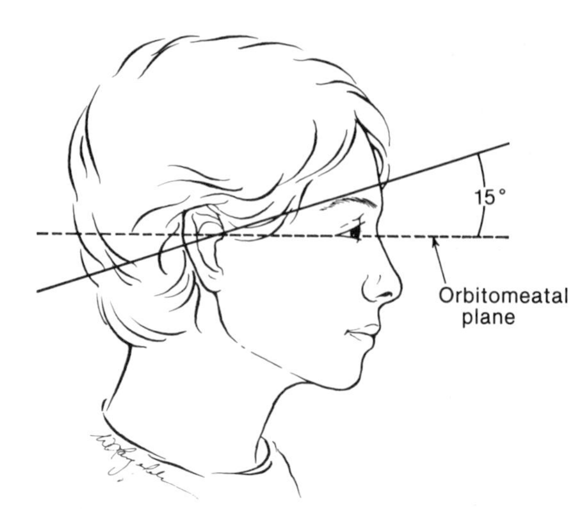

Figure 5-1. The angulation of the cross-sectional views commonly displayed in CT scans of the cranium. The CT scans displayed in Figures 5-2 through 5-6 are all angled as shown. The orbitomeatal plane extends along a line running from the lateral canthi of the orbits to the external auditory canals. (See section I B 1).

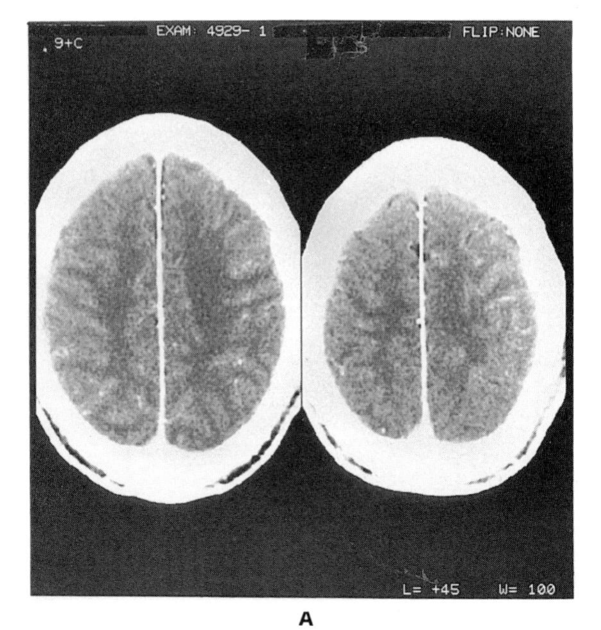

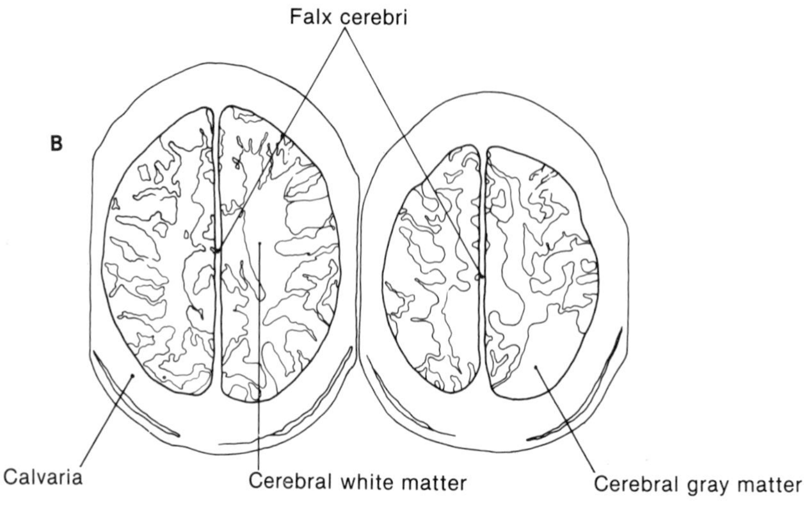

Figure 5-2. (*A*) CT scan which images the cranium above the level of the lateral ventricles and (*B*) its schematic representation. (See section I B 2.)

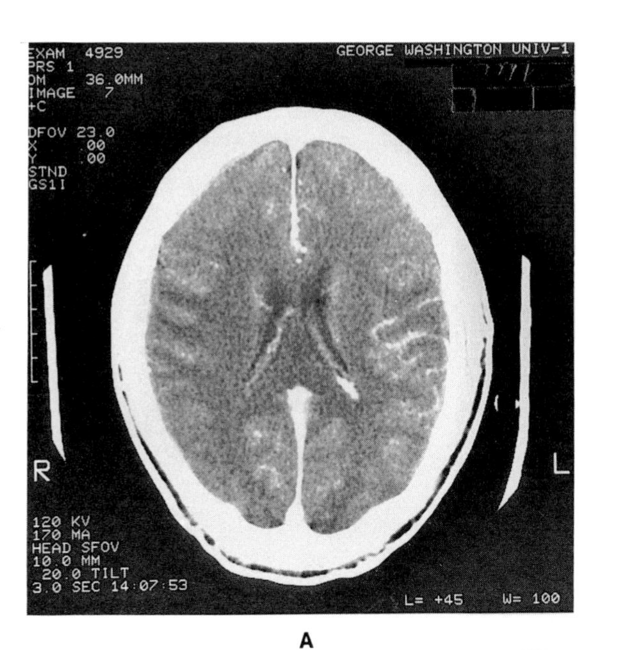

A

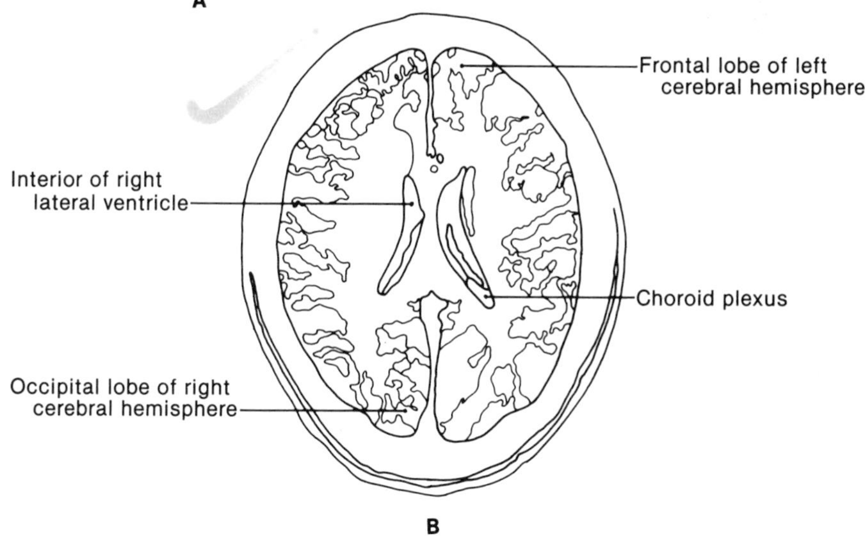

B

Figure 5-3. (*A*) CT scan which images the cranium at the level of the bodies of the lateral ventricles and (*B*) its schematic representation. (See section I B 3.)

b. The anterior and posterior parts of the **falx cerebri** are shown separating, respectively, the **frontal and occipital lobes** of the cerebral hemispheres.

4. **CT scans which image the cranium at the level of the third ventricle** (Figure 5-4)
   a. The CSF-filled interior of the **third ventricle** appears as a centrally located, midline dark band.
   b. The **pineal gland** may appear as a roughly globular radiopaque body directly posterior to the third ventricle.
   c. The **anterior horns of the lateral ventricles** appear as a pair of dark curved bands directly anterior to the third ventricle.

5. **CT scans which image the cranium at the level of the circle of Willis** (Figure 5-5). Scans at this level show one or more of the following arteries that either contribute to or are associated with the circle of Willis:
   a. Anterior cerebral arteries
   b. Middle cerebral arteries
   c. Posterior communicating arteries
   d. Posterior cerebral arteries

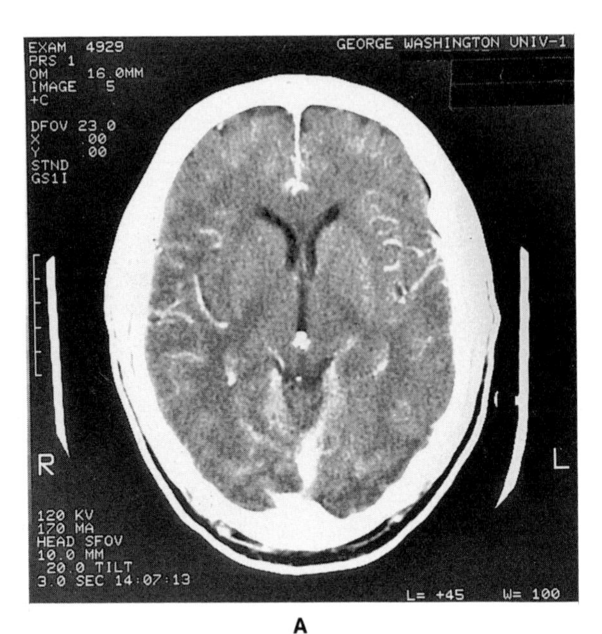

A

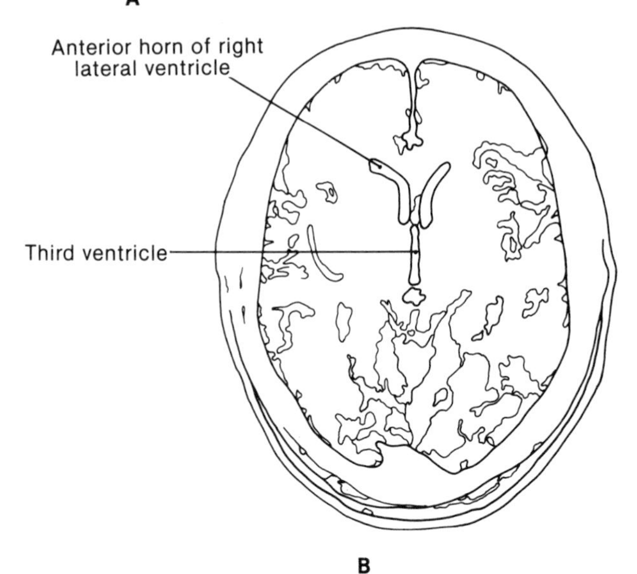

B

Figure 5-4. (*A*) CT scan which images the cranium at the level of the third ventricle and (*B*) its schematic representation. (See section I B 4.)

6. CT scans which image the base of the skull at the level of the anterior floor of the cranial cavity anteriorly and the petrous part of the temporal bone posterolaterally (Figure 5-6). Scans at this level show the following structures:

a. Interior of the frontal sinuses
b. Cribriform plate of the ethmoid bone overlying the nasal cavities
c. Orbital plates of the frontal bone overlying the orbital cavities
d. Interior of the sphenoid sinuses
e. Temporal lobes of the cerebral hemispheres in the middle cranial fossa
f. Interior of the mastoid air cells
g. Cerebellum in the posterior cranial fossa
h. Interior of the fourth ventricle, a dark, inverted U-shape

C. Clinical and radiographic features of cerebrovascular disease and injury

1. Thrombotic and embolic obstructions of a cerebral artery (stroke). Thrombotic or embolic obstruction of a cerebral artery produces infarction in the region supplied by the artery.

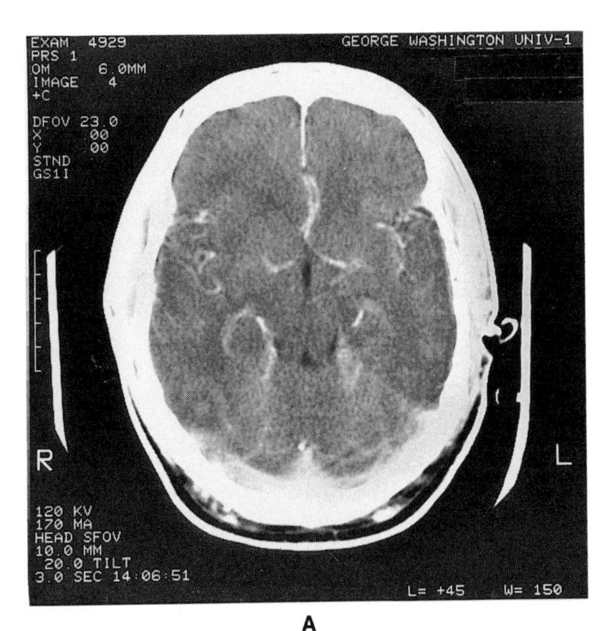

A

Figure 5-5. (*A*) CT scan which images the cranium at the level of the circle of Willis and (*B*) its schematic representation. The arteries that either contribute to or are associated with the circle of Willis are not always sufficiently highlighted with contrast material to permit unambiguous identification. (See section I B 5.)

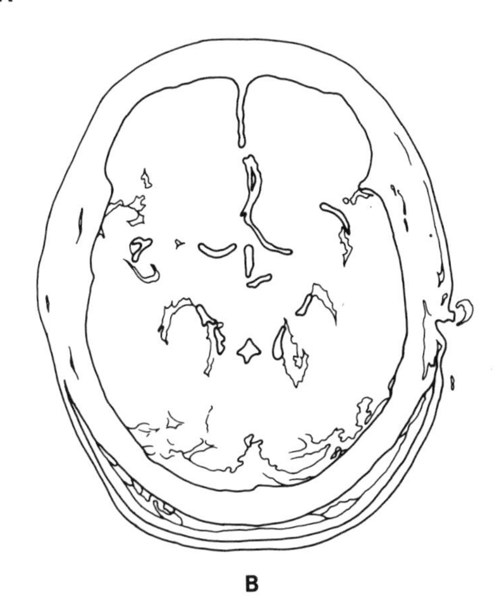

B

a. The ischemic region commonly displays decreased radiopacity within 6 to 24 hours following the vascular accident.

b. If there is no further change in the status of the thrombus or embolus, the radiopacity of the affected region progressively decreases to that of the CSF, which ultimately replaces the infarcted brain tissue.

2. Intracranial hematomas. Intracranial hematomas may be intracerebral, intracerebellar, subdural, or epidural.

a. Features common to all types of intracranial hematomas

(1) A region of an acute intracranial hemorrhage is more radiopaque than the surrounding or adjacent brain tissue. If the hematoma clots and ages without further hemorrhage, the hematoma progressively decreases in radiopacity, ultimately becoming less radiopaque than the adjacent or surrounding brain tissue.

(2) Depending on its size and location, a unilateral intracranial hematoma can laterally displace midline structures to the contralateral side or compress the ipsilateral lateral ventricle.

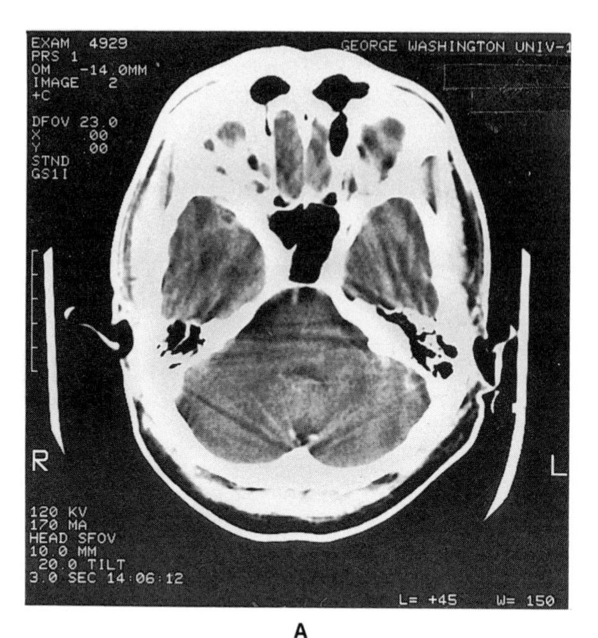

A

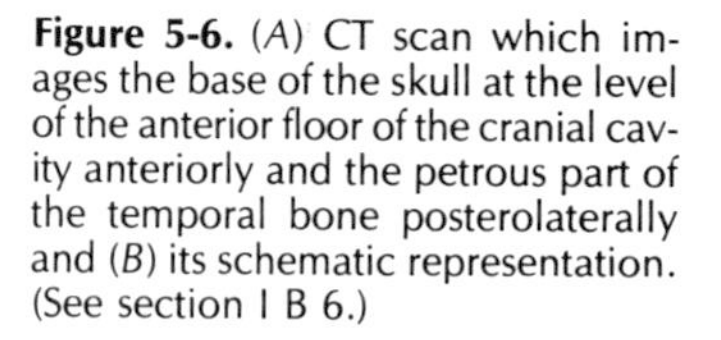
Figure 5-6. (*A*) CT scan which images the base of the skull at the level of the anterior floor of the cranial cavity anteriorly and the petrous part of the temporal bone posterolaterally and (*B*) its schematic representation. (See section I B 6.)

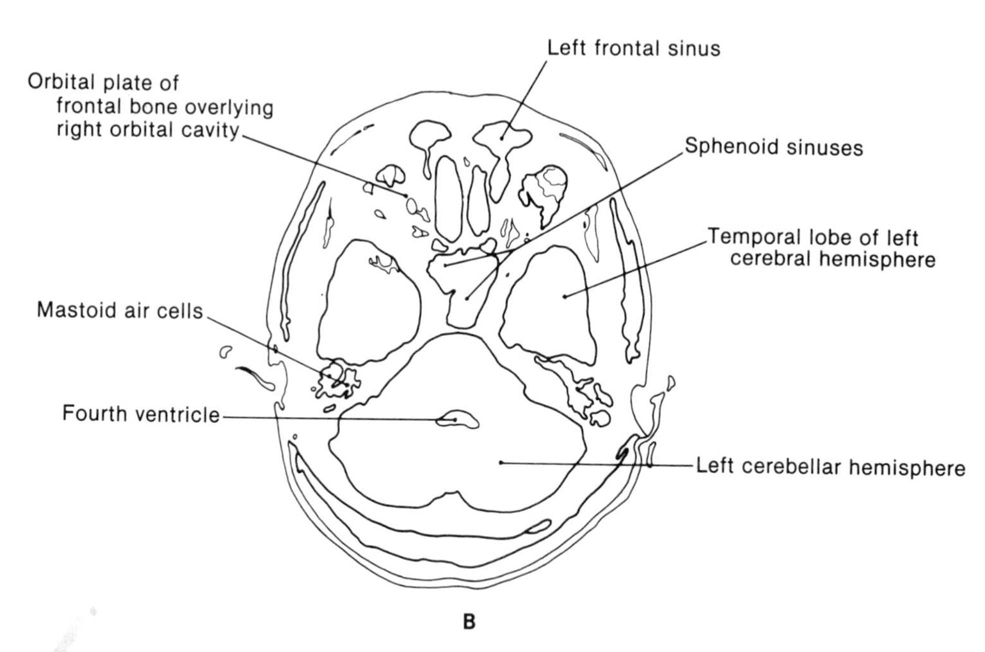

B

b. Subdural hematomas

(1) Hemorrhage into the space between a cerebral or cerebellar surface and the dura mater superficial to the surface produces a subdural hematoma.

(2) Whereas the outer margin of a subdural hematoma is commonly defined radiographically by the smooth, curved outline of the dura mater, the inner margin generally assumes the grooved outline of the adjacent cerebral or cerebellar surface.

(3) Subdural hematomas do not generally cross the falx cerebri.

c. Epidural hematomas

(1) Hemorrhage into the space between the dura mater and the inner bony surface of the cranial cavity produces an epidural hematoma.

(2) Epidural hematomas are commonly lens-shaped. Radiographically, the outer and inner margins of the hematoma are generally both smooth; this is because the outer margin commonly faces the smooth bony inner surface of the skull, and the inner margin faces the smooth depressed surface of the dura mater deep to the hematoma.

II. FACE

A. Anatomy of the face

1. Nasal cavity

a. Skeletal foundation

(1) The cribriform plate of the **ethmoid bone** forms the **roof** of each nasal cavity.

(2) The medial wall, or **nasal septum**, consists of the following:
   (a) The **septal cartilage plate** anteriorly
   (b) The perpendicular plate of the **ethmoid bone** posterosuperiorly
   (c) The **vomer bone** posteroinferiorly

(3) The **lateral wall** bears three **bony shelves** which project medially into the nasal cavity.
   (a) The **superior** and **middle conchae** are parts of the ethmoid bone.
   (b) The **inferior concha** is an individual bone of the skull.

(4) The palatine process of the **maxillary bone** and the horizontal plate of the **palatine bone** form the **floor** of each nasal cavity.

b. Passageways

(1) Three curved passageways in the nasal cavity—the **superior**, **middle**, and **inferior meatuses**—extend beneath the superior, middle, and inferior conchae, respectively.

(2) One curved passageway, the **sphenoethmoidal recess**, passes above the superior concha.

c. Paranasal sinuses (paired right and left)

(1) The **maxillary sinus**, in the maxillary bone, is the largest paranasal sinus. It drains its mucus into the middle meatus.

(2) The **frontal sinus**, in the frontal bone, drains into the middle meatus.

(3) The ethmoid bone houses **anterior**, **middle**, and **posterior ethmoid air cells**. The anterior and middle air cells drain into the middle meatus, and the posterior air cells drain into the superior meatus.

(4) The **sphenoid sinus**, in the sphenoid bone, lies anteroinferior to the hypophyseal fossa. It drains into the sphenoethmoidal recess.

d. Innervation of the nasal cavity

(1) **Sensory**
   (a) **Olfactory nerve**
      (i) The cell bodies of the olfactory nerve reside in the epithelial lining of the sphenoethmoidal recess.
      (ii) Afferent fibers pass through the perforations in the cribriform plate of the ethmoid bone to enter the anterior cranial fossa, and there merge to form the **olfactory bulb**, from which the **olfactory tract** extends posteriorly to the brain.
   (b) **Trigeminal nerve.** Branches of the **ophthalmic** and **maxillary divisions** of the trigeminal nerve provide sensory innervation, respectively, to the epithelial lining of the anterior one-third and posterior two-thirds of the nasal cavity.

(2) **Autonomic**
   (a) The **pterygopalatine ganglion** provides postganglionic parasympathetic secretomotor fibers to the mucosal glands of the nasal cavity.
   (b) The **facial nerve**, via its **greater petrosal nerve**, provides the preganglionic parasympathetic fibers which synapse within the pterygopalatine ganglion.

2. Orbital cavity

a. Skeletal foundation

(1) The orbital plate of the **frontal bone** forms the **roof** of each orbital cavity.

(2) Proceeding from the anterior rim to the posterior limit, the **medial wall** consists of the following:
   (a) Frontal process of the **maxillary bone**
   (b) **Lacrimal bone**
   (c) Orbital plate of the **ethmoid bone**
   (d) Body of the **sphenoid bone**

(3) The **lateral wall** is formed anteriorly by the frontal process of the **zygomatic (malar) bone** and posteriorly by the greater wing of the **sphenoid bone**.

(4) The orbital plate of the **maxillary bone** forms the **floor** of each orbital cavity.

b. Extraocular muscles of the orbital cavity

(1) **Levator palpebrae superioris** elevates the upper eyelid. The muscle is composed of both skeletal and smooth muscle fibers.

(2) Six muscles determine the orientation of the eyeball.

(a) **Superior rectus** moves the eyeball from its primary position to an orientation in which the cornea faces superiorly and medially.
(b) **Medial rectus** moves the eyeball from its primary position to an orientation in which the cornea faces directly medially.
(c) **Inferior rectus** moves the eyeball from the primary position to an orientation in which the cornea faces inferiorly and medially.
(d) **Lateral rectus** moves the eyeball from its primary position to an orientation in which the cornea faces directly laterally.
(e) **Superior oblique** moves the eyeball from its primary position to an orientation in which the cornea faces inferiorly and laterally.
(f) **Inferior oblique** moves the eyeball from its primary position to an orientation in which the cornea faces superiorly and laterally.

c. Intraocular muscles of the orbital cavity
(1) **Ciliaris** lessens the tension in the suspensory ligaments of the lens; this action focuses the lens on objects closer to the eyeball.
(2) **Sphincter pupillae** constricts the pupil.
(3) **Dilator pupillae** dilates the pupil.

d. Lacrimal gland
(1) The lacrimal gland lies in the superolateral aspect of the orbital cavity.
(2) Its watery secretion flows inferomedially across the front of the eyeball and is collected by the **lacrimal canaliculi** at the medial canthus of the eye.
(a) The **lacrimal sac** drains the lacrimal canaliculi and in turn is drained by the nasolacrimal duct.
(b) The **nasolacrimal duct** drains into the inferior meatus of the nasal cavity.

e. Innervation of the eye
(1) **Optic nerve.** The cell bodies of the optic nerve reside in the ganglionic layer of the retina. Their afferent fibers converge at the back of the eyeball to form the optic nerve.
(2) **Oculomotor nerve.** The oculomotor nerve innervates the following muscles:
(a) The skeletal muscle fibers of levator palpebrae superioris
(b) Superior rectus
(c) Medial rectus
(d) Inferior rectus
(e) Inferior oblique
(3) **Trochlear nerve.** The trochlear nerve innervates superior oblique.
(4) **Ophthalmic division of the trigeminal nerve.** The orbital cavity transmits the three branches of the ophthalmic division of the trigeminal nerve: the **nasociliary**, **frontal**, and **lacrimal nerves**. Collectively, these branches provide sensory innervation for
(a) The epithelial lining of the anterior one-third of the nasal cavity
(b) The skin of the uppermost part of the face; specifically, that covering the forehead, the upper eyelids, and the bridge and tip of the nose
(5) **Abducent nerve.** The abducent nerve innervates lateral rectus.
(6) **Autonomic innervation**
(a) The **ciliary ganglion** provides postganglionic parasympathetic fibers to innervate ciliaris and sphincter pupillae; the **oculomotor nerve** provides the preganglionic parasympathetic fibers which synapse within the ciliary ganglion.
(b) The **pterygopalatine ganglion** provides postganglionic parasympathetic secretomotor fibers to the lacrimal gland; the **facial nerve**, via its **greater petrosal nerve**, provides the preganglionic parasympathetic fibers which synapse within the pterygopalatine ganglion.
(c) Postganglionic sympathetic fibers from the **superior cervical ganglion** innervate dilator pupillae and the smooth muscle fibers of levator palpebrae superioris.

3. Ear

a. Divisions
(1) **Outer ear.** The **auricle** collects the sound vibrations in the air that impinge upon a person, and the **external auditory meatus** conducts the vibrations to the tympanic membrane.
(2) **Middle ear.** By convention, the middle ear is described as a cavity, the **tympanic** or **middle ear cavity**, bordered by six **walls**: lateral, anterior, medial, and posterior walls, roof, and floor.
(a) **Lateral wall.** The **tympanic membrane** forms most of the lateral wall of the tympanic cavity. The manubrium of the **malleus** is attached to the tympanic membrane.

(b) **Anterior wall**

(i) The lateral end of the **auditory (eustachian) tube** opens into the anterior wall of the tympanic cavity. The auditory tube, opening medially into the nasopharynx, provides for equilibrium of air pressure across the tympanic membrane.

(ii) **Tensor tympani** originates from the anterior wall. Tensor tympani dampens excessive vibrations of the tympanic membrane.

(c) **Medial wall.** The medial wall has two openings:

(i) The **oval window**, in which lies the base of the **stapes**

(ii) The **round window**, which is covered by the **secondary tympanic membrane**

(d) **Posterior wall**

(i) The **mastoid** antrum opens into the posterior wall of the tympanic cavity.

(ii) **Stapedius** originates from the posterior wall of the tympanic cavity. Stapedius prevents excessive medial displacement of the stapes when tensor tympani contracts to dampen tympanic membrane vibrations.

(e) **Roof.** The roof of the tympanic cavity underlies the temporal lobe of the cerebral hemisphere.

(f) **Floor.** The floor of the tympanic cavity overlies the internal jugular vein.

(g) **Ossicles.** The **malleus, incus**, and **stapes** transmit vibrations of the tympanic membrane to the endolymph of the cochlea.

(3) **Inner ear.** The inner ear is a **bony labyrinth** divisible into three major parts:

(a) The **cochlea** is the snail-shell–shaped, anterior part of the bony labyrinth; it houses the organ of hearing.

(b) The **vestibule** is the central part of the bony labyrinth; the oval window opens into the vestibule.

(c) The three **semicircular canals** form the posterior part of the bony labyrinth; they house the organ of equilibrium.

b. Innervation

(1) **Sensory**

(a) The **vestibular** and **cochlear** portions of the **vestibulocochlear nerve** originate from the sensory organs housed by the semicircular canals and the cochlea, respectively.

(b) Branches of the mandibular division of the **trigeminal nerve** and the **vagus nerve** provide sensory innervation to the skin covering the outer surface of the tympanic membrane; the **tympanic plexus**, which is a plexus largely derived from the **glossopharyngeal nerve**, provides sensory innervation to the mucous membrane covering the inner surface of the tympanic membrane.

(2) **Motor**

(a) Tensor tympani is innervated by a branch of the mandibular division of the **trigeminal nerve**.

(b) Stapedius is innervated by the **facial nerve**.

4. Temporal and infratemporal regions

a. Parotid gland

(1) The parotid gland is the largest salivary gland. It has superficial and deep parts: the **superficial part** lies superficial to the masseter muscle; its **deep part** lies between the ramus of the mandible anteriorly and the external acoustic meatus posteriorly.

(2) The **parotid duct** emerges from the anterior border of the gland, extends anteriorly across the superficial surface of masseter, and finally turns medially to pierce buccinator and open into the vestibule of the oral cavity opposite the upper second molar.

(3) **Structures within the parotid gland**

(a) Most of the **parotid lymph nodes** lie within the parotid gland.

(b) The terminal part of the **facial nerve** extends through the parotid gland.

(i) The facial nerve ramifies into temporal, zygomatic, buccal, mandibular, and cervical branches.

(ii) These branches provide motor innervation to the **muscles of facial expression**.

(c) The **retromandibular vein** forms within the parotid gland from the union of the superficial temporal and maxillary veins.

(d) The **external carotid artery** terminally bifurcates within the parotid gland into the **superficial temporal** and **maxillary arteries**.

b. Mandible and temporomandibular joint (TMJ)

(1) The articular disk of the TMJ divides the joint cavity into superior and inferior cavities.

(a) Raising and lowering of the mandible occur in the **inferior cavity**, via the articulation between the articular disk and the head of the mandible.

(b) Protraction and retraction of the mandible occur in the **superior cavity**, via the articulation of the articular disk with the mandibular fossa and articular tubercle of the zygomatic process of the temporal bone.

(2) **Muscles of mastication**

(a) **Temporalis** can raise and retract the mandible.

(b) **Masseter** can raise the mandible.

(c) **Medial pterygoid** can raise the mandible.

(d) **Lateral pterygoid** can protract and lower the mandible.

c. **Innervation**

(1) **Sensory.** The major sensory branches of the **mandibular division** of the **trigeminal nerve** arise in the infratemporal fossa; these branches are the

(a) Buccal branch

(b) Lingual nerve

(c) Inferior alveolar nerve

(d) Auriculotemporal nerve

(2) **Motor.** The muscles of mastication are innervated by branches of the **mandibular division** of the **trigeminal nerve**.

(3) **Autonomic**

(a) The **otic ganglion** provides postganglionic parasympathetic secretomotor fibers to the parotid gland.

(b) The **glossopharyngeal nerve**, via its **lesser petrosal nerve**, provides the preganglionic parasympathtic fibers which synapse within the otic ganglion.

5. **Oral cavity**

a. **Palate**

(1) **Hard palate.** The anterior part of the palate has a bony foundation, and thus is called the **hard palate**. The palatine process of the **maxillary bone** and the horizontal plate of the **palatine bone** form the bony foundation of the hard palate.

(2) **Soft palate.** The posterior part of the palate has a fibromuscular foundation, and thus is called the **soft palate**. The **muscles** of the soft palate are

(a) **Tensor veli palatini**, which can tense the anterior part of the soft palate

(b) **Levator veli palatini**, which can raise the posterior part of the soft palate

(c) **Musculus uvula**, which raises the uvula and deviates it toward the ipsilateral side

(d) **Palatoglossus**, which extends into the tongue [see section II A 5 b (2) (d)]

(e) **Palatopharyngeus**, which can raise the pharynx

b. **Tongue**

(1) **Intrinsic muscles.** The intrinsic muscles of the tongue are the **four pairs of muscles** (vertical, transverse, superior longitudinal, and inferior longitudinal) which extend only within the tongue; their actions define the shape of the tongue.

(2) **Extrinsic muscles.** The extrinsic muscles of the tongue extend into the tongue from sites above and below the tongue; their actions move the tongue within or out of the oral cavity.

(a) **Genioglossus** extends posterosuperiorly into the tongue from the posterior surface of the mandible near the midline. It is the only extrinsic muscle which can protrude the tongue from the oral cavity; in so doing, each genioglossus also deviates the tip of the tongue toward the contralateral side.

(b) **Hyoglossus** extends anterosuperiorly into the tongue from the hyoid bone. It retracts and lowers the tongue.

(c) **Styloglossus** extends anteroinferiorly into the tongue from the styloid process of the temporal bone. It retracts and raises the tongue.

(d) **Palatoglossus** extends anteroinferiorly into the tongue from the soft palate. It retracts and raises the tongue.

c. **Submandibular and sublingual glands**

(1) The **submandibular gland** is the second largest salivary gland. Its **superficial** and **deep parts** lie, respectively, inferior and superior to the floor of the mouth. The **submandibular duct** opens into the oral cavity beneath the tongue.

(2) The **sublingual gland** is the smallest salivary gland; it lies beneath the tongue. Its secretions are released into the oral cavity via a variable number of small ducts.

d. **Floor of the mouth.** The paired **mylohyoid muscles** form the floor of the oral cavity.

e. **Innervation**

(1) **Sensory**

(a) The **maxillary division** of the **trigeminal nerve** provides sensory innervation to

(i) All of the epithelial lining of the palate except that of the uvula

(ii) The skin of the midregion of the face; specifically, that overlying the lower eyelids, the maxillary bone, the upper dental arch and upper gum, and the upper lip

(b) The **mandibular division** of the **trigeminal nerve** provides sensory innervation to
(i) The anterior two-thirds of the tongue
(ii) The floor of the mouth underlying the anterior two-thirds of the tongue
(iii) The skin of the lowest region of the face; specifically, that overlying the lower dental arch and lower gum, the lower lip, the chin, and the lower margin of the body of the mandible

(c) The **glossopharyngeal nerve** provides sensory innervation to
(i) The uvula
(ii) The posterior one-third of the tongue

(d) **Taste sensation**
(i) The **facial nerve** (via its **chorda tympani branch**) provides taste sensation to the **anterior two-thirds** of the tongue.
(ii) The **glossopharyngeal nerve** provides taste sensation to the **posterior one-third** of the tongue.

(2) **Motor**
(a) The cranial part of the **accessory nerve** (via the **pharyngeal plexus**) innervates all the muscles of the soft palate except tensor veli palatini, which is innervated by the mandibular division of the **trigeminal nerve**.
(b) The **hypoglossal nerve** innervates all the intrinsic tongue muscles and all the extrinsic tongue muscles except palatoglossus, which is innervated by the cranial part of the **accessory nerve**.
(c) Mylohyoid is innervated by the mandibular division of the **trigeminal nerve**.

(3) **Autonomic**
(a) The **submandibular ganglion** provides postganglionic parasympathetic secretomotor fibers to the submandibular and sublingual glands.
(b) The **facial nerve**, via its **chorda tympani branch**, provides the preganglionic parasympathetic fibers which synapse within the submandibular ganglion.

B. Major features of radiographs of the face

1. **Waters' view.** A Waters' radiograph of the face provides an angled frontal projection of the facial skeleton (Figure 5-7).
   a. The radiograph provides a cross-sectional view of the anterior upper part of each **nasal cavity**.
      (1) The **medial border** of the nasal cavity represents the septal cartilage and perpendicular plate of the ethmoid bone.
      (2) The **lateral border** is a bony arch consisting of
         (a) The nasal bone
         (b) The frontal process of the maxillary bone
   b. The **frontal sinuses** are projected superolateral to the bony arches of the nasal cavities.
   c. The poorly defined images of the **conchae** are superimposed upon the spaces of the ethmoid air cells.
   d. Two distinct curved lines mark the floor of each **orbital cavity**.
      (1) The **superior line** represents the palpable lower half of the **orbital rim**.
      (2) The **inferior line** represents the **posterior part** of the **floor of the orbital cavity**; the **discontinuity** in the lateral part of the inferior line marks the **infraorbital groove**.
   e. The radiograph shows the **zygomaticofrontal** and **zygomaticotemporal sutures**, and provides foreshortened views of the frontal and temporal processes of the **zygomatic bone**.
   f. The radiograph provides a relatively unobstructed, angled frontal projection of the **maxillary sinuses**.

2. **Lateral radiograph** (Figure 5-8). The lateral radiograph provides partially superimposed views of the following structures:
   a. Frontal sinuses
   b. Orbital plates of the frontal bone
   c. Anterior and posterior clinoid processes of the sella turcica
   d. Sphenoid sinuses
   e. Ethmoid air cells
   f. Maxillary sinuses (maxillary antra)

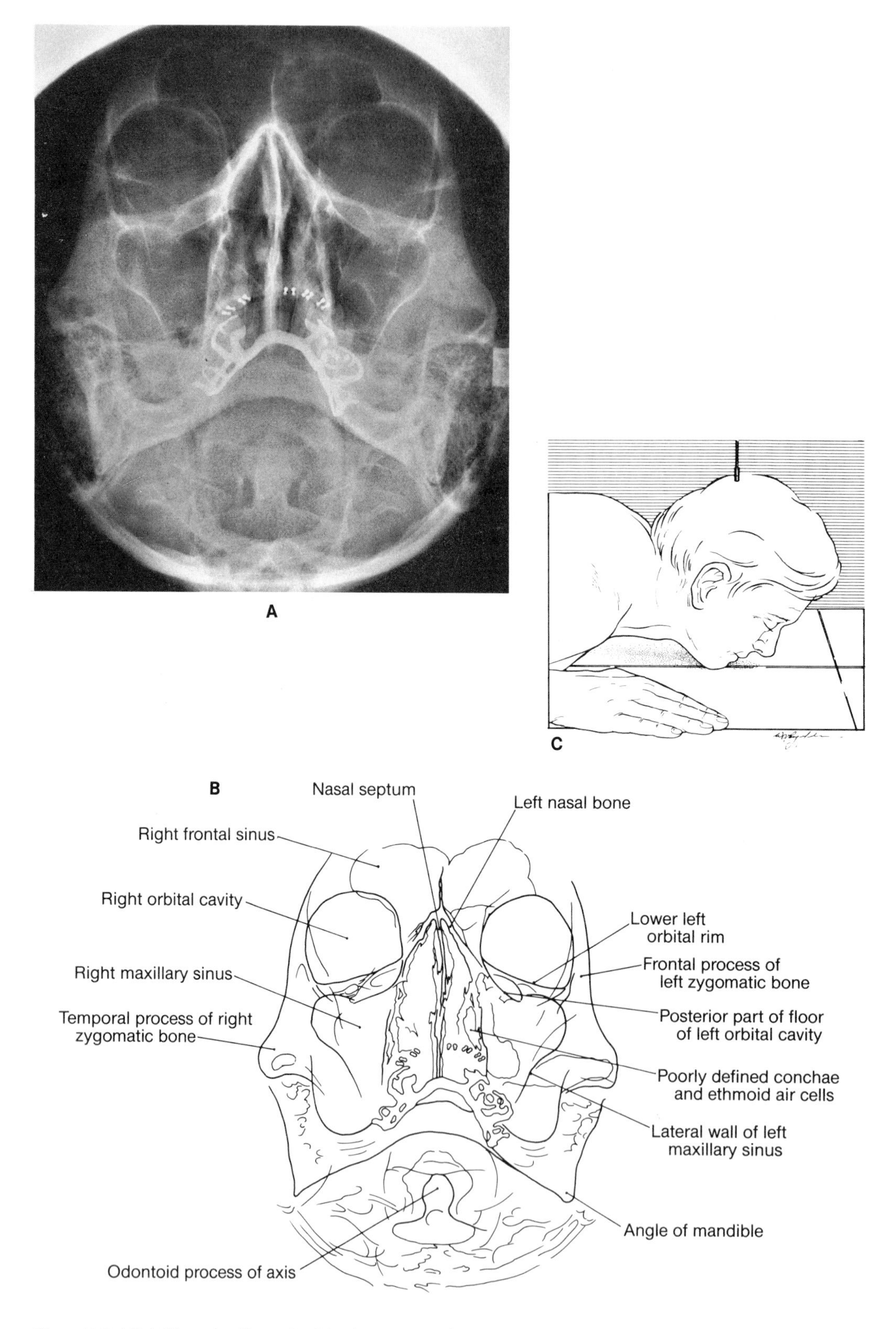

Figure 5-7. (*A*) A Waters' radiograph of the face, (*B*) its schematic representation, and (C) the orientation of the patient's head relative to the x-ray beam and film cassette for the radiograph. (See section II B 1.)

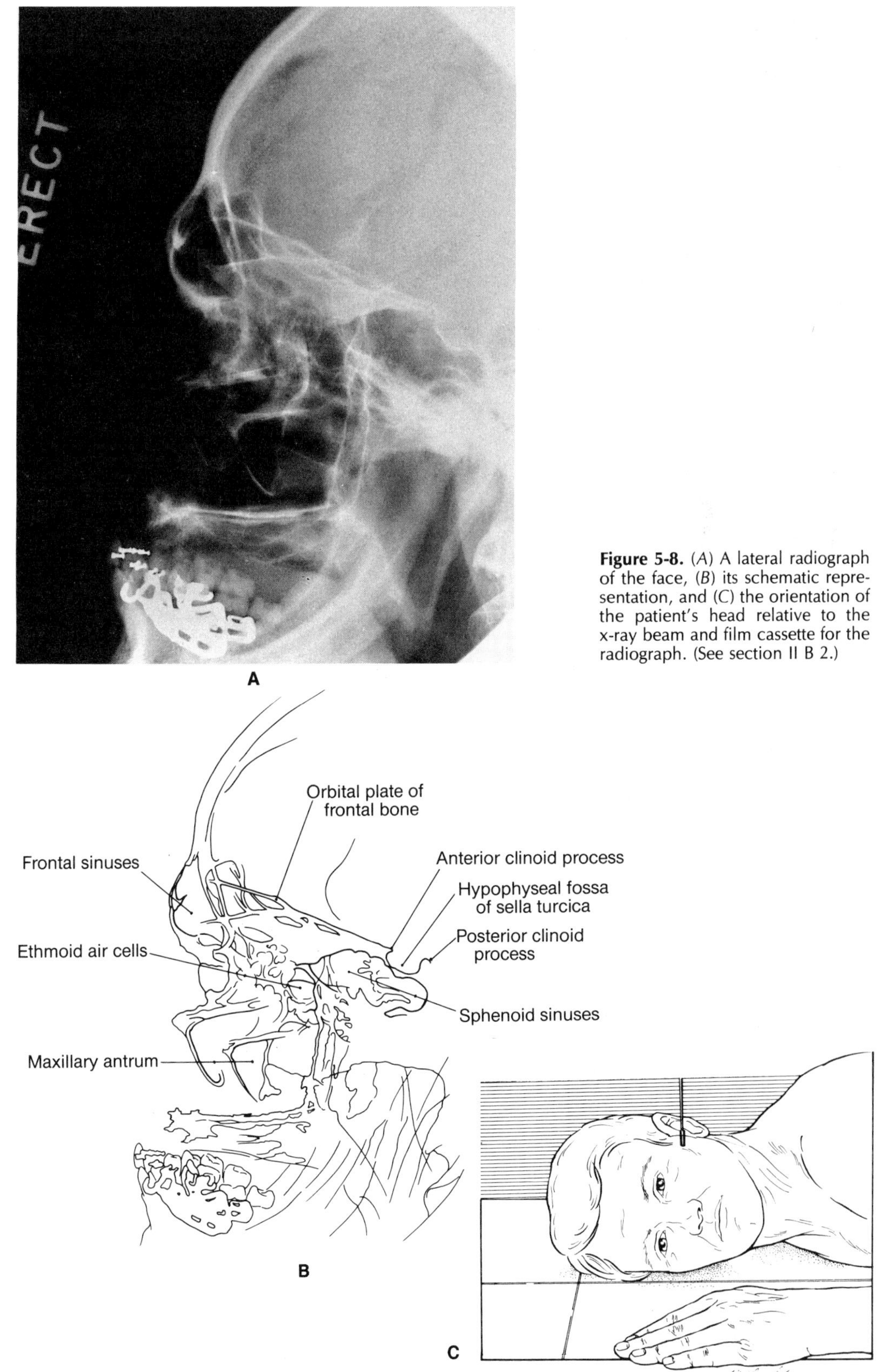

Figure 5-8. (*A*) A lateral radiograph of the face, (*B*) its schematic representation, and (*C*) the orientation of the patient's head relative to the x-ray beam and film cassette for the radiograph. (See section II B 2.)

C. Clinical and radiographic features of maxillofacial fractures. Radiologic evaluation of traumatic injury to the midfacial region begins with an examination of plain films of the facial skeleton. Of these plain films, the **Waters' and lateral radiographs** commonly provide the best views for detecting fractures in the midfacial region.

1. Maxillary fractures

a. Etiology and clinical features

(1) Maxillary fractures result from a severe blow to the midfacial region, such as that which may be sustained in an automobile accident when the midfacial region strikes the steering wheel.

(2) Maxillary fractures may be accompanied by compromise of the upper airway and severe hemorrhage.

(3) Physical examination commonly reveals mobile maxillary bones.

b. Radiographic features

(1) Le Fort classification and its limitations

(a) Maxillary fractures are generally classified according to a scheme proposed by Le Fort, who observed that fractures of the maxillary bones and surrounding bones of the midfacial skeleton tend to be representative of one of three common patterns.

(b) However, many maxillary fractures cannot be appropriately characterized by the Le Fort scheme.

(c) Furthermore, the type of Le Fort fracture on one side of the face is frequently different from that on the other side.

(2) Fracture lines characteristic of a Le Fort I fracture (Figure 5-9)

(a) The **hallmark of a Le Fort I fracture** is a maxillary fracture which

(i) Begins anteromedially at the lower lateral edge of the anterior nasal aperture

(ii) Cuts through the medial and lateral walls of the maxillary sinus

(iii) Extends posteriorly through the maxillary bone

(b) The fracture commonly **continues** posteriorly through the lower parts of the pterygoid plates of the sphenoid bone.

(c) In the **midline**, it is common for the fracture to extend horizontally backward through the lower part of the vomer bone.

(d) In sum, **bilateral Le Fort I fractures** typically separate the upper dental arch from the upper facial skeleton.

(3) Fracture lines characteristic of a Le Fort II fracture (Figure 5-10)

(a) The **hallmark of a Le Fort II fracture** is a maxillary fracture which

(i) Begins anteromedially along the upper part of the nasomaxillary suture

(ii) Extends inferolaterally through the medial and inferior walls of the orbital cavity

(iii) Cuts through the lateral wall of the maxillary sinus

(iv) Extends posteriorly through the maxillary bone

(b) The fracture commonly **continues** posteriorly through the midregions of the pterygoid plates of the sphenoid bone.

(c) In the **midline**, it is common for the fracture to begin in the nasal bone and then cut through the perpendicular plate of the ethmoid bone and the vomer bone as it extends posteriorly through the nasal septum.

(d) In sum, **bilateral Le Fort II fractures** typically separate a pyramid-shaped nasomaxillary fragment from the upper facial skeleton.

(4) Fracture lines characteristic of a Le Fort III fracture (Figure 5-11)

(a) The **hallmarks of a Le Fort III fracture** are

(i) A **maxillary fracture** near the frontomaxillary suture

(ii) Fractures that extend posteriorly through the medial and lateral walls of the orbital cavity

(iii) A **frontal or zygomatic fracture** near the zygomaticofrontal suture

(iv) A **fracture of the zygomatic arch** near the zygomaticotemporal suture

(b) The fracture commonly **continues** posteriorly through the pterygoid process or the uppermost parts of the pterygoid plates of the sphenoid bone.

(c) In the **midline**, it is common for the fracture to begin in the nasal bone and then cut through the nasal spine of the frontal bone, the perpendicular plate of the ethmoid bone, and the vomer bone as it extends posteriorly through the nasal septum.

(d) In sum, **bilateral Le Fort III fractures** typically separate a nasal, maxillary, and zygomatic bone complex from the cranial part of the skull.

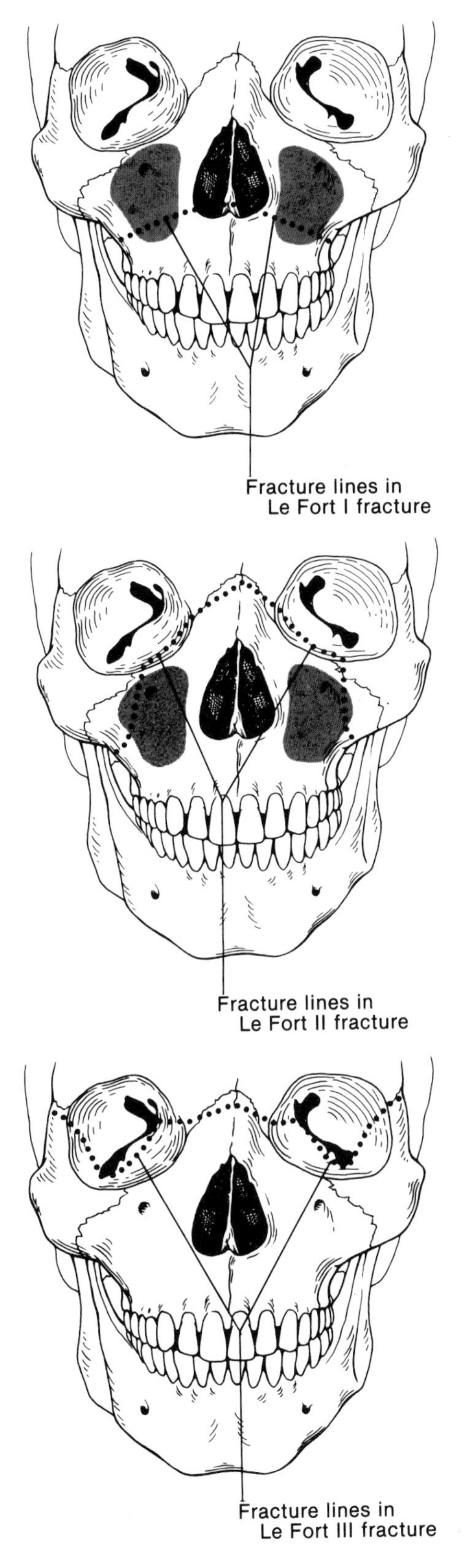

Figure 5-9. A schematic drawing of the fracture lines characteristic of a Le Fort I fracture. The *shaded areas* indicate the locations of the maxillary sinuses. [See section II C 1 (b) (2).]

Figure 5-10. A schematic drawing of the fracture lines characteristic of a Le Fort II fracture. The *shaded areas* indicate the locations of the maxillary sinuses. [See section II C 1 (b) (3).]

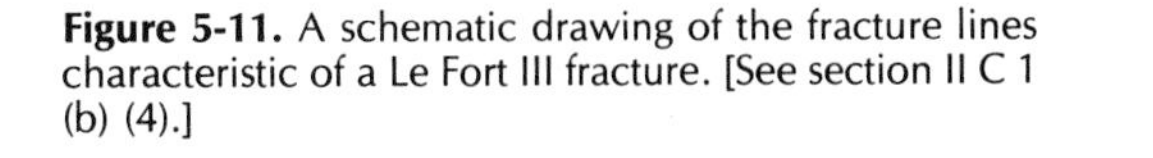

Figure 5-11. A schematic drawing of the fracture lines characteristic of a Le Fort III fracture. [See section II C 1 (b) (4).]

(5) **Other radiographic features of Le Fort fractures**
(a) **Hemorrhage** into a maxillary sinus may produce an air–fluid level in the sinus on an upright film.
(b) The presence of an air-density region in the periorbital soft tissues indicates a fracture which has opened the orbital cavity to the nasal cavity or a paranasal sinus.

2. **Orbital floor fractures**
a. **Etiology and clinical features**
(1) Orbital floor (orbital "blow-out") fractures generally result from a blow to the orbital rim by a convex object whose diameter is slightly greater than that of the orbital rim, such as a baseball.
(2) The blow fractures the orbital plate of the maxillary bone, and commonly herniates orbital contents into the underlying maxillary sinus.
(3) Diplopia may result as a consequence of either entrapment of inferior rectus or inferior oblique or increased tension on these muscles.
b. **Radiographic features**
(1) The Waters' radiograph shows disruption and displacement of the line representing the posterior part of the floor of the orbital cavity.
(2) Both Waters' and lateral radiographs show
(a) An air–fluid level in the maxillary sinus on upright films if there has been hemorrhage into the sinus
(b) A water-density region in the upper part of the maxillary sinus if orbital contents have herniated through the floor of the orbital cavity

III. NECK

A. Anatomy of the neck

1. **Layers of the deep cervical fascia**
a. **Investing layer.** The investing layer is the most superficial layer of deep cervical fascia.
(1) The investing layer extends from the base of the skull to the root of the neck.
(2) The investing layer forms the lateral wall of the posterior triangle of the neck.
(3) The sternocleidomastoid and trapezius muscles and the parotid gland are embedded within the investing layer.
b. **Prevertebral layer**
(1) The **axillary sheath** is a tubular extension of the prevertebral layer.
(2) The prevertebral layer extends inferiorly into the superior mediastinum.
c. **Pretracheal layer**
(1) The pretracheal layer binds the thyroid gland posteriorly to the larynx and trachea.
(2) The pretracheal layer extends inferiorly into the superior mediastinum.
d. **Carotid sheath.** The carotid sheath envelops the following structures:
(1) Common and internal carotid arteries
(2) Internal jugular vein
(3) Vagus nerve
(4) Some of the deep cervical lymph nodes

2. **Cervical vertebrae**
a. The **first** and **second** cervical vertebrae are commonly called the **atlas** and **axis**, respectively.
(1) When the head is nodded forward and backward in the sagittal plane, most of the movement consists of the occipital condyles rocking forward and backward atop the superior articular facets of the atlas.
(2) When the head is rotated to either side, most of the movement consists of the head and atlas rotating in unison about the odontoid process (dens) of the axis.
b. The spinous process of the **seventh cervical** vertebra is commonly the **highest palpable** vertebral spinous process.

3. **Muscles**
a. **Sternocleidomastoid.** Sternocleidomastoid turns the face to the contralateral side and directs it upward. When both sternocleidomastoids act together, they anteriorly flex the neck. Sternocleidomastoid is innervated by the spinal part of the accessory nerve.
b. **Suprahyoid muscles**
(1) The suprahyoid muscles consist of
(a) Mylohyoid [see sections II A 5 d and e (2) (c)]

(b) Geniohyoid, which is innervated by spinal cord segment C1
(c) Stylohyoid, which is innervated by the facial nerve
(d) The anterior and posterior bellies of digastric, which are innervated by the mandibular division of the trigeminal nerve and by the facial nerve, respectively

(2) The suprahyoid muscles act during the early phase of the swallowing reflex to raise the floor of the mouth and the tongue; this action assists in the rapid transfer of food from the oral cavity into the oropharynx.

c. Infrahyoid muscles

(1) The infrahyoid muscles consist of
(a) Thyrohyoid, which is innervated by spinal cord segment C1
(b) Sternohyoid, sternothyroid, and both bellies of omohyoid, all of which are innervated by spinal cord segments C1, C2, and C3 (via the ansa cervicalis)

(2) The infrahyoid muscles, acting together, serve either as antagonists of the suprahyoid muscles or as fixators of the hyoid for the actions of the suprahyoid muscles.

d. Scalenus anterior and medius

(1) Scalenus anterior and medius are lateral flexors of the neck and accessory muscles of respiration. They are innervated by branches derived from the anterior rami of the lower six cervical spinal nerves.

(2) **Relationships**
(a) As the divisions of the brachial plexus and the subclavian artery pass over the first rib, they pass between scalenus anterior and medius.
(b) As the subclavian vein passes over the first rib, it passes anterior to scalenus anterior.

4. Arteries

a. Subclavian arterial system

(1) The **first part** of the subclavian artery is the part that lies **medial to scalenus anterior**; its **branches** include the following:
(a) Internal thoracic artery
(b) Vertebral artery
(c) Thyrocervical trunk, whose branches are the following:
(i) Inferior thyroid artery
(ii) Transverse cervical artery
(iii) Suprascapular artery

(2) The **second part** of the subclavian artery is the part that lies **posterior to scalenus anterior**; its only **branch** is the **costocervical trunk**, which bifurcates into the superior intercostal and deep cervical arteries.

(3) The **third part** of the subclavian artery is the part that lies **lateral to scalenus anterior**; it has no branches but continues as the axillary artery.

b. Carotid arterial system

(1) **Common carotid artery**
(a) The common carotid artery extends superiorly from the root of the neck to the upper border of the thyroid cartilage, at which point it bifurcates into the **internal** and **external carotid arteries**.
(b) The **pulse** of the common carotid artery can be palpated against the side of the thyroid cartilage, immediately deep to the anterior border of sternocleidomastoid.

(2) **Internal carotid artery.** The internal carotid artery ascends in the neck up to the base of the skull, which it enters via the carotid canal.

(3) **External carotid artery**
(a) The external carotid artery gives rise to six **branches** prior to its terminal bifurcation:
(i) Superior thyroid artery
(ii) Lingual artery
(iii) Facial artery, whose **pulsations** are palpable at the point where the artery crosses the lower margin of the body of the mandible
(iv) Ascending pharyngeal artery
(v) Occipital artery
(vi) Posterior auricular artery
(b) The external carotid artery ends within the parotid gland by dividing into the **superficial temporal** and **maxillary arteries**; the **pulsations** of the superficial temporal artery are palpable in front of the ear where the artery ascends superficially over the zygomatic process of the temporal bone.

(4) Carotid sinus
- **(a)** The carotid sinus is commonly located at the origin of the internal carotid artery, near the site at which the pulse of the common carotid artery can be palpated against the side of the thyroid cartilage.
- **(b)** The carotid sinus has **baroreceptors** from the glossopharyngeal nerve.
  - **(i)** Stimulation of these baroreceptors initiates an autonomic reflex that helps to regulate blood pressure levels (in part by decreasing the rate of the heartbeat).
  - **(ii)** Massage of the carotid sinus can produce increases in blood pressure sufficient to stimulate the barorecpetors, and can thereby decrease the rate of the heartbeat.

(5) Carotid body
- **(a)** The carotid body is located between the origins of the internal and external carotid arteries.
- **(b)** The carotid body has **chemoreceptors** (from the glossopharyngeal nerve); their stimulation initiates an autonomic reflex that helps to regulate blood gas levels (in part by increasing the rate of the heartbeat).

5. Jugular veins

a. Internal jugular vein. The internal jugular vein descends in the neck from its origin at the jugular foramen to its union with the subclavian vein to form the **brachiocephalic vein**. The **facial vein** is the major tributary of the internal jugular vein.

b. External jugular vein
- **(1)** The external jugular vein begins via the union of the posterior division of the retromandibular vein with the posterior auricular vein.
- **(2)** It descends from its origin superficial to sternocleidomastoid.
- **(3)** In the lower part of the neck, the external jugular vein pierces the investing layer of deep cervical fascia before uniting with the subclavian vein.

6. Cervical plexus. The cervical plexus arises from the anterior rami of C1, C2, C3, and C4. The major **branches** of the cervical plexus (with their segmental derivation in parentheses) are as follows:
- **a.** Superior root (C1) and inferior root (C2 and C3) of the ansa cervicalis
- **b.** Lesser occipital nerve (C2)
- **c.** Greater auricular nerve (C2 and C3)
- **d.** Transverse cutaneous nerve of the neck (C2 and C3)
- **e.** Supraclavicular nerves (C3 and C4)
- **f.** Phrenic nerve (C3, C4, and C5)

7. Larynx

a. Muscles
- **(1)** The **posterior cricoarytenoids** are the only abductors of the vocal folds.
- **(2)** The **lateral cricoarytenoids** are the chief adductors of the vocal folds.
- **(3)** The **transverse arytenoid** and the **oblique arytenoids** act during deglutition to draw the arytenoid cartilages together and to draw the epiglottis backward and downward over the laryngeal inlet.
- **(4)** The **cricothyroids** are the chief tensors of the vocal folds.
- **(5)** The **thyroarytenoids** are the chief relaxors of the vocal folds.

b. Innervation

(1) Sensory
- **(a)** The **internal laryngeal nerve** provides sensory innervation to the mucous membrane lining the interior of the larynx from the laryngeal inlet to the level of the glottis.
- **(b)** The **recurrent laryngeal nerve** provides sensory innervation to the mucous membrane lining the interior of the infraglottic region of the larynx.

(2) Motor. The **recurrent laryngeal nerve** innervates all of the aforementioned muscles of the larynx except cricothyroid, which is innervated by the **external laryngeal nerve**.

8. Pharynx

a. Divisions. The pharynx is divided for descriptive purposes into three regions:
- **(1)** Nasopharynx
- **(2)** Oropharynx
- **(3)** Laryngopharynx (or hypopharynx)

b. Muscles
- **(1)** Three muscles constrict segments of the pharynx during deglutition.

(a) The **superior constrictor** originates from the posterior borders of the buccinator muscles; it constricts the pharynx in the vicinity of the border region between the nasopharynx and oropharynx.
(b) The **middle constrictor** originates from the hyoid bone; it constricts the pharynx in the vicinity of the border region between the oropharynx and laryngopharynx.
(c) The **inferior constrictor** originates from the thyroid and cricoid cartilages of the larynx; it constricts the lower part of the laryngopharynx.

(2) Three muscles elevate the pharynx during deglutition and phonation.
(a) **Palatopharyngeus** pulls up upon the pharynx from the soft palate.
(b) **Salpingopharyngeus** pulls up upon the pharynx from the auditory tube.
(c) **Stylopharyngeus** pulls up upon the pharynx from the styloid process of the temporal bone.

c. Innervation

(1) Sensory
(a) The maxillary division of the **trigeminal nerve** provides almost all of the sensory innervation to the epithelial lining of the nasopharynx.
(b) The **glossopharyngeal nerve** provides sensory innervation to the epithelial lining of the oropharynx and the uppermost posterior part of the laryngopharynx.
(c) The **vagus nerve** provides sensory innervation to the remainder of the epithelial lining of the laryngopharynx. In particular, the vagus nerve provides sensory innervation to the epithelial lining of two pairs of recesses:
(i) The **valleculae** (the paired spaces between the tongue and epiglottis)
(ii) The **piriform recesses** (the paired spaces at the level of the cricoid cartilages between the laryngeal inlet and the lateral wall of the pharynx)

(2) **Motor.** The cranial root of the **accessory nerve** (via the **pharyngeal plexus**) innervates all the muscles of the pharynx except stylopharyngeus, which is innervated by the **glossopharyngeal nerve**.

9. Thyroid gland

a. The **upper poles** of the gland's **lateral lobes** extend up to the oblique line of the thyroid cartilage, and the **lower poles** of the lateral lobes extend down to the fourth or fifth tracheal ring. The **isthmus** generally lies anterior to the second, third, and fourth tracheal rings.

b. Ligation of the superior and inferior **thyroid arteries** during a thyroidectomy risks inadvertent injury to the respective adjacent external laryngeal and recurrent laryngeal nerves.

c. On each side, the superior and middle **thyroid veins** drain into the ipsilateral internal jugular vein, and the inferior thyroid vein drains into the left brachiocephalic vein.

10. Parathyroid glands. Most individuals have four parathyroid glands; on each side, the **superior parathyroid gland** generally lies behind the midregion of the lateral lobe of the thyroid gland, and the **inferior parathyroid gland** usually lies behind the inferior pole of the lateral lobe of the thyroid gland.

B. Major features of the lateral neck film. The lateral neck film provides for examination principally of the cervical vertebrae, hyoid bone, and soft tissues and airways of the neck (Figure 5-12). The radiograph also images the bony and soft tissues of the face, the lower part of the skull, and the uppermost part of the thorax.

1. Bones of the neck

a. **Cervical vertebrae.** The radiograph provides a lateral view of the following:
(1) Anterior and posterior arches of the **atlas**
(2) Odontoid process (dens) of the **axis** (projecting up to the level of the atlas)
(3) **Bodies and lateral structures** of the second through seventh cervical vertebrae
(4) Water-density spaces cast by the **intervertebral disks** between the lower six cervical vertebrae
(5) Water-density **joint cartilage spaces** between the superior and inferior articular facets of some cervical vertebrae
(6) Bifid **spinous processes** of the second through sixth cervical vertebrae
(7) **Spinous process** of the seventh cervical vertebra

b. **Hyoid bone.** The radiograph shows the hyoid bone embedded in the water-density shadow cast by the soft tissues of the anterior part of the neck. The **body** of the hyoid lies at about the level of the body of the fourth cervical vertebra; the superimposed **greater wings** of the hyoid can be seen to extend posterosuperiorly from the body.

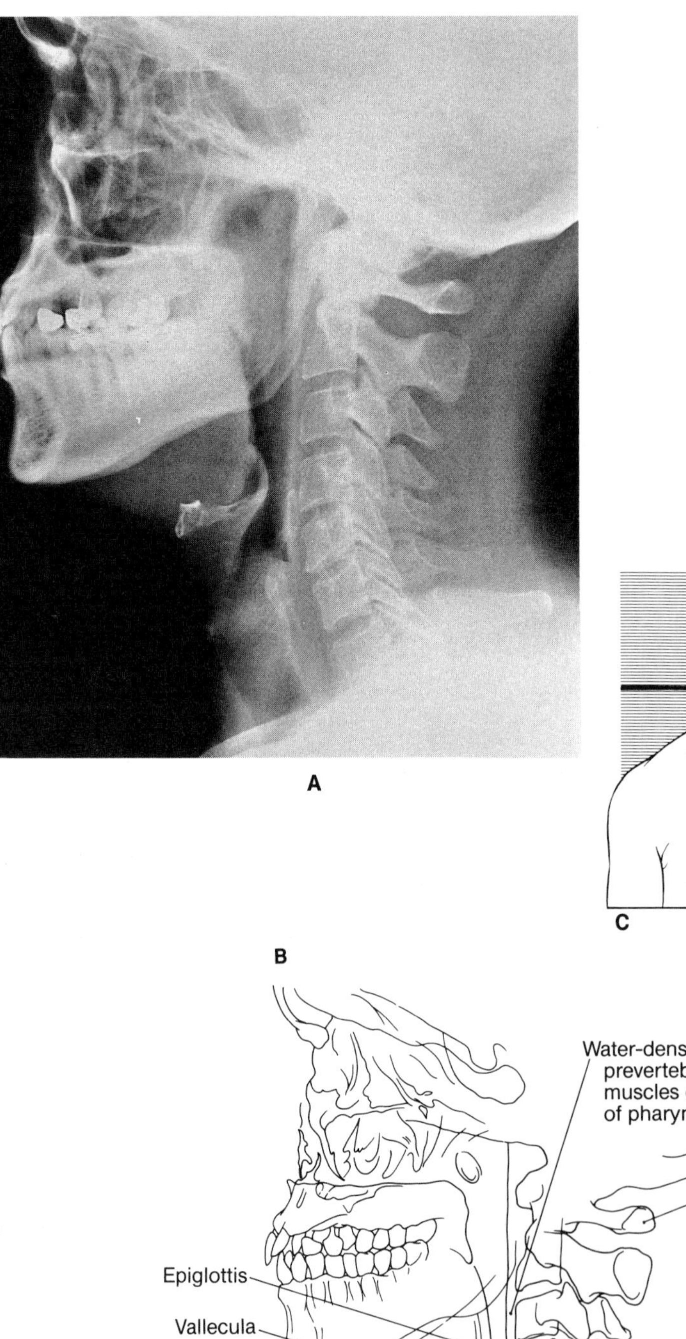

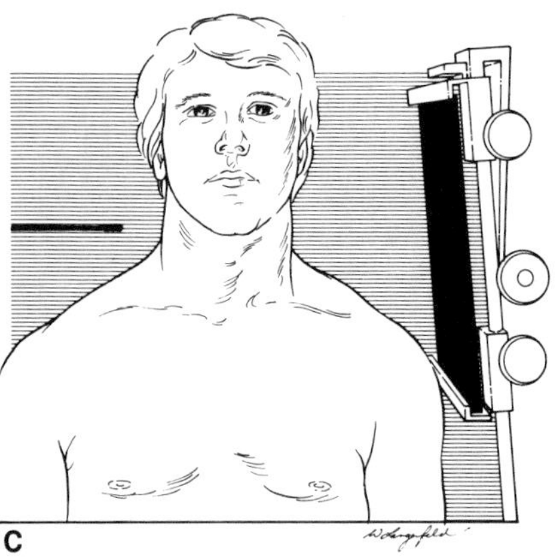

Figure 5-12. (*A*) A lateral radiograph of the neck, (*B*) its schematic representation, and (*C*) the orientation of the patient's head and neck relative to the x-ray beam and film cassette for the radiograph. (See section III B.)

2. Soft tissues of the neck

a. The water-density soft tissues of the neck outline the air-density passageways of the oropharynx, laryngopharynx, larynx, and upper trachea.

b. The **epiglottis** casts a water-density shadow which projects posterosuperiorly from the back of the tongue. The epiglottic shadow has the shape and proportions of an infant's partially flexed finger.

c. The air-density space between the posterior surface of the tongue and the epiglottic shadow represents the **valleculae**.

d. The **laryngeal cartilages** and **tracheal rings** tend to calcify with increasing age.

e. **Muscles and associated soft tissues**

(1) **Prevertebral muscles** and the muscle tissue of the **posterior wall of the pharynx** account for the water-density shadow in front of the anterior arch of the atlas and the bodies of the second through fourth cervical vertebrae.

(2) The soft tissues of the **posterolateral part of the larynx** add to this water-density shadow at the levels of the fifth and sixth cervical vertebrae; this addition accounts for the abrupt anterior protrusion of the shadow at the level of the intervertebral disk between the fourth and fifth cervical vertebrae.

f. The lower part of the air-density region extending posteroinferiorly from the epiglottic shadow to the shadow of the soft tissues of the posterolateral part of the larynx represents the superimposed **piriform recesses**.

g. At the level of the fifth cervical vertebra, the superimposed **laryngeal ventricles** may produce a lens-shaped region in the laryngeal passageway that appears more radiolucent than the passageway itself.

h. The air-density **tracheal lumen** begins near the level of the intervertebral disk between the sixth and seventh cervical vertebrae.

i. The walls of the **esophagus** are generally too closely approximated to show the slit-like esophageal lumen in the prevertebral water-density shadow in the lower part of the neck.

C. Clinical and radiographic features of cervical vertebral fractures and of epiglottitis

1. Fractures of the axis

a. **Fractures of the odontoid process (dens)**

(1) **Etiology.** Fracture of the odontoid process can occur as a consequence of either hyperflexion or hyperextension of the neck.

(2) **Radiographic features**

(a) The three most common types of odontoid fractures are those which extend

(i) Obliquely through the upper part of the process

(ii) Transversely through the base of the process

(iii) Obliquely through both the base of the process and the body of the axis

(b) Of the above three categories, transverse fractures through the base of the odontoid process are the least stable; they require surgical intervention to ensure adequate reunion.

b. **Fractures of the pedicles of the axis**

(1) **Etiology.** Fracture of the axis' pedicles occurs as a consequence of hyperextension of the neck. The injury is often called a **hangman's fracture** since it commonly occurs during execution by hanging.

(2) **Radiographic features.** A lateral radiograph of the neck shows the following points:

(a) The fracture generally passes anterior to the inferior articular facets of the axis.

(b) The body of the axis may be anteriorly subluxated relative to the underlying body of the third cervical vertebra.

2. Fractures of the third through seventh cervical vertebrae

a. **Burst (compression) fractures**

(1) **Etiology.** Burst fractures occur as a consequence of severe compression of the neck.

(2) **Radiographic features.** A lateral radiograph of the neck shows the following points:

(a) A burst fracture passes vertically through the body of the vertebra.

(b) The posterior fragment is commonly posteriorly displaced.

b. **Teardrop fractures (a specific form of burst fractures)**

(1) **Etiology.** Teardrop fractures occur as a consequence of hyperflexion of the neck.

(2) **Radiographic features**

(a) Teardrop fractures are so named because a lateral radiograph of the neck shows a teardrop-shaped fragment from the anteroinferior part of the body of the fractured cervical vertebra anteroinferiorly displaced from the vertebra.

(b) The fractured cervical vertebra is frequently posteriorly subluxated.

(c) One or more posterior parts of the cervical vertebra, such as its spinous process, may also be fractured.

3. Epiglottitis

a. Etiology and clinical features

(1) Epiglottitis is an acute inflammation of the epiglottis and the aryepiglottic folds caused by bacterial infection. Although it most commonly occurs in children aged 1 to 9 years, it can also afflict adults.

(2) Epiglottitis begins with a sore throat which quickly progresses to inspiratory stridor (i.e., noisy breathing upon inspiration), drooling, and difficulty and pain in swallowing. At this stage epiglottitis becomes a **life-threatening condition**.

(a) Hence, the patient should not be submitted to any procedure which makes breathing more difficult. In particular, an examiner should not attempt to visualize the epiglottis with a tongue depressor, since this can elicit the gag reflex, initiating a sudden closure of the laryngeal inlet (because the edematous epiglottis adheres to the similarly edematous aryepiglottic folds).

(b) Accordingly, from the moment at which epiglottitis is tentatively diagnosed until the time that endotracheal intubation has been performed (and antibiotic treatment commenced), the patient must have access at all times to medical personnel with the skills and equipment necessary to establish an emergency airway.

b. Radiographic features. Epiglottitis is positively diagnosed upon examination of a lateral radiograph of the neck's soft tissues. A positive finding is an enlarged, poorly defined epiglottic shadow; edema accounts for both the enlargement and the blurring of the shadow's outline.

STUDY QUESTIONS

Directions: Each question below contains five suggested answers. Choose the **one best** response to each question.

1. In CT scans of the cranium at the level of the bodies of the lateral ventricles, taken at an angle of 15° relative to the orbitomeatal plane, all of the following structures are normally imaged EXCEPT the

(A) corpus callosum
(B) pineal gland
(C) choroid plexus (if filled with blood bearing a radiopaque substance)
(D) frontal lobes of the cerebral hemispheres
(E) occipital lobes of the cerebral hemispheres

2. In CT scans which image the base of the skull at the level of the anterior floor of the cranial cavity anteriorly and the petrous part of the temporal bone posterolaterally, all of the following structures are normally imaged EXCEPT the

(A) interior of the frontal sinuses
(B) cribriform plate of the ethmoid bone
(C) interior of the sphenoid sinuses
(D) occipital lobes of the cerebral hemispheres
(E) interior of mastoid air cells

3. All of the following bony structures are fractured in a typical Le Fort I fracture EXCEPT

(A) the medial wall of the maxillary sinus
(B) the lateral wall of the maxillary sinus
(C) the lower parts of the pterygoid plates of the sphenoid bone
(D) the vomer bone
(E) the nasal bone

4. All of the following bony structures are typically fractured in both Le Fort II and Le Fort III fractures EXCEPT

(A) the medial wall of the orbital cavity
(B) the lateral wall of the orbital cavity
(C) the nasal bone
(D) the perpendicular plate of the ethmoid bone
(E) the vomer bone

5. All of the following statements regarding a lateral radiograph of the bony and soft tissues of the neck are true EXCEPT

(A) the upper part of the odontoid process of the axis lies at the level of the atlas
(B) the epiglottis casts a water-density shadow which projects posterosuperiorly from the back of the tongue
(C) the water-density shadow in front of the anterior arch of the atlas and the bodies of the second through fourth cervical vertebrae represents in part the muscle tissue of the posterior wall of the pharynx
(D) the soft tissues of the posterior part of the larynx cast a water-density shadow at the level of the intervertebral disk between the fourth and fifth cervical vertebrae
(E) the air-density lumen of the esophagus is visible in the lower part of the neck

6. The middle meningeal artery enters the cranial cavity via the

(A) foramen rotundum
(B) foramen ovale
(C) foramen spinosum
(D) carotid canal
(E) hypoglossal canal

7. All of the following structures are transmitted from the cranial cavity into the neck via the jugular foramen EXCEPT the

(A) cranial part of the accessory nerve
(B) spinal part of the accessory nerve
(C) glossopharyngeal nerve
(D) vagus nerve
(E) transverse sinus

8. Branches of the subclavian artery supply all of the following structures EXCEPT the

(A) external intercostal muscle of the second intercostal space
(B) thyroid gland
(C) regions of the brain
(D) submandibular gland
(E) supraspinatus muscle

9. The ophthalmic division of the trigeminal nerve provides sensory innervation to all of the following surface areas EXCEPT the

(A) skin of the upper eyelid
(B) skin of the lower eyelid
(C) epithelial lining of the anterior one-third of the nasal cavity
(D) skin of the forehead
(E) skin at the tip of the nose

10. Which of the following muscles are the chief tensors of the vocal folds?

(A) Cricothyroids
(B) Lateral cricoarytenoids
(C) Posterior cricoarytenoids
(D) Thyroarytenoids
(E) Oblique arytenoids

Directions: Each question below contains four suggested answers of which **one or more** is correct. Choose the answer

A if **1, 2, and 3** are correct
B if **1 and 3** are correct
C if **2 and 4** are correct
D if **4** is correct
E if **1, 2, 3, and 4** are correct

11. True statements regarding epiglottitis include which of the following?

(1) It can occur in adults
(2) The afflicted individual exhibits inspiratory stridor
(3) The afflicted individual exhibits pain upon swallowing
(4) A lateral radiograph of the soft tissues of the neck can provide definitive evidence of epiglottitis

12. Which of the following cranial nerves would provide sensory innervation for either the skin over the lateral side of the tympanic membrane or the mucous membrane over the medial side of the tympanic membrane?

(1) Glossopharyngeal nerve
(2) Mandibular division of the trigeminal nerve
(3) Vagus nerve
(4) Vestibulocochlear nerve

13. Muscles which can protrude the tip of the tongue include

(1) styloglossus
(2) hyoglossus
(3) palatoglossus
(4) genioglossus

14. True statements regarding the external jugular vein include which of the following?

(1) The external jugular vein is formed by the union of the superficial temporal and maxillary veins
(2) In the upper part of the neck, the external jugular vein lies superficial to the sternocleidomastoid muscle
(3) In the lower part of the neck, the external jugular vein pierces the pretracheal layer of deep cervical fascia
(4) The external jugular vein ends by uniting with the subclavian vein

15. True statements regarding the carotid sinus include which of the following?

(1) The carotid sinus has baroreceptors that are sensitive to blood pressure levels
(2) The carotid sinus is innervated by the glossopharyngeal nerve
(3) The carotid sinus is located near the site at which the pulse of the common carotid artery can be palpated against the side of the thyroid cartilage
(4) Massage of the carotid sinus will generally slow down the rate of the heartbeat

16. Postganglionic sympathetic fibers provide motor innervation to which of the following muscles in the orbital cavity?

(1) Ciliaris
(2) Levator palpebrae superioris
(3) Sphincter pupillae
(4) Dilator pupillae

17. Parasympathetic fibers from the facial nerve synapse within which of the following ganglia?

(1) Ciliary ganglion
(2) Pterygopalatine ganglion
(3) Otic ganglion
(4) Submandibular ganglion

Directions: Each question below contains four suggested answers. Choose the **one best** response to each question.

18. True statements regarding the radiopacities of intracranial hematomas in CT scans include which of the following?

(A) An acute intracranial hemorrhage is more radiopaque than the adjacent or surrounding brain tissue
(B) The radiopacity of an intracranial hemorrhage is never equivalent to that of the adjacent or surrounding brain tissue
(C) Both statements
(D) Neither statement

19. True statements regarding the appearance of extracerebral (i.e., epidural and subdural) hematomas in CT scans include which of the following?

(A) A lens-shaped extracerebral hematoma is more likely to be an epidural than a subdural hematoma
(B) The inner margin of a subdural hematoma is generally grooved
(C) Both statements
(D) Neither statement

20. True statements regarding a teardrop fracture of a lower cervical vertebra include which of the following?

(A) The fractured cervical vertebra is frequently anteriorly subluxated
(B) Both the body and spinous process of the cervical vertebra may be fractured
(C) Both statements
(D) Neither statement

21. Which of the following fractures of the axis can occur as a consequence of hyperextension of the neck?

(A) Fracture of the odontoid process of the axis
(B) Fracture of the pedicles of the axis
(C) Both fractures
(D) Neither fracture

22. True statements regarding the superior oblique muscle of the eye include which of the following?

(A) When it alone acts on the eye, it moves the eye from the primary position to an orientation in which the cornea faces inferiorly and medially
(B) It is innervated by the abducent nerve
(C) Both statements
(D) Neither statement

23. True statements regarding a lateral radiograph of the soft tissues of the neck include which of the following?

(A) The air-density space between the posterior surface of the tongue and the epiglottic shadow represents the valleculae
(B) The lower part of the air-density region extending posteroinferiorly from the epiglottic shadow to the shadow of the soft tissues of the posterolateral part of the larynx represents the superimposed piriform recesses
(C) Both statements
(D) Neither statement

24. True statements regarding the soft palate include which of the following?

(A) The cranial part of the accessory nerve innervates all the muscles of the soft palate
(B) If the muscles of the soft palate are unilaterally paralyzed, the uvula deviates toward the side of paralysis when the person opens the mouth and says ''Ah''
(C) Both statements
(D) Neither statement

25. True statements regarding the thyroid gland include which of the following?

(A) The isthmus of the thyroid gland generally lies anterior to the second, third, and fourth tracheal rings
(B) The inferior thyroid vein on each side drains into the internal jugular vein
(C) Both statements
(D) Neither statement

ANSWERS AND EXPLANATIONS

1. The answer is B. [*I B 3; Figure 5-3*] When taken at an angle of 15° relative to the orbitomeatal plane, CT scans at the level of the bodies of the lateral ventricles image the parts of the corpus callosum which lie between the bodies of the lateral ventricles. The choroid plexus that lines the posterior margin of each lateral ventricle is rendered highly radiopaque if a radiopaque substance is intravenously administered before the CT scans are taken. The scans show the anterior and posterior parts of the falx cerebri intervening between the frontal and occipital lobes of the cerebral hemispheres, respectively. The pineal gland is not imaged since it lies below the level of these CT scans.

2. The answer is D. [*I B 6; Figure 5-6*] When angulated 15° from the orbitomeatal plane and taken at the level of the anterior floor of the cranial cavity anteriorly and the petrous part of the temporal bone posteriorly, CT scans of the base of the skull image the cribriform plate of the ethmoid bone and the orbital plates of the frontal bone, as these bony parts form most of the anterior floor of the cranial cavity. The angulated CT scans also image the interior of the frontal sinuses and that of the sphenoid sinuses, as the frontal and sphenoid sinuses lie, respectively, just above and just below the anterior cranial fossa. The CT scans also image the interior of the mastoid air cells, as these air cells lie within the petrous part of the temporal bone, posterior to the tympanic cavity. The CT scans skirt just beneath the tentorium cerebelli in the posterior part of the cranial cavity, and thus image the cerebellar hemispheres and not the occipital lobes of the cerebral hemispheres.

3. The answer is E. [*II C 1 b (2) (a)–(c); Figure 5-9*] In a typical Le Fort I fracture, the medial and lateral walls of the maxillary sinus and the lower parts of the pterygoid plates are fractured. In the midline, the vomer bone is fractured just above its inferior margin. The nasal bone is not fractured, as there typically are no fractures along the uppermost parts of the medial and lateral walls of the nasal cavity.

4. The answer is B. [*II C 1 b (3), (4); Figures 5-10 and 5-11*] Typically Le Fort II and Le Fort III fractures both exhibit a fracture in the midline which extends posteriorly from the nasal bone through the perpendicular plate of the ethmoid bone to the upper part of the vomer bone. The two types of fractures also both typically extend laterally through the nasal bone near the frontomaxillary suture into the medial wall of the orbital cavity; however, laterally from this point onward, the two types of fractures differ. Whereas the Le Fort II fracture typically curves inferolaterally through the floor of the orbital cavity and then the lateral wall of the maxillary sinus, the Le Fort III fracture typically extends posterolaterally toward the apex of the orbital cavity and then laterally through the lateral wall of the orbital cavity, the frontal or zygomatic bones near the zygomaticofrontal suture, and the zygomatic arch near the zygomaticotemporal suture.

5. The answer is E. [*III B 1 a (1), (2), 2 b, e, h, i; Figure 5-12*] The odontoid process (dens) of the axis extends superiorly from the body of the axis to a spot directly posterior to the anterior arch of the atlas. The water-density shadow of the epiglottis, which has the shape of an infant's partially flexed finger, projects posterosuperiorly from the back of the tongue. Prevertebral muscles and the muscle tissue of the pharyngeal constrictors account for the water-density shadow in front of the upper four cervical vertebrae. The water-density shadow of the soft tissues of the posterior part of the larynx account for the abrupt anterior protrusion of the prevertebral water-density shadow at the level of the intervertebral disk between the fourth and fifth cervical vertebrae. The tracheal lumen is visible, but the slit-like lumen of the esophagus is not apparent because it is too thin. However, the luminal border of the esophagus can be visualized if coated with a barium sulfate suspension (only rarely is air seen in the lower cervical esophagus).

6. The answer is C. [*I A 2 b (3) (e)*] The middle meningeal artery enters the cranial cavity via the foramen spinosum, an opening in the middle cranial fossa—specifically, in the greater wing of the sphenoid bone. The middle meningeal artery is the major source of blood supply to the meninges of the brain. Upon entering the cranial cavity, the middle meningeal artery bifurcates into anterior and posterior branches; the anterior branch passes directly deep to the pterion, the H-shaped group of sutures on the side of the skull uniting the frontal bone, parietal bone, squamous part of the temporal bone, and greater wing of the sphenoid bone. Severe blows to the side of the head can rupture the anterior or posterior branches of the middle meningeal artery; the arterial branches commonly rupture at sites superficial to the dura mater, and thus produce epidural hemorrhages.

The foramen rotundum transmits the maxillary division of the trigeminal nerve from the cranial cavity to the pterygopalatine fossa. The foramen ovale transmits the mandibular division of the trigeminal nerve from the cranial cavity to the infratemporal fossa. The carotid canal transmits the internal carotid artery into the base of the skull. The hypoglossal canal transmits the hypoglossal nerve from the cranial cavity to the neck.

7. The answer is E. [*I A 2 c (3) (b)*] The jugular foramen transmits the glossopharyngeal nerve, the vagus nerve, and the cranial and spinal parts of the accessory nerve. The jugular foramen is also the site at which the internal jugular vein begins as a continuation of the sigmoid sinus. The transverse sinuses extend along the posterior margin of the tentorium cerebelli.

8. The answer is D. [*III A 4 a (1), (2)*] The internal thoracic artery, which is a branch of the first part of the subclavian artery, gives rise to the anterior intercostal arteries of the upper five intercostal spaces; the external intercostal muscle of the second intercostal space is supplied by the anterior and posterior intercostal arteries of the second intercostal space. The thyroid gland is supplied by the superior and inferior thyroid arteries; the inferior thyroid artery is a branch of the thyrocervical trunk, which, in turn, is a branch of the first part of the subclavian artery. The brain is supplied by the internal carotid and vertebral arteries; the vertebral artery is a branch of the first part of the subclavian artery. The supraspinatus muscle is supplied by the suprascapular artery, which is a branch of the thyrocervical trunk. The lingual artery, which is a branch of the external carotid artery, supplies the submandibular gland.

9. The answer is B. [*II A 2 e (4)*] The ophthalmic division of the trigeminal nerve provides sensory innervation to the uppermost surface areas of the head and face. These surface areas include the anterior half of the scalp over the top of the skull; the skin of the forehead, the upper eyelids, and the bridge and tip of the nose; the epithelial lining of the anterior one-third of the nasal cavity; and the bulbar conjunctiva of the eye. The maxillary division of the trigeminal nerve provides sensory innervation to the skin of the lower eyelids.

10. The answer is A. [*III A 7 a (4)*] The cricothyroids and thyroarytenoids are, respectively, the chief tensors and relaxors of the vocal folds. The lateral and posterior cricoarytenoids are, respectively, the chief adductors and abductors of the vocal folds. The oblique arytenoids act in concert with the transverse arytenoid to bring the arytenoid cartilages closer together and to pull the epiglottis backward and downward over the laryngeal inlet during the act of swallowing. All of these laryngeal muscles except cricothyroid are innervated by the recurrent laryngeal nerve, which is a branch of the vagus nerve. Cricothyroid is innervated by the external laryngeal nerve; this nerve is a branch of the superior laryngeal nerve, which, in turn, is a branch of the vagus nerve. The vagus nerve thus provides motor innervation to all of the laryngeal muscles.

11. The answer is E (all). [*III C 3*] Although epiglottitis generally occurs in childhood, it can also afflict adolescents and even adults. The edematous epiglottis and aryepiglottic folds narrow the laryngeal inlet, and thereby produce inspiratory stridor. Swallowing is difficult and painful because the inflamed epiglottis and aryepiglottic folds are brought into contact with each other and with the surrounding tissues. A diagnosis of epiglottitis is confirmed if a lateral radiograph of the soft tissues of the neck shows an enlarged and blurred epiglottic shadow; both the enlargement and the blurring are due to the edema.

12. The answer is A (1, 2, 3). [*II A 3 b (1)*] The glossopharyngeal nerve provides sensory innervation to the mucous membrane that covers the medial side of the tympanic membrane. Branches of the mandibular division of the trigeminal nerve and the vagus nerve provide sensory innervation to the skin that covers the lateral side of the tympanic membrane. The sensory innervation provided by the vagus nerve is the anatomic basis for the fact that washing of the external acoustic meatus and tympanic membrane can initiate a reflex vagal stimulation of the cardiac plexus which decreases the rate of the heartbeat. The vestibulocochlear nerve does not provide any sensory innervation to the epithelial linings of the tympanic membrane.

13. The answer is D (4). [*II A 5 b (2) (a)*] Genioglossus is the only muscle which can protrude the tip of the tongue out of the oral cavity. Each genioglossus also deviates the tip of the tongue toward the contralateral side. These two actions of genioglossus form the basis of the clinical test used to detect unilateral paralysis of tongue muscles. If a normal person is asked to stick the tongue out of the oral cavity, the tip of the tongue will be located in the midline since the thrust to the right side by the left genioglossus is equally counteracted by the thrust to the left side by the right genioglossus. However, if a person suffering from paralysis of the tongue muscles on the left side is asked to stick out the tongue, the tip of the tongue will deviate toward the left side, since the paralyzed left genioglossus does not counteract the actions of the functional right genioglossus.

14. The answer is C (2, 4). [*III A 5 b*] The union of the posterior auricular vein with the posterior division of the retromandibular vein forms the external jugular vein. In the upper part of the neck, the external jugular vein lies superficial to the sternocleidomastoid muscle. In the lower part of the neck, the vein pierces the investing layer of deep cervical fascia before uniting with the subclavian vein. The attachment to the investing layer tends to keep the external jugular vein always open. Consequently, if the vein is cut anywhere above its attachment to the investing layer, there is the risk that a pulmonary air embolism will occur as a result of air being sucked into the vein during inspiration.

15. The answer is E (all). [*III A 4 b (4)*] The carotid sinus is commonly located at the origin of the internal carotid artery; alternatively, it may be located at the end of the common carotid artery. Since massage of the carotid sinus for 5 to 10 seconds will generally decrease the rate of the heartbeat, such massage is sometimes used in the differential diagnosis and treatment of tachycardias. However, carotid sinus massage in very elderly patients may cause cardiac arrest. Moreover, carotid sinus massage should not be attempted in patients with occlusive carotid disease, as the massage may loosen an atheromatous plaque and produce a cerebral embolism (i.e., a stroke).

16. The answer is C (2, 4). [*II A 2 e (6)*] Postganglionic parasympathetic fibers from the ciliary ganglion provide motor innervation for ciliaris and sphincter pupillae; their concurrent contraction during the examination of a relatively close object is called the accommodation reflex. The superior cervical ganglion provides the postganglionic sympathetic fibers that supply motor innervation to dilator pupillae and to the smooth muscle fibers of levator palpebrae superioris; disruption or abolishment of these postganglionic sympathetic fibers produces Horner's syndrome. Horner's syndrome is characterized by ptosis (drooping of the upper eyelid because of partial denervation of levator palpebrae superioris), meiosis (pupil constriction because dilator pupillae cannot counteract sphincter pupillae), and anhydrosis (absence of sweating on the affected side of the face because of denervation of the sweat glands).

17. The answer is C (2, 4). [*II A 1 d (2) (b), 2 e (6), 4 c (3), 5 e (3) (b)*] The facial nerve, via its greater petrosal nerve, provides the preganglionic parasympathetic fibers which synapse within the pterygopalatine ganglion. The facial nerve, via its chorda tympani, provides the preganglionic parasympathetic fibers which synapse within the submandibular ganglion. The oculomotor nerve and the lesser petrosal branch of the glossopharyngeal nerve provide the preganglionic parasympathetic fibers which synapse, respectively, within the ciliary and otic ganglia.

18. The answer is A. [*I C 2 a (1)*] An intracranial hemorrhage is initially more radiopaque than the adjacent or surrounding brain tissue. If there is no further hemorrhage at the affected site, the radiopacity of the hematoma progressively decreases until its radiopacity is less than that of the adjacent brain tissue. Consequently, there is a period during which the radiopacity of the hematoma approximates that of the adjacent brain tissue.

19. The answer is C. [*I C 2 b (2), c (2)*] The shape and margins of epidural and subdural hematomas vary with respect to their location and extent. A lens-shaped extracerebral hematoma is more likely to be an epidural than a subdural hematoma because an epidural hemorrhage is commonly confined to a limited region between the concave surface of the inner plate of a skull bone and the underlying, smoothly depressed area of the dura mater, whereas a subdural hemorrhage is generally free to dissipate within the subdural space. A subdural hemorrhage generally has a grooved inner margin because the hemorrhage tends to fill the sulci of the brain surface it faces.

20. The answer is B. [*III C 2 b (2) (b), (c)*] A teardrop fracture of a lower cervical vertebra generally occurs as a consequence of hyperflexion of the neck. Both the body of the vertebra and its spinous process may be fractured. The hallmark of a teardrop fracture is anteroinferior displacement of a teardrop-shaped fragment from the anteroinferior part of a cervical vertebra's body. Attendant disruption of the ligamentum flavum and anterior longitudinal ligament at the level of the fracture render the injured part of the vertebral column unstable. The spinal cord may be injured because of posterior subluxation of the fractured vertebra and pressure exerted by anterior protrusion of the ligamentum flavum.

21. The answer is C. [*III C 1 a (1), b (1)*] Fractures of the pedicles of the axis occur as a consequence of hyperextension of the neck; fractures of the odontoid process can occur as a consequence of either hyperextension or hyperflexion of the neck. The least stable odontoid process fractures are those which extend transversely through the base of the process. Fractures of the axis' pedicles may be associated with anterior subluxation of the body of the axis.

22. The answer is D. [*II A 2 b (6), e (3)*] Superior oblique is innervated by the trochlear nerve. The abducent nerve innervates lateral rectus. When superior oblique alone acts on the eye, it moves the eye from the primary position to an orientation in which the cornea faces inferiorly and laterally. However, when superior oblique's innervation is clinically tested, the patient is asked first to look at the nose (that is, to move the eyeball so that the cornea faces directly medially) and then to look downward. This is because when the cornea faces directly medially, superior oblique is the only extraocular muscle which can then direct the cornea to face inferiorly also.

23. The answer is C. [*III B 2 c, f; Figure 5-12*] The piriform recesses and the valleculae can be seen as air-density regions in a lateral neck film. The valleculae are seen between the posterior surface of the tongue and the epiglottic shadow. The piriform recesses are the lower part of the air-density region extending posteroinferiorly from the epiglottic shadow to the shadow of the soft tissues of the posterolateral part of the larynx. The piriform recesses and the valleculae are the most common sites at which small chicken and fish bones are entrapped in the pharynx. The piriform recesses are common sites of entrapment because these spaces transmit food boli and liquids during deglutition. The piriform recesses are the spaces lateral to the laryngeal inlet at and just above the level of the arytenoid cartilages. The valleculae are located between the posterior surface of the tongue and the epiglottis.

24. The answer is D. [*II A 5 a (2) (c), e (2) (a)*] The cranial part of the accessory nerve (via the pharyngeal plexus) innervates all the muscles of the soft palate except tensor veli palatini, which is innervated by the mandibular division of the trigeminal nerve. Musculus uvula and levator veli palatini are the prime movers for raising the soft palate when phonating or swallowing; musculus uvula also deviates the uvula to the ipsilateral side. Normally, when a person opens the mouth and says "Ah," the soft palate rises with the uvula in the midline. By contrast, if musculus uvula and levator veli palatini are unilaterally paralyzed, the uvula deviates away from the side of paralysis when the person opens the mouth and says "Ah."

25. The answer is A. [*III A 9 a, c*] The inferior thyroid vein on each side drains inferiorly into the left brachiocephalic vein. The isthmus of the thyroid gland generally lies anterior to the second, third, and fourth tracheal rings. A tracheotomy, which is an incision through the anterior wall of the cervical part of the trachea, is commonly performed to establish a protected airway in individuals with laryngeal obstruction (such as that which may suddenly occur from closure of the laryngeal inlet because of epiglottitis). Elective (i.e., nonemergency) tracheotomies are not usually performed above the isthmus of the thyroid gland (i.e., through the first tracheal ring) because of the risk of inadvertent damage to the tissues of the infraglottic region of the larynx; such injury can produce subglottic stenosis and a resulting dyspnea postoperatively. Tracheotomies are preferably performed below the level of the isthmus; this approach encounters the anterior jugular veins superficially and the inferior thyroid veins and a possible thyroid ima artery deeply. A thyroid ima artery is a branch of the aortic arch that supplies the thyroid gland.

Challenge Exam

In each of the following radiographic cases, one to four unlabeled radiographs are presented with a brief statement of the patient's history. In all but three of the cases, the reader's assignment is to discern if there are abnormal findings in the radiographs. Except for most of the orthopedic radiographs of the extremities, the radiographic evidence is insufficient to render a diagnosis. In three of the cases, the reader will find instructions to identify normal abdominal and pelvic viscera in radiographs taken after contrast material was introduced into the patient's gastrointestinal tract or urinary system.

Immediately following the page or pages bearing the unlabeled radiographs the reader will find a written explanation of any abnormal findings, accompanied by labeled radiographs (in a few cases, the anatomic basis of the abnormal findings has not been previously discussed in the text).

Case 1

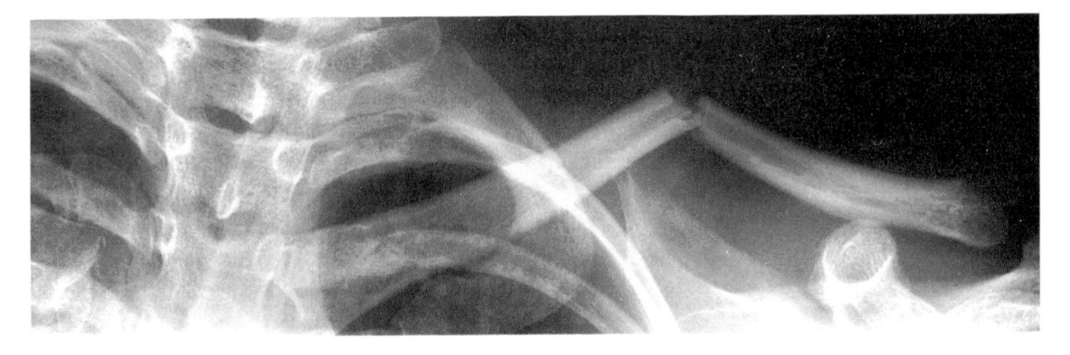

AP view of the left clavicle of a 25-year-old woman who has sustained injuries in an automobile accident.

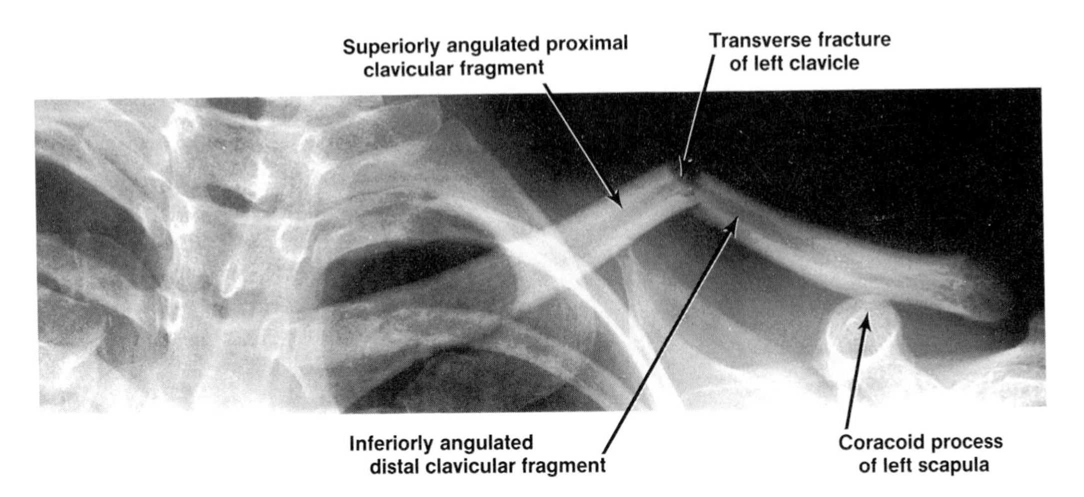

Case 1 discussion. [*Chapter 1 I C 3*] The radiograph shows a simple transverse fracture of the middle third of the left clavicle. The clavicle is the most commonly fractured bone of the body. When the upper limb is used to brace the body, forces are transmitted from the limb to the trunk of the body. In particular, forces are transmitted from the humerus to the scapula via the shoulder joint, from the scapula to the clavicle via the coracoclavicular ligament, then medially along the clavicle, and finally from the clavicle to the body trunk, generally via the costoclavicular ligament. Bracing of the body with the upper limb commonly occurs during accidental collisions and falls; such bracing can impose stresses on the clavicle sufficient to fracture it.

The clavicle serves as a strut that both elevates and posterolaterally displaces the shoulder region. Consequently, when the clavicle is fractured, the shoulder region tends to be displaced inferiorly, anteriorly, and medially from its normal position. The inferior displacement of the shoulder region accounts for the inferior angulation of the distal fragment of the clavicle. The upward pull of the sternocleidomastoid muscle commonly angulates the proximal fragment of the clavicle superiorly.

Case 2

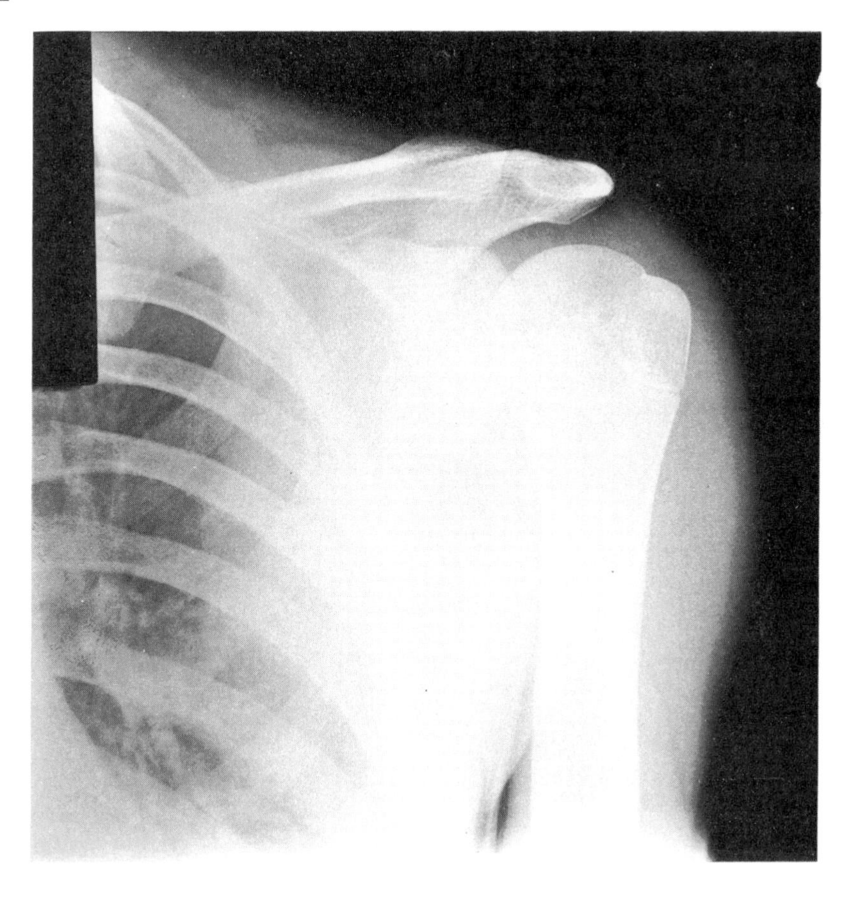

AP views of the left and right shoulders of a 16-year-old boy who fell down on his right shoulder. Ten-pound weights were being held at the time that the radiographs were taken.

continued on next page

Case 2 *continued*

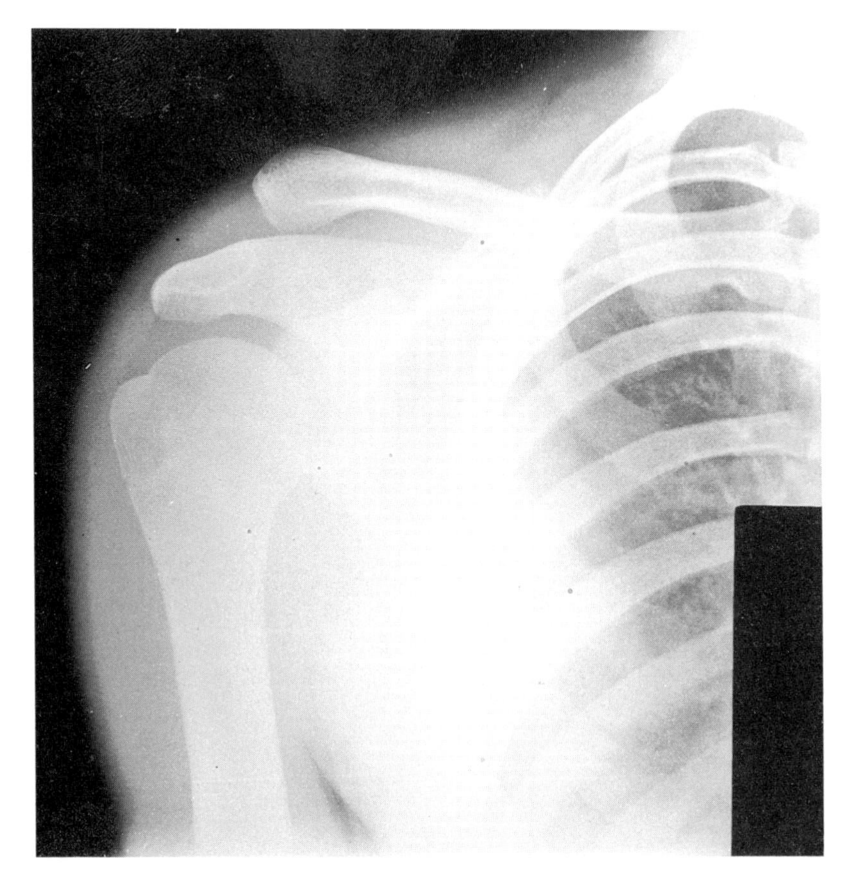

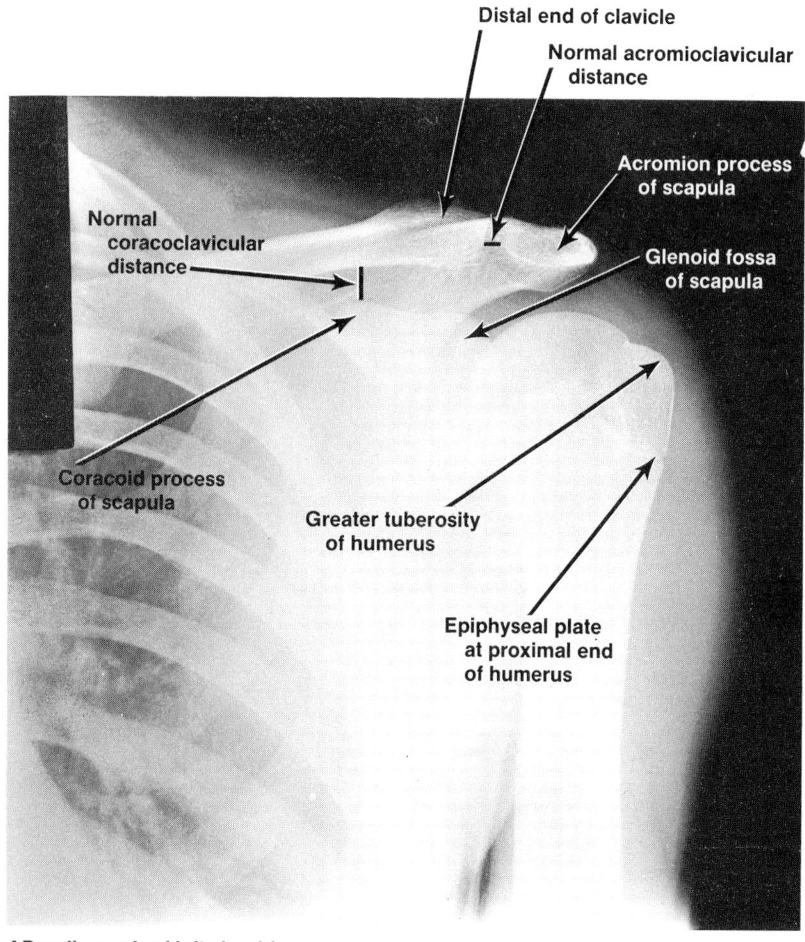

AP radiograph of left shoulder

Case 2 discussion. [*Chapter 1 I C 1 c*] Comparison of the left and right radiographs shows a grade III shoulder separation on the right side. A grade III shoulder separation is an injury in which there is dislocation of the acromioclavicular joint because of severe disruption of both the capsule of the acromioclavicular joint and the coracoclavicular ligament. The clavicle can no longer adequately prop up the shoulder region, since the principal ligamentous attachments suspending the scapula from the clavicle are disrupted. Consequently, the scapula is commonly inferiorly displaced, especially if the upper limb is made to bear the extra burden of a weight strapped around the wrist. The radiographic criteria of a grade III shoulder separation are that the acromioclavicular and coracoclavicular distances are each about 50% greater on the injured side than on the contralateral, uninjured side.

The proximal epiphyseal plate of the humerus is visible on each side. The proximal humeral epiphysis fuses with the humeral shaft at approximately 20 years of age.

continued on next page

Case 2 discussion *continued*

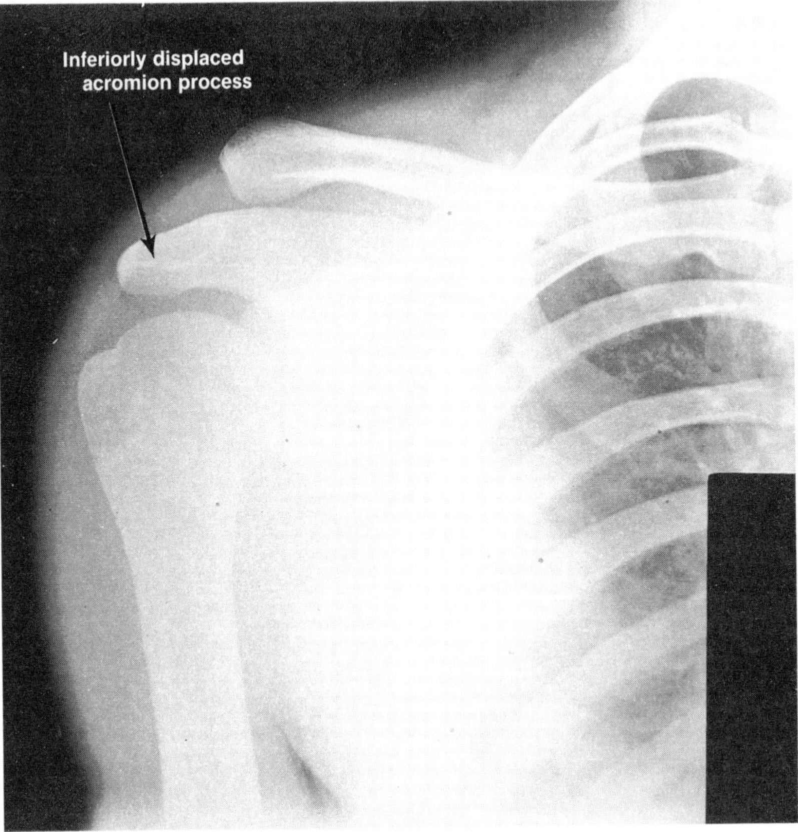

AP radiograph of right shoulder

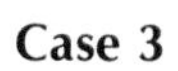

Case 3

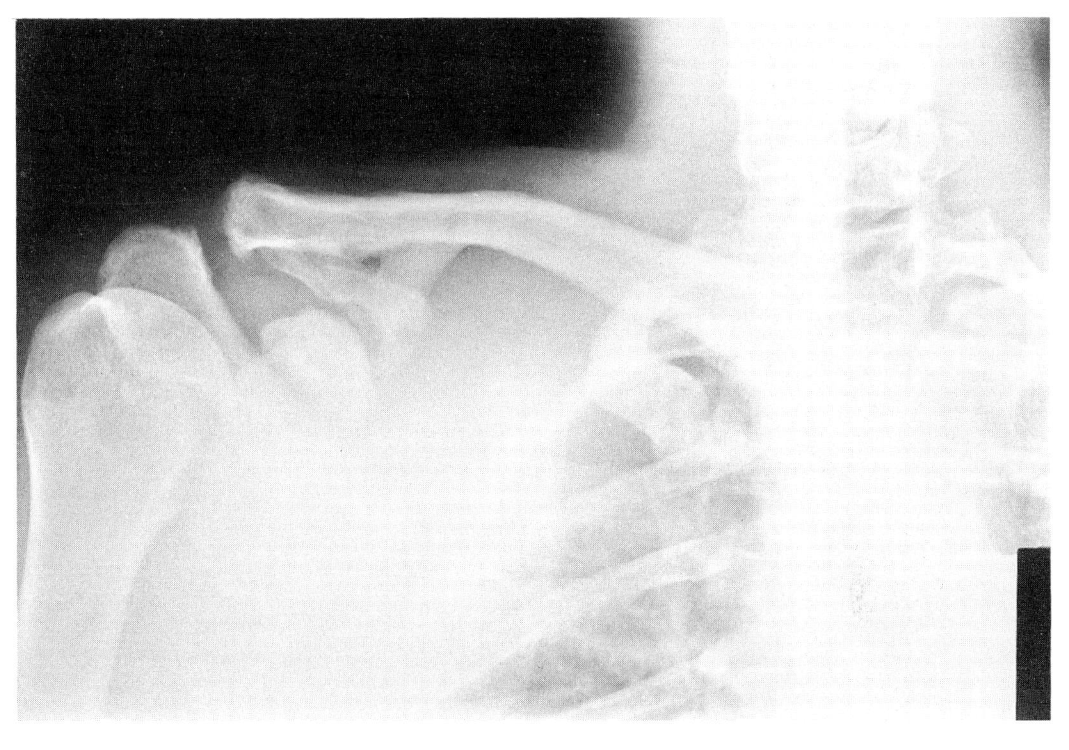

AP view of the right shoulder of a 27-year-old man who has sustained repetitive shoulder separations on the right side.

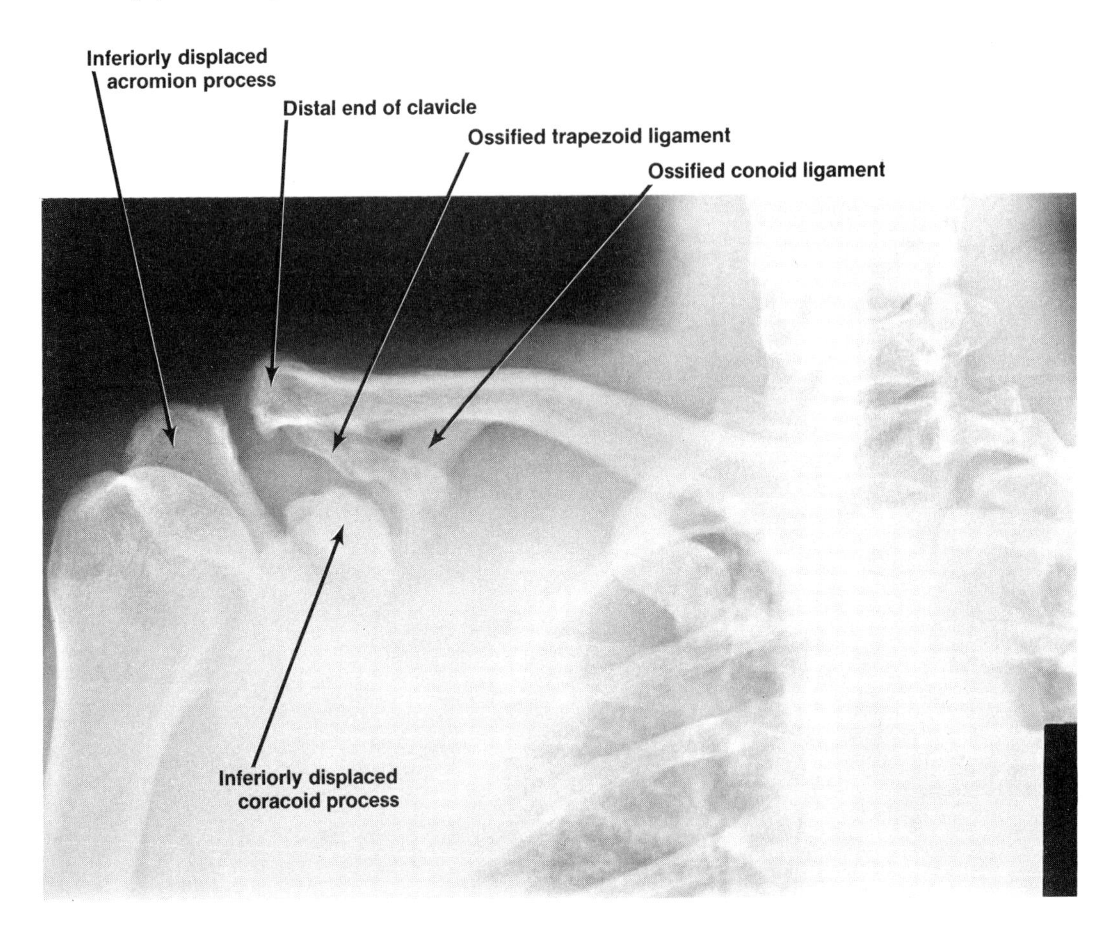

Case 3 discussion. [*Chapter 1 I C 1 c*] The radiograph shows a grade III shoulder separation on the right side with ossification of the two parts of the coracoclavicular ligament (i.e., the trapezoid and conoid ligaments). The coracoclavicular ligament is an accessory ligament of the acromioclavicular joint. It has lateral and medial parts. The lateral part, the trapezoid ligament, lies almost horizontal as it extends anterolaterally from the coracoid process to the clavicle. The medial part, the conoid ligament, extends posteromedially from the coracoid process to the clavicle. The radiograph shows the coracoid process separated from the ossified trapezoid and conoid ligaments.

The coracoclavicular ligament is the strongest nonmuscular structure binding the two bones of the pectoral girdle, namely the scapula and clavicle, and commonly transmits almost all forces between the two bones. The ligament also serves as the center of rotation for movements about the acromioclavicular joint.

Case 4

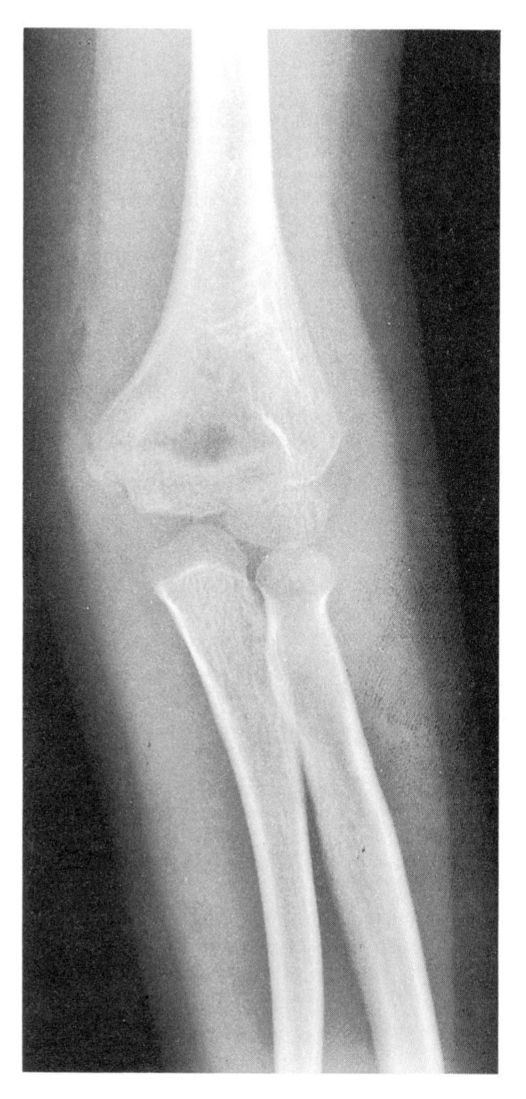

AP and lateral views of the elbow of a 7-year-old girl who fell on her outstretched hand.

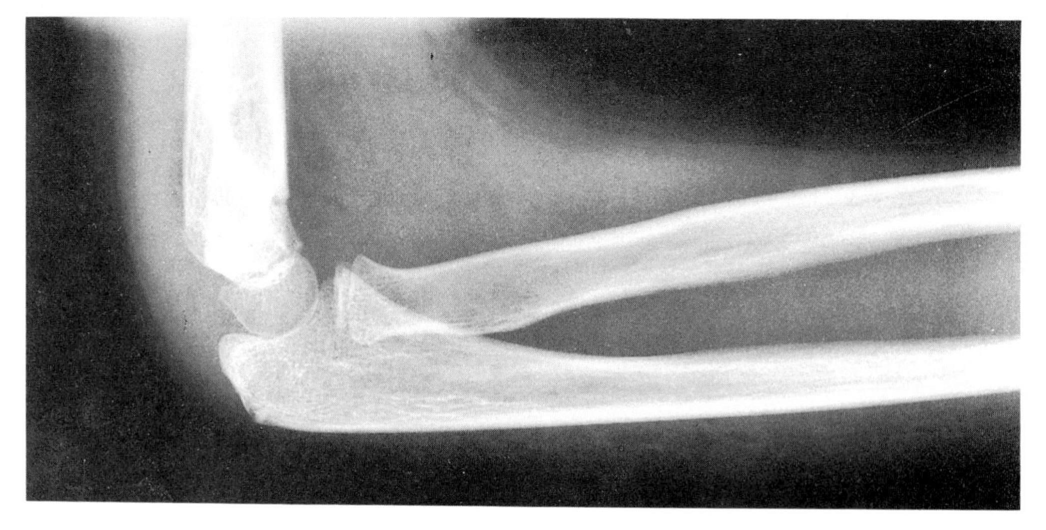

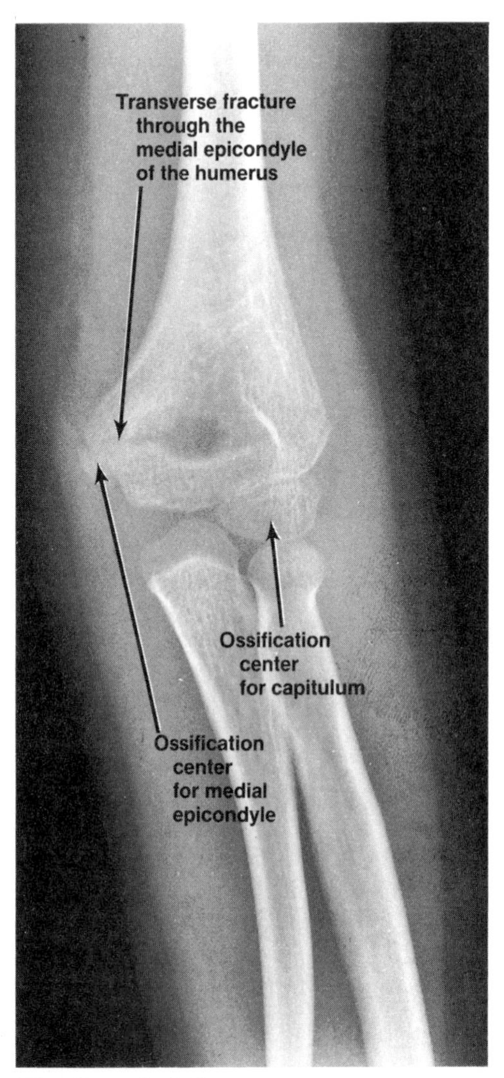

AP radiograph of elbow

Case 4 discussion. [*Chapter 1 II C 2*] The AP radiograph shows a transverse fracture through the medial epicondyle of the humerus. As expected, one can see the ossification centers for the capitulum and for the medial epicondyle (which appear, respectively, during the first 6 months after birth and at 4 to 6 years of age), and there are no ossification centers for the trochlea and lateral epicondyle (which appear, respectively, at ages 8 to 9 years and 11 to 12 years). The AP radiograph shows that there is not any marked medial or lateral angular displacement of the distal humeral epiphysis, as the carrying angle of the elbow is within the normal range. Evidence of subtle angular displacement of the distal humeral epiphysis would require comparison with the carrying angle of the contralateral, uninjured elbow (whose AP radiograph is not available).

The lateral radiograph shows the transverse fracture at the distal end of the humerus and, as expected, both the sail sign and the positive posterior fat pad sign (both of which are due to effusion of the elbow joint synovial cavity). There is no evidence of subtle anterior or posterior displacement of the distal humeral epiphysis, because there is no malalignment of the capitulum with respect to the anterior humeral and midhumeral lines. There is also no evidence of disruption of the radiocapitellar line.

In summary, the radiographs show a transverse fracture through only the distal end of the humerus; there is no evidence of a fracture through the distal humeral epiphyseal plate. The principal potential complication of this distal humeral fracture is Volkmann's contracture, a condition in which the forearm muscles suffer ischemic atrophy because of edema in the elbow region.

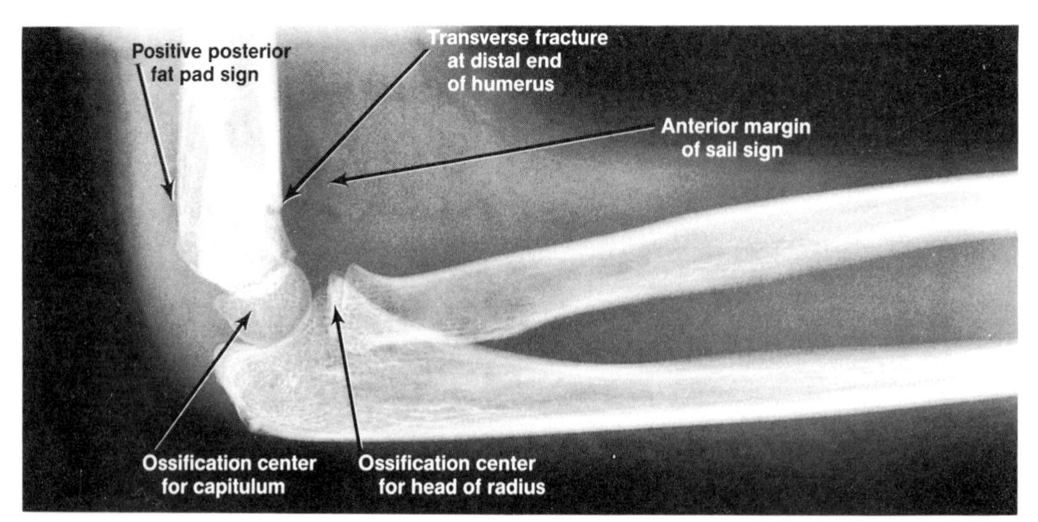

Lateral radiograph of elbow

Case 5

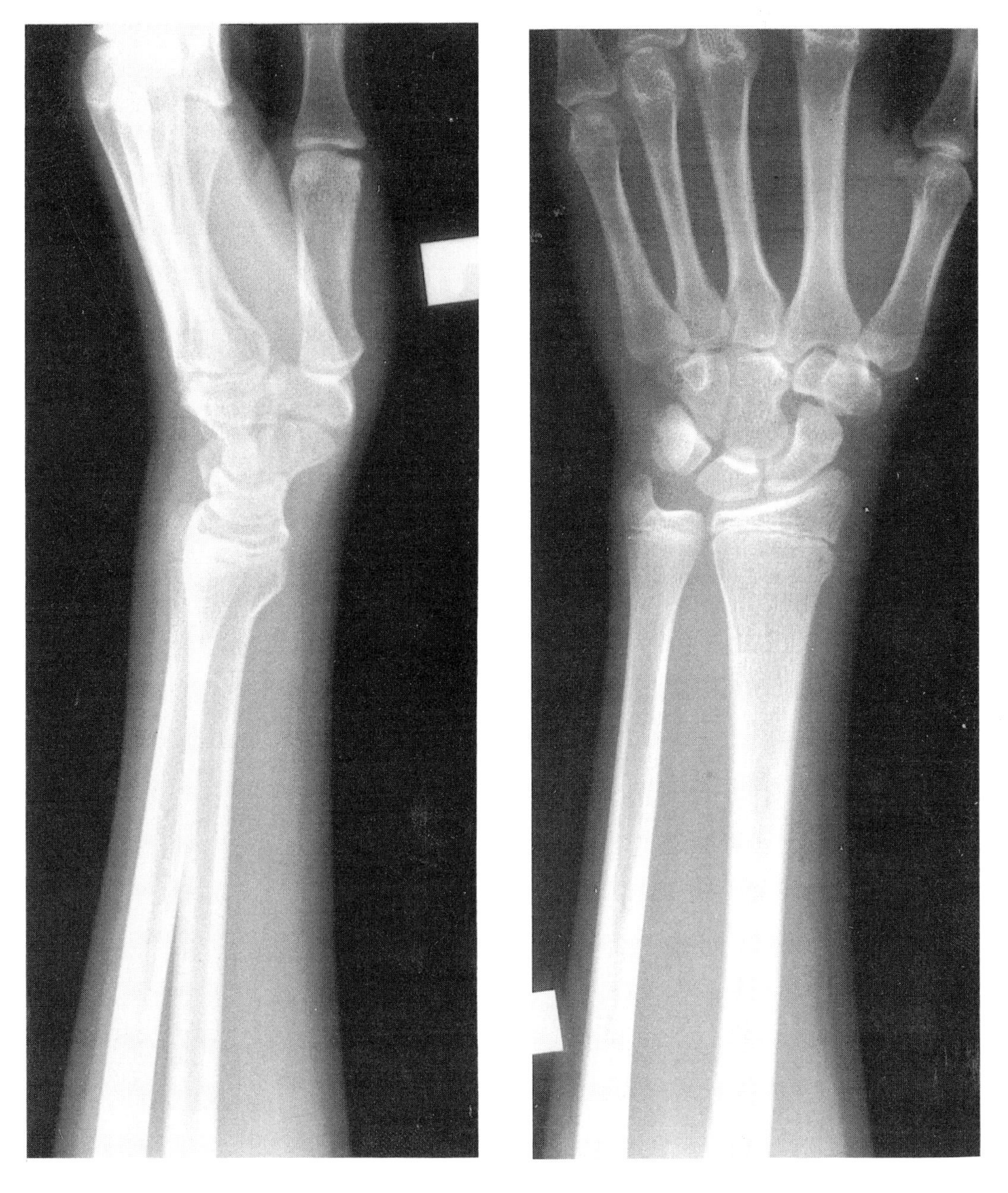

Lateral and AP views of the distal forearm of a 13-year-old boy who fell on his outstretched hand.

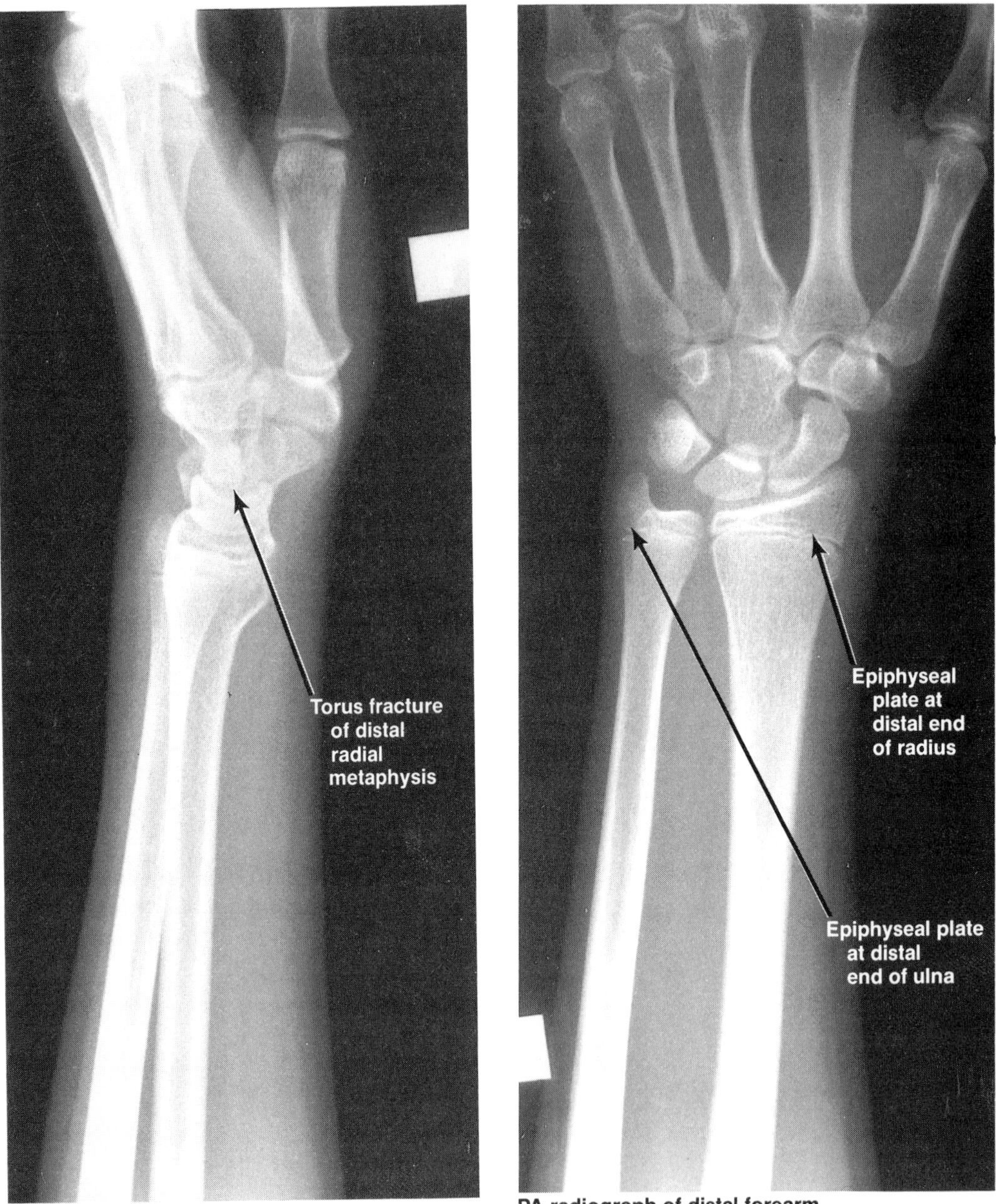

Lateral radiograph of distal forearm

PA radiograph of distal forearm

Case 5 discussion. [*Chapter 1 III C 2 b (1), (2)*] The lateral radiograph shows a torus fracture along the anterior margin of the distal radial metaphysis. A hard fall on an outstretched hand is a common mechanism by which this fracture is produced in children. The epiphyses at the distal ends of the radius and ulna fuse with their respective metaphyses at 17 to 19 years of age.

The bones of children are relatively supple and easily bent because of their comparatively high content of organic matter relative to mineral matter. Accordingly, when the long bones of the extremities of an infant or young child are subject to unbearable stress, the cortical bone of the shaft, or diaphysis, is more likely to bend or buckle than shatter.

Case 6

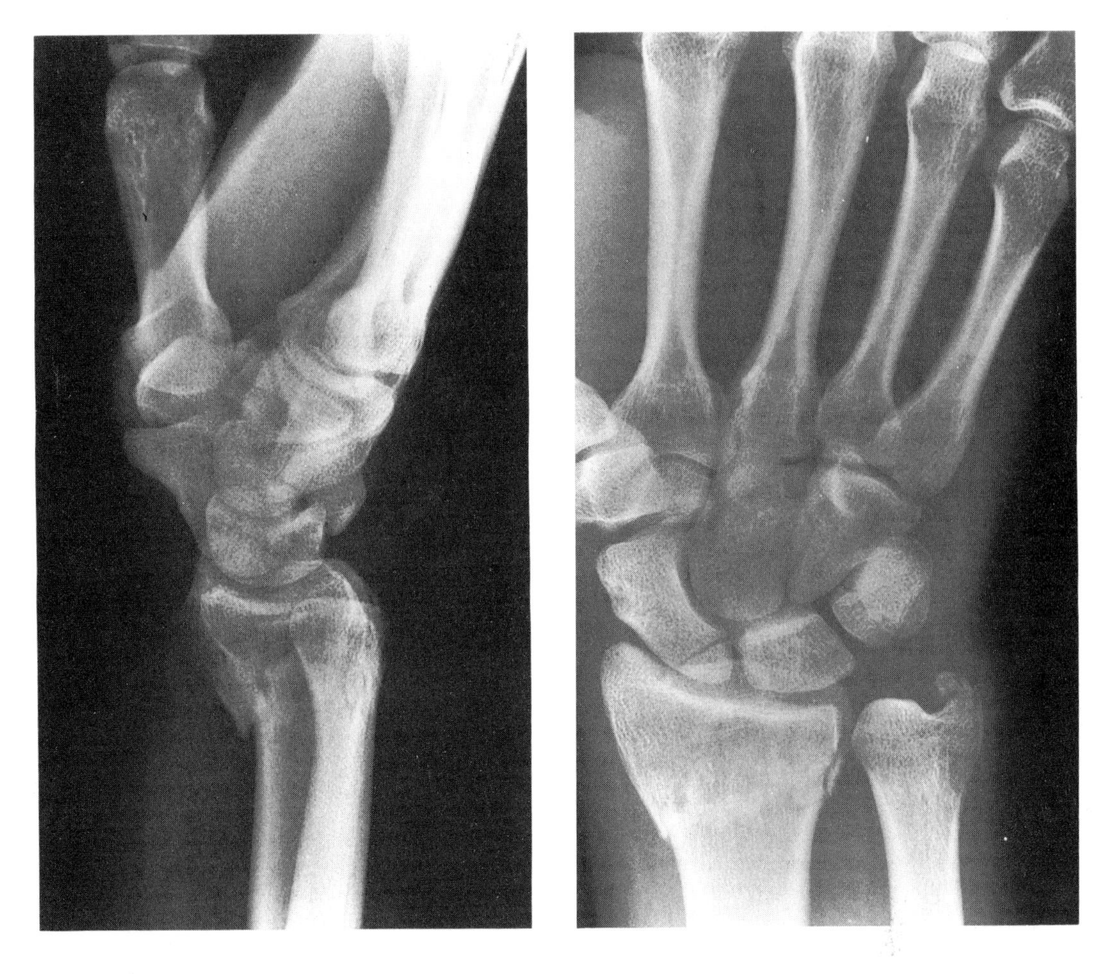

Lateral and PA views of the wrist of a 32-year-old man who fell on the dorsum of his hand.

Case 6 discussion. [*Chapter 1 II C 3; III C 2 d*] The lateral radiograph shows a comminuted fracture extending transversely through the distal radius.

The PA radiograph shows evidence of four fractures: (1) the transverse fracture of the distal radius, (2) a fracture of the styloid process of the ulna, (3) a transverse fracture through the proximal pole of the scaphoid, and (4) a fracture along the medial margin of the triquetrum. Most scaphoid fractures occur in the bone's waist.

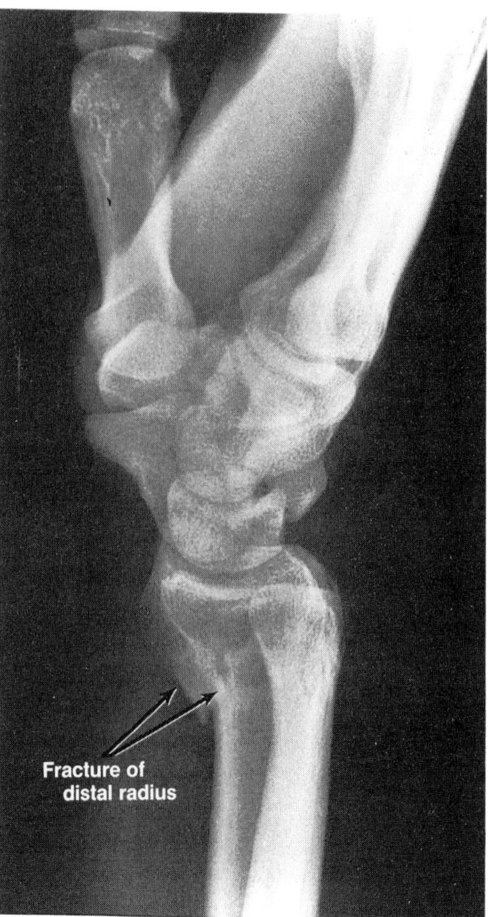

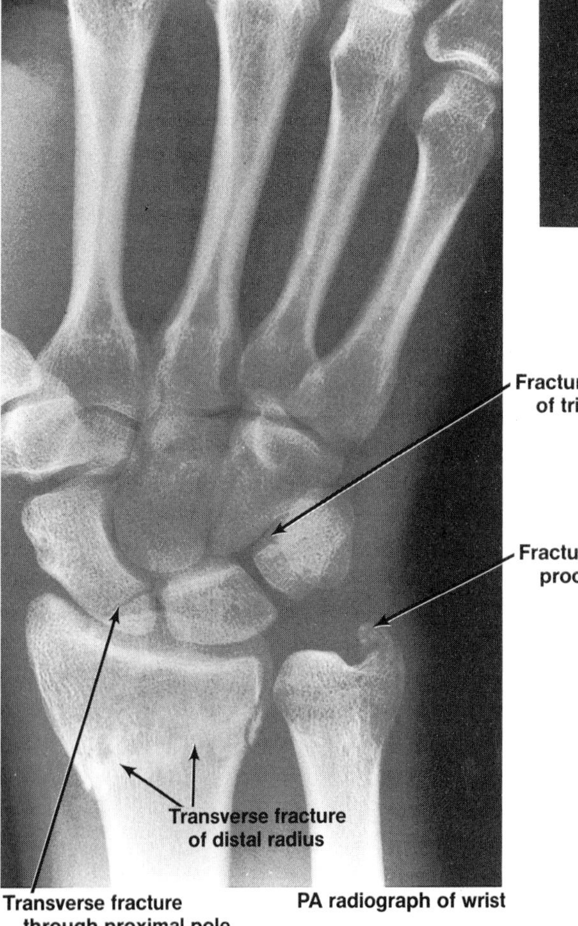

PA radiograph of wrist

Case 7

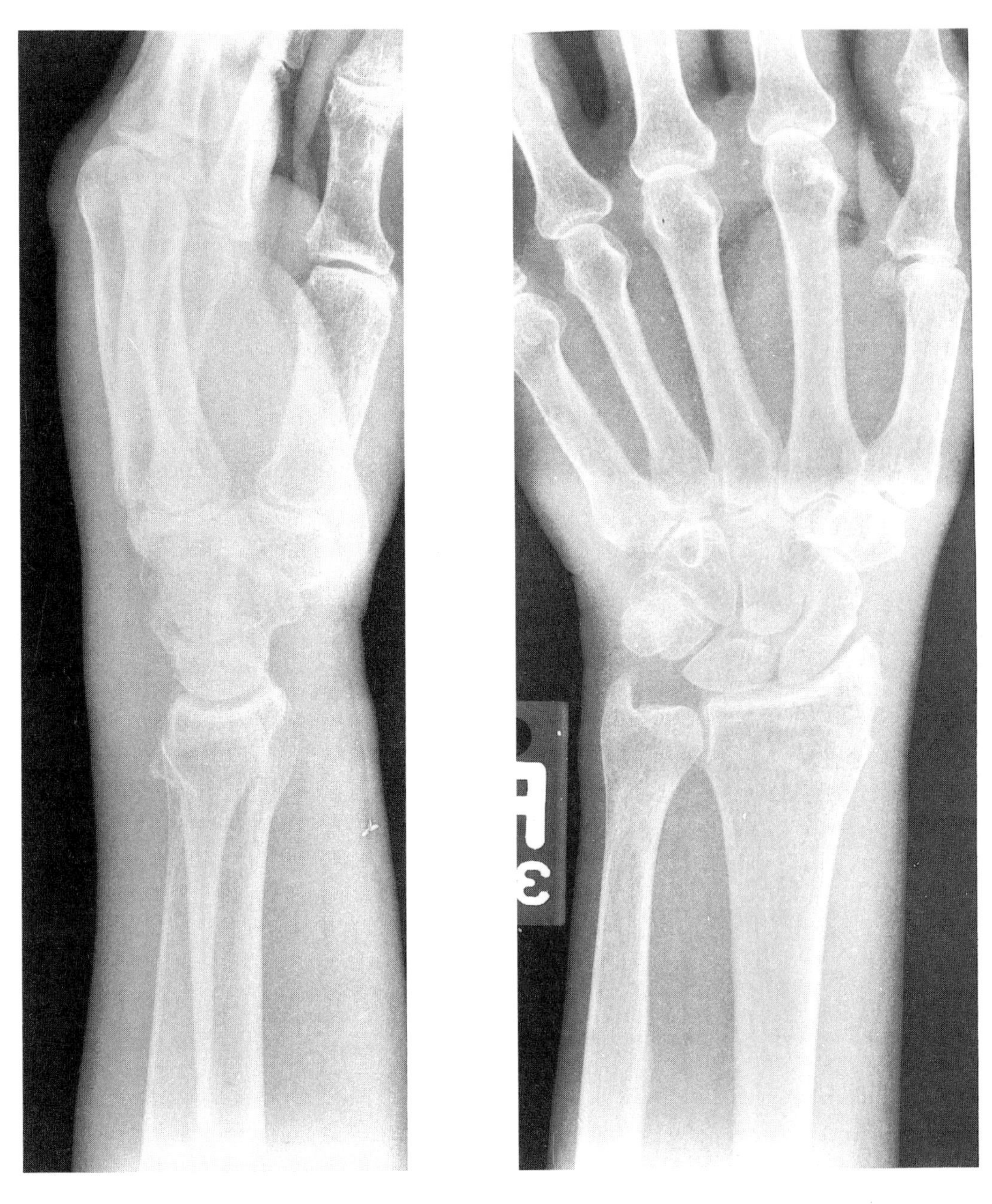

Lateral and PA views of the wrist of a 67-year-old woman who fell on her outstretched hand.

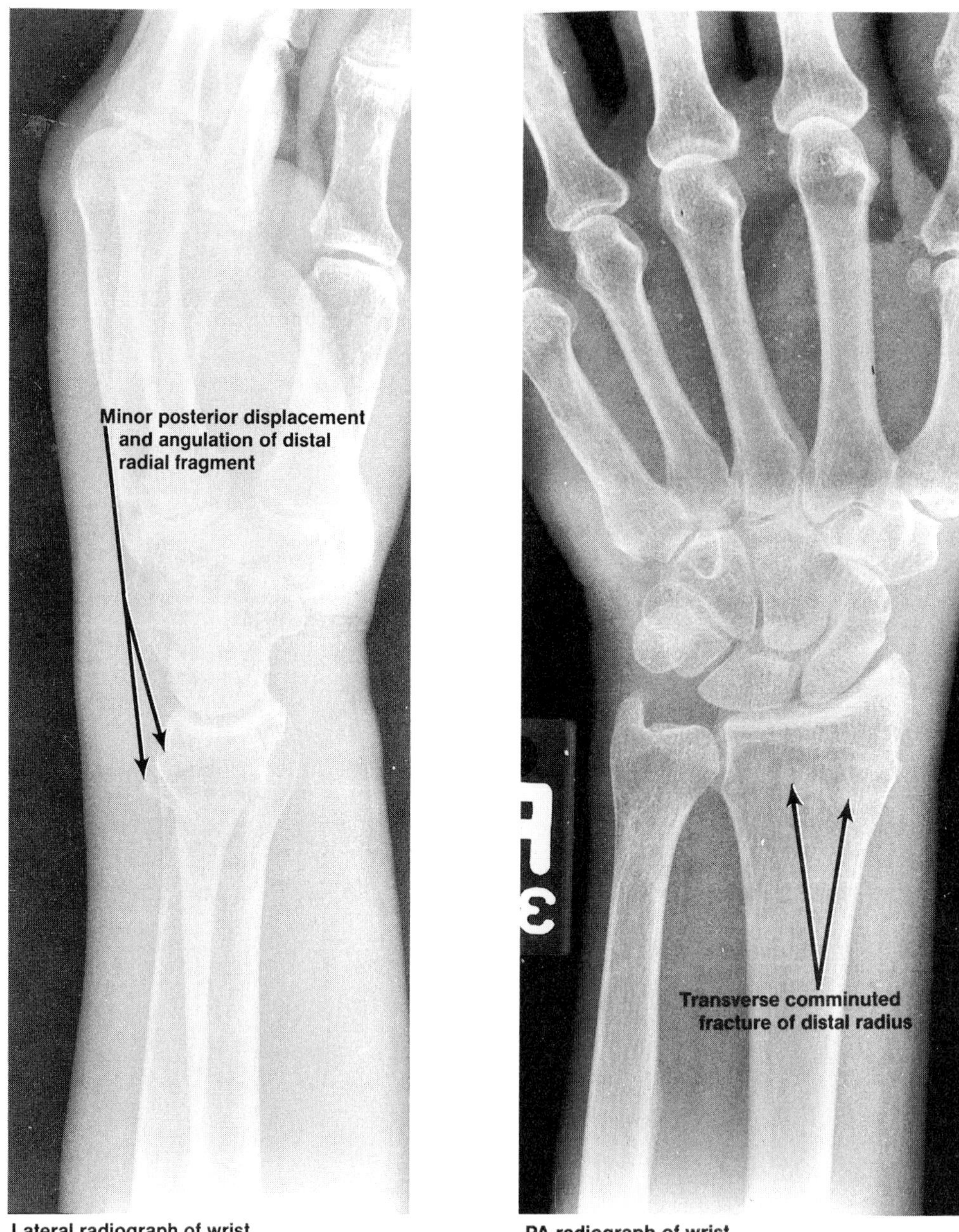

Lateral radiograph of wrist

PA radiograph of wrist

Case 7 discussion. [*Chapter 1 III C 2 c*] The lateral radiograph shows a Colles' fracture of the distal radius. The lateral and PA views together show a fracture that extends transversely through the distal radius; there is impaction of the fragments with minor posterior displacement and angulation. Colles' fractures most commonly occur in adults 50 years of age and older.

Case 8

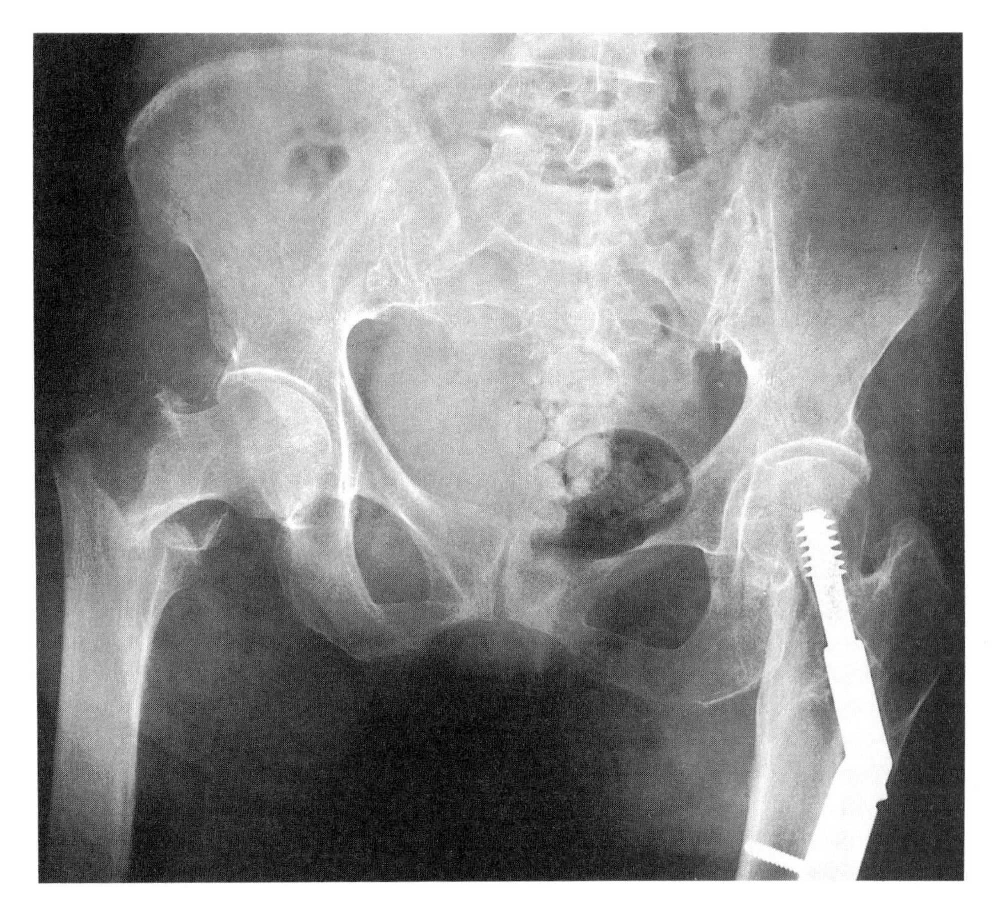

AP view of the pelvis of a 76-year-old woman who tripped and fell.

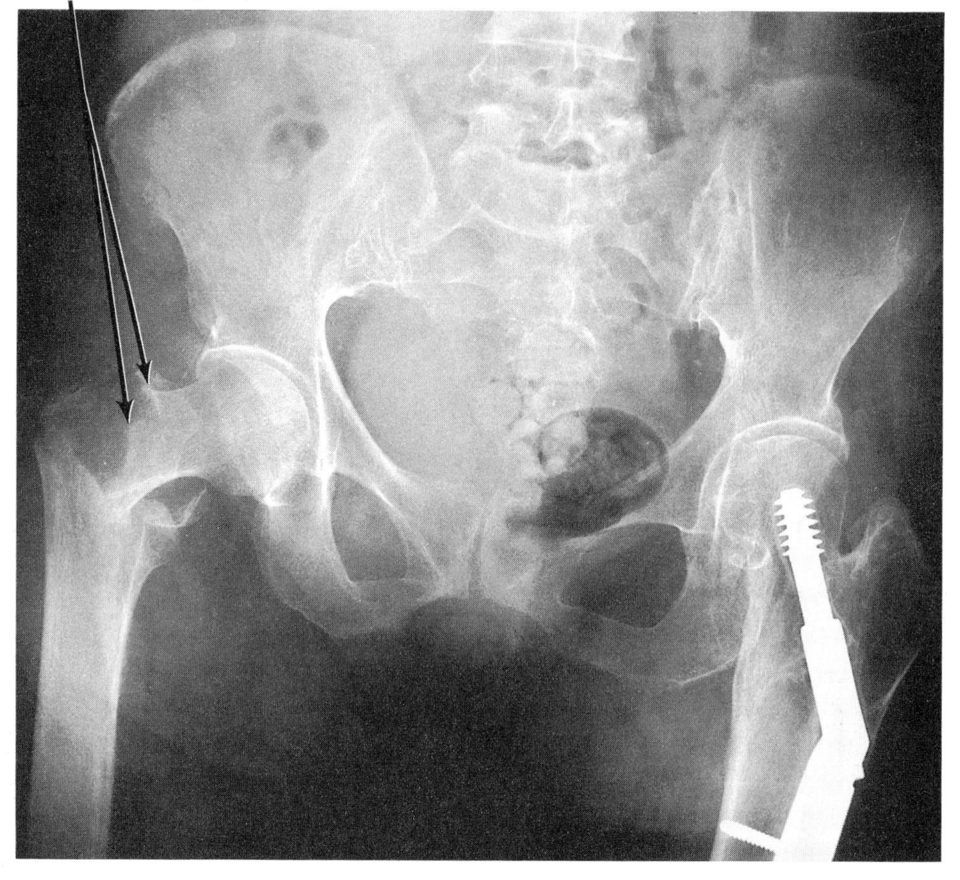

Case 8 discussion. (*Chapter 2 I C 3 a*] The radiograph shows a comminuted intertrochanteric fracture of the right hip. The axial pull of the thigh muscles in concert with the medial pull of the adductors has displaced the femoral shaft proximally and medially, and thus forced the hip into a varus position. Intertrochanteric fractures (which are extracapsular hip fractures) generally do not compromise blood supply to the head of the femur; accordingly, nonunion and avascular necrosis of the femoral head are infrequently encountered as postreduction complications.

The radiograph shows a previous left hip fracture that has been reduced and fixed with a compression nail and plate.

Case 9

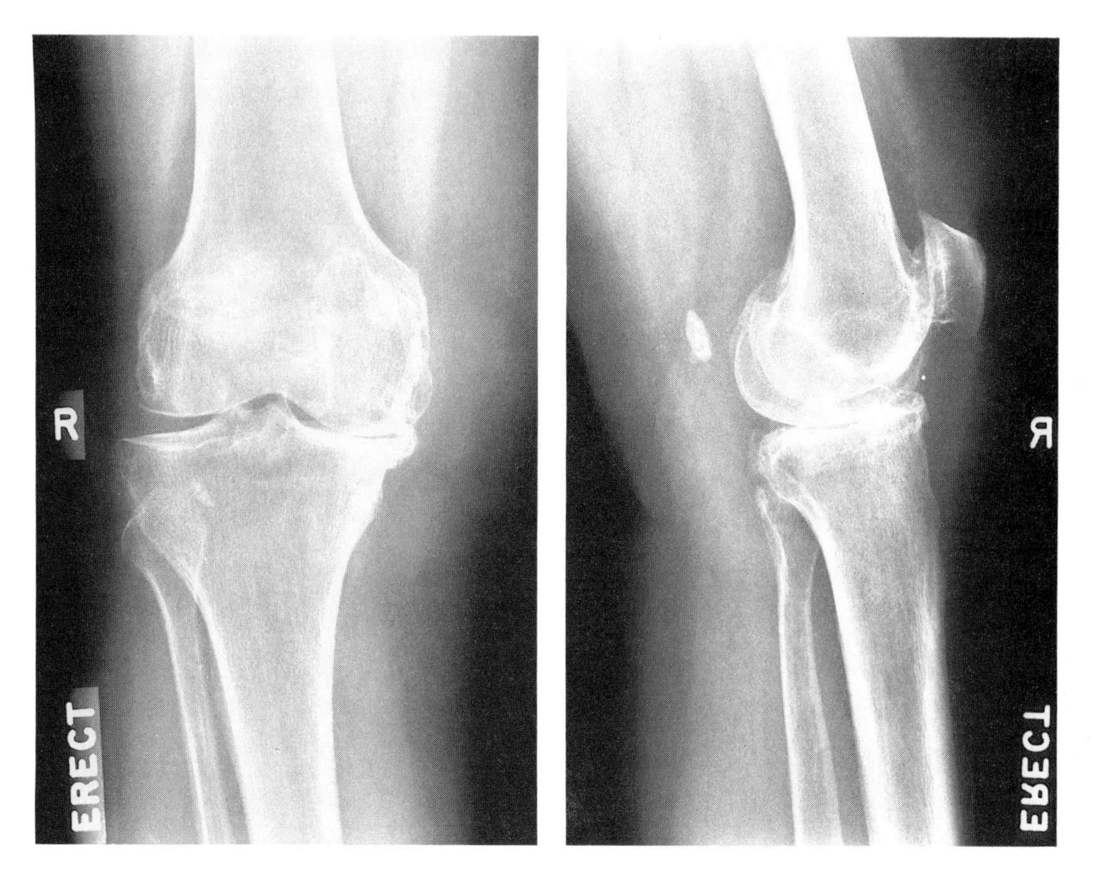

AP and lateral views of the right knee of a 73-year-old woman with pain in the right knee.

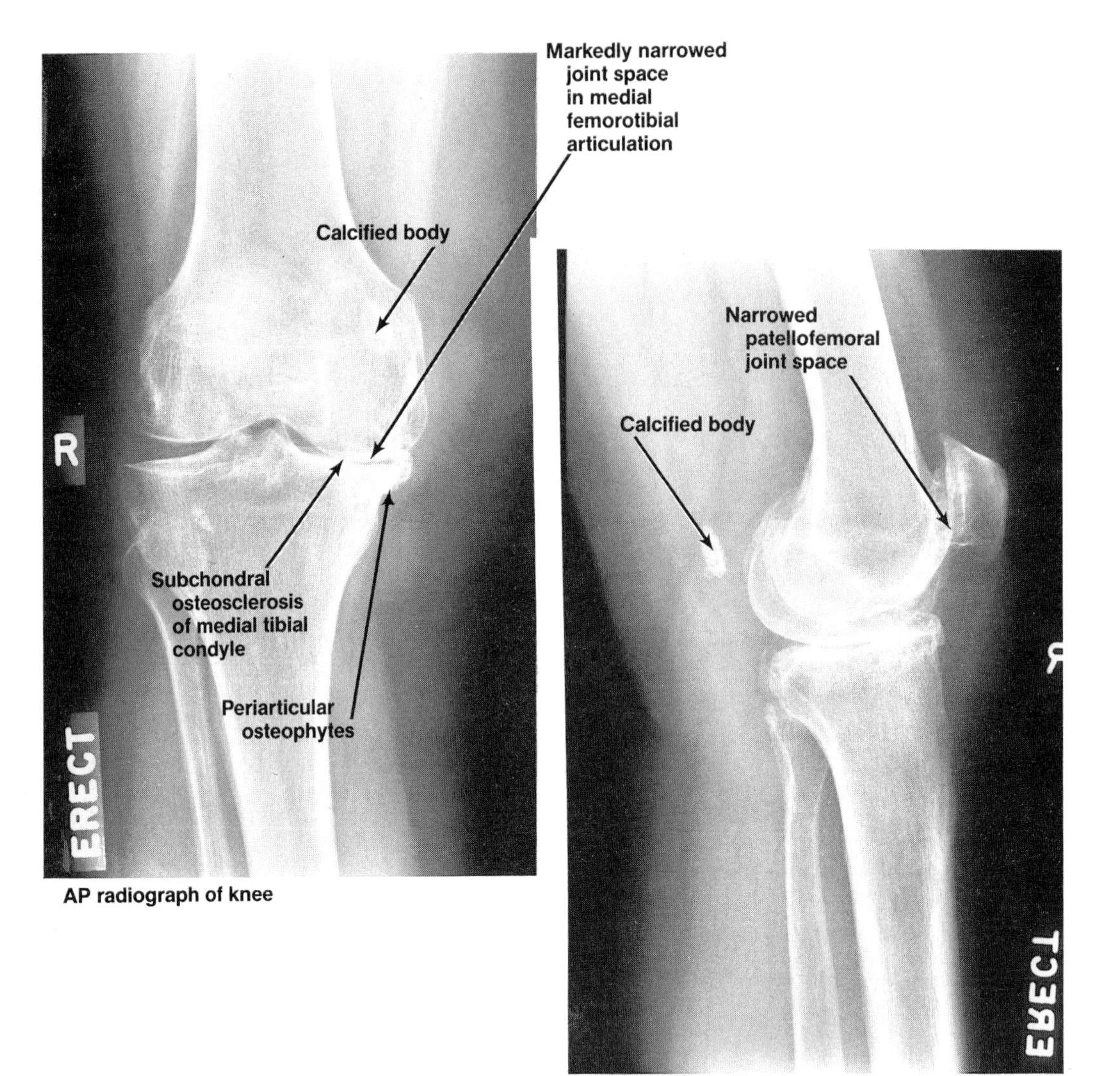

AP radiograph of knee

Lateral radiograph of knee

Case 9 discussion. [*Chapter 2 II E 8 a, b*] The radiographs show evidence of osteoarthritis of the right knee. A common etiology for osteoarthritis of the knee joint is development of a varus or valgus deformity at the knee. In a varus deformity, increased stress is applied across the medial femorotibial articulation; in a valgus deformity, the increased stress is applied across the lateral femorotibial articulation. In either deformity, the stress produces subchondral osteosclerosis in the underlying tibial condyle and loss of its articular cartilage. Other common findings are periarticular osteophytes (a consequence of subchondral bone formation and remodeling) and subchondral cysts.

The radiographs were taken with the patient standing upright, so as to show the configuration of the knee when weight-bearing. The pertinent findings exhibited in the radiographs are as follows:

(1) The AP view shows a varus deformity at the knee. There is a marked loss of articular cartilage in the medial femorotibial articulation, as evidenced by the almost obliterated space between the medial femoral and medial tibial condyles. Such localized narrowing of a joint cartilage space is characteristic of osteoarthritis.

(2) There is subchondral osteosclerosis of the medial tibial condyle, as evidenced by the fact that the subchondral bone of the medial tibial condyle is more radiopaque than that of the lateral tibial condyle.

(3) The AP view shows periarticular osteophytes along the medial margin of the medial tibial plateau.

(4) The lateral view suggests that there is also narrowing of the patellofemoral joint space.

(5) The AP and lateral radiographs together show a calcified body behind the medial part of the distal femur; this calcified body is not a fabella.

Case 10

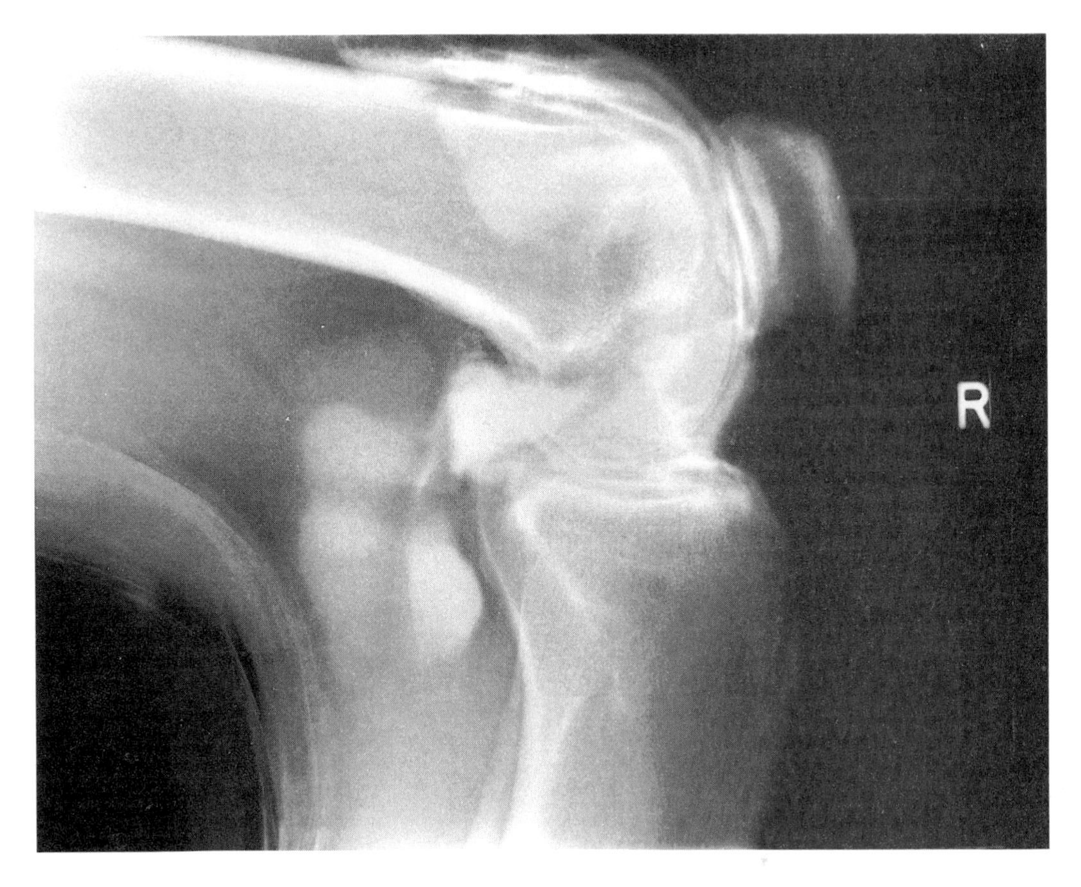

Lateral view of an arthrogram of the right knee of a 45-year-old man with a painful swelling in the popliteal fossa of the right knee.

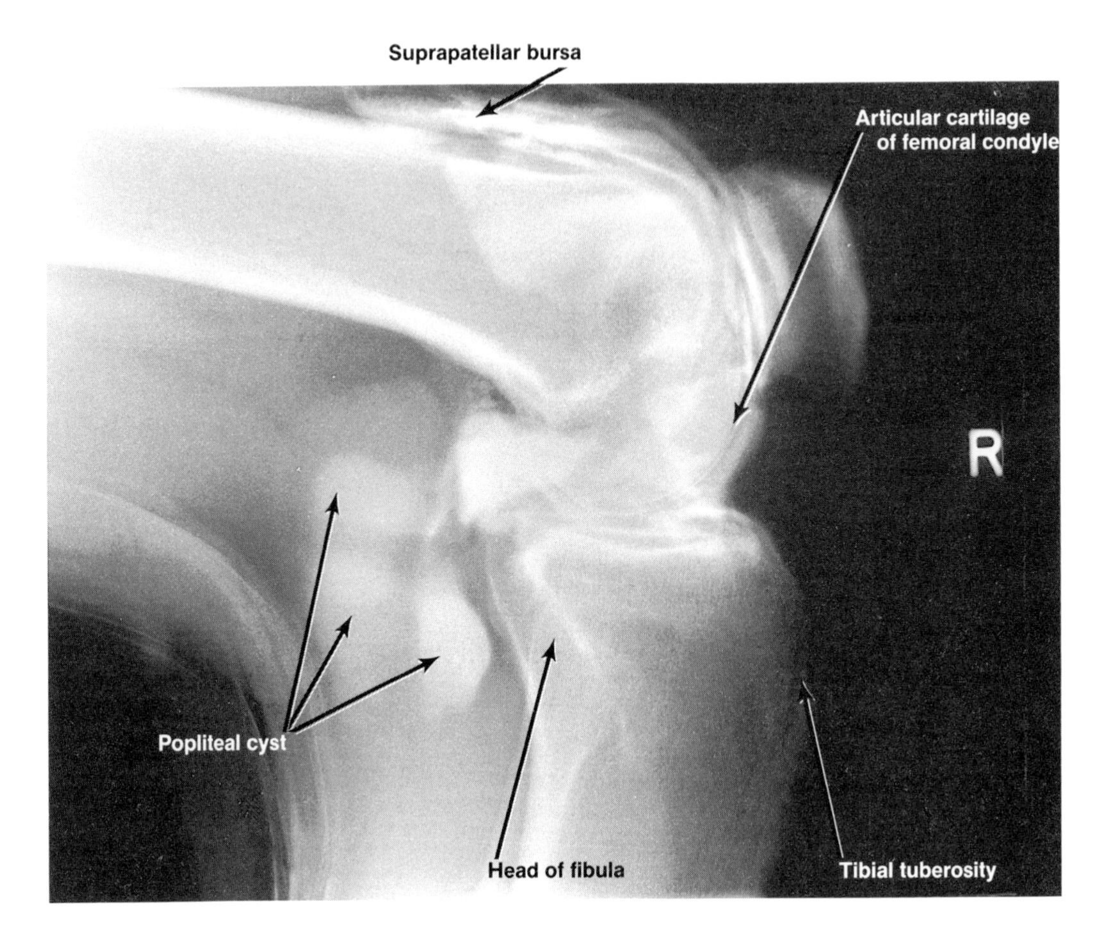

Case 10 discussion. [*Chapter 2 II A 2 a (3) (a)*] The radiograph shows a popliteal (or Baker's) cyst of the right knee. Most popliteal cysts represent a distended gastrocnemius or semimembranosus bursa or a fluid-filled cyst lined with fibrous tissue. Since most popliteal cysts communicate with the synovial cavity of the knee joint, diagnosis may be confirmed by an arthrogram of the knee, which involves injecting a radiopaque solution into the knee joint's synovial cavity and taking multiple projections of the knee.

Popliteal cysts are a common complication of rheumatoid arthritis. Most popliteal cysts are asymptomatic, but rupture of the cyst and dissection of its fluid contents into either the lower posterior thigh or upper calf may produce acute pain. The signs and symptoms of a painful popliteal cyst resemble those of thrombophlebitis; diagnosis of an inflamed thrombotic vein in the popliteal fossa may be confirmed by venograms or a Doppler study.

Case 11

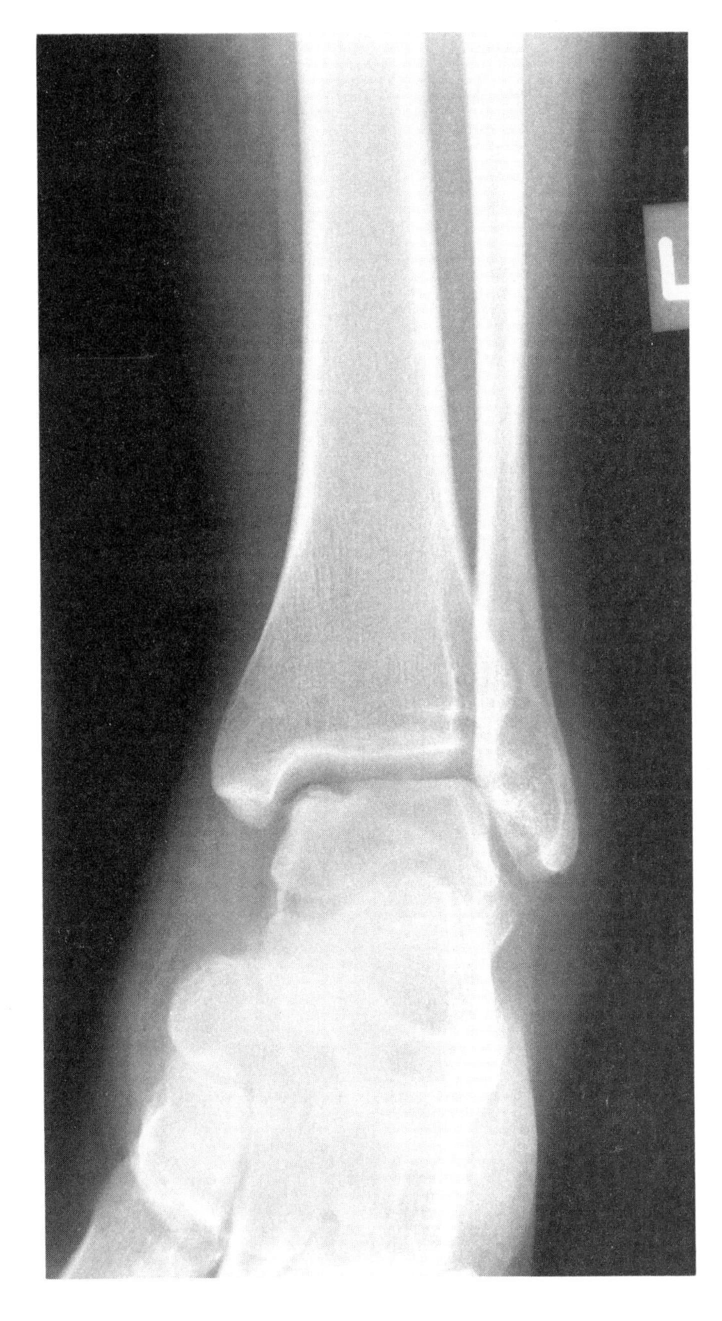

AP view of the left ankle of a 33-year-old professional dancer with pain in her left ankle.

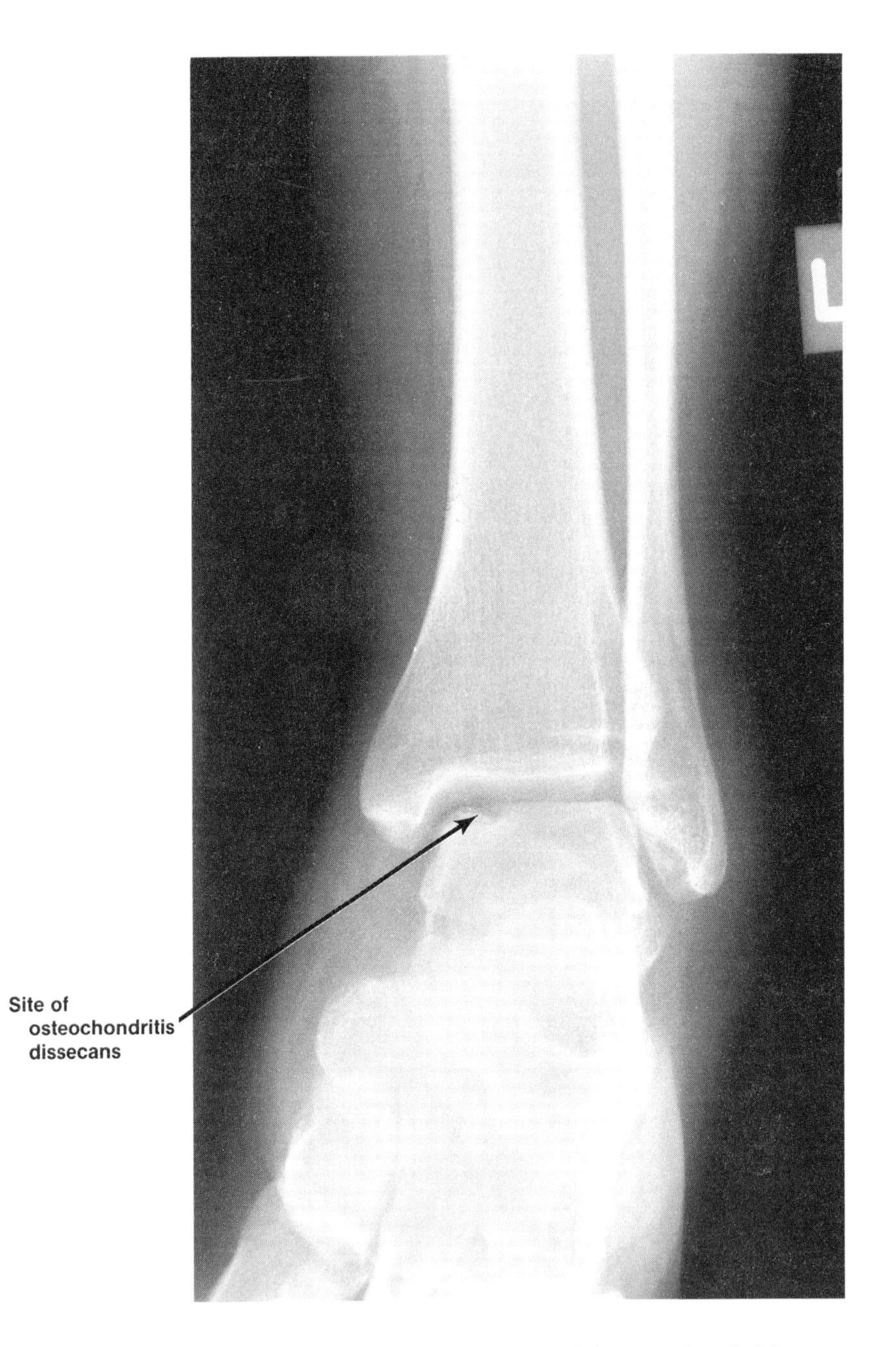

Case 11 discussion. [*Chapter 2 II E 6*] The radiograph shows a subtle osteochondral fracture near the medial margin of the dome of the talus which has progressed to osteochondritis dissecans of the talus. (In the knee, which is the most common site of osteochondritis dissecans, most of the lesions occur in the lateral aspect of the medial femoral condyle). The radiograph of the dancer's ankle shows that there is no dislodgement of the osteochondral fragment. The radiograph does not show uniformly wide joint spaces within the ankle joint nor colinearity between the floor of the fibular notch of the tibia and the lateral margin of the body of the talus; this is because the patient's foot was not internally rotated for a mortise radiograph of the ankle.

Case 12

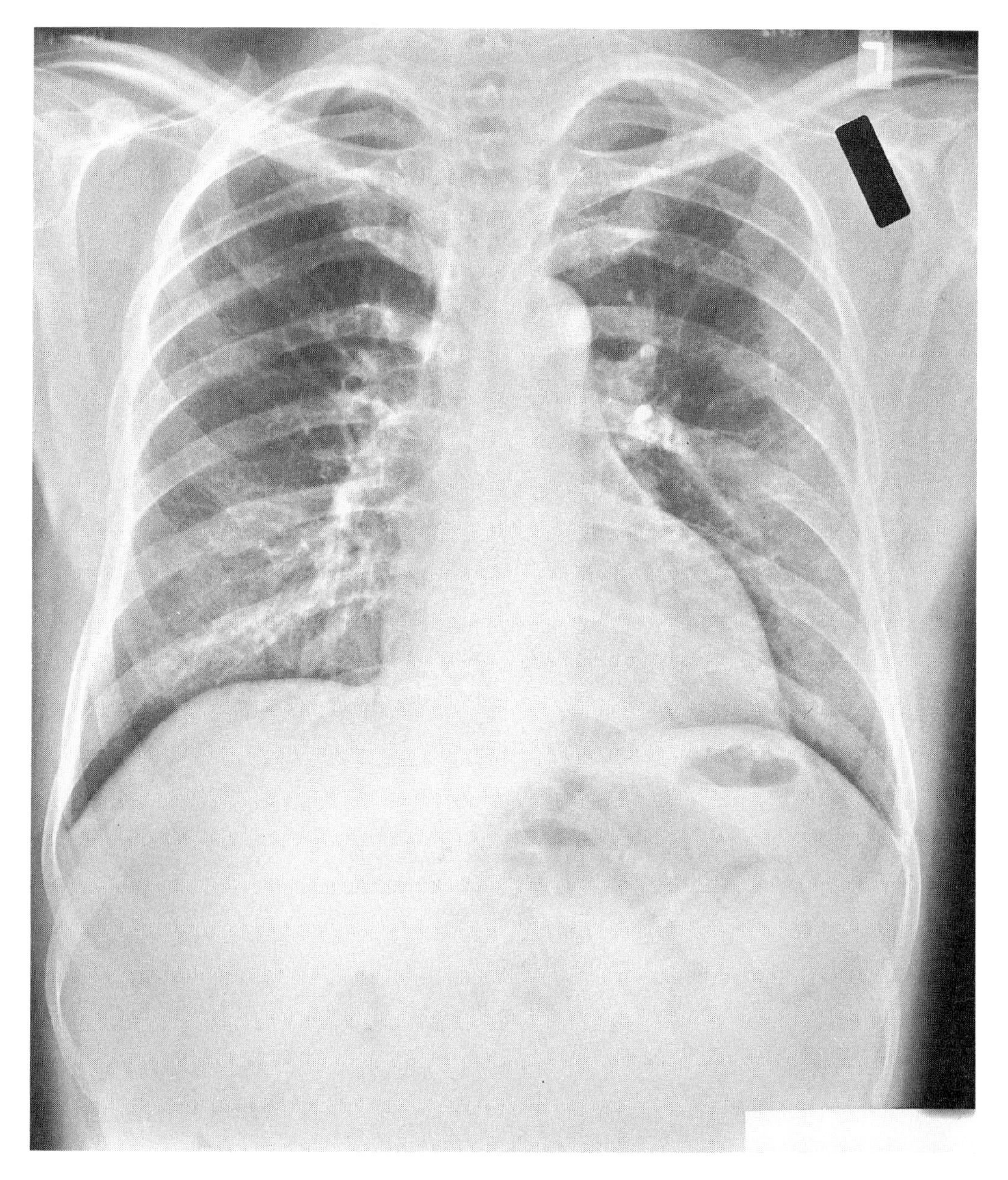

PA and lateral chest films taken during the annual physical examination of a 64-year-old man.

continued on next page

Case 12 *continued*

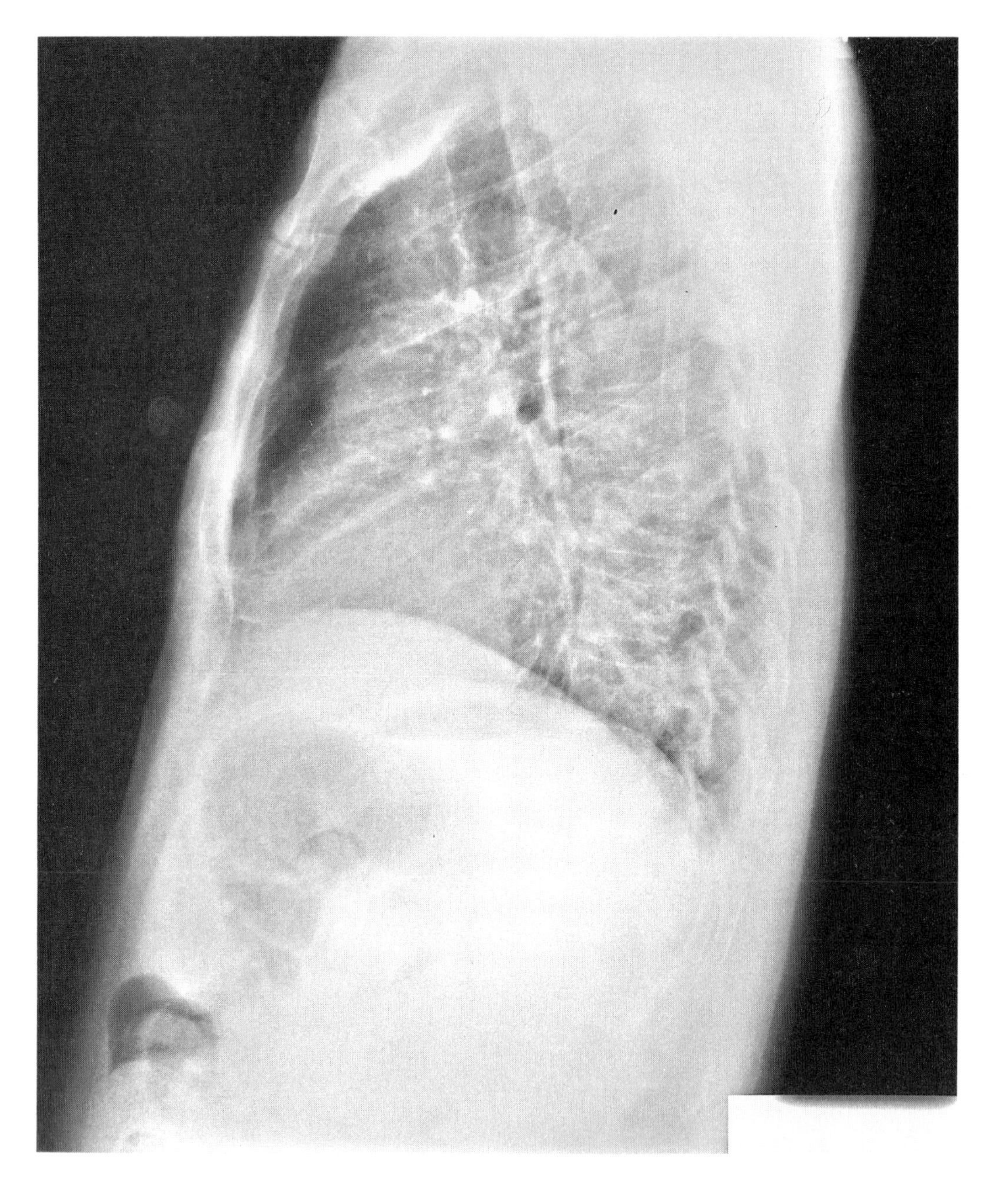

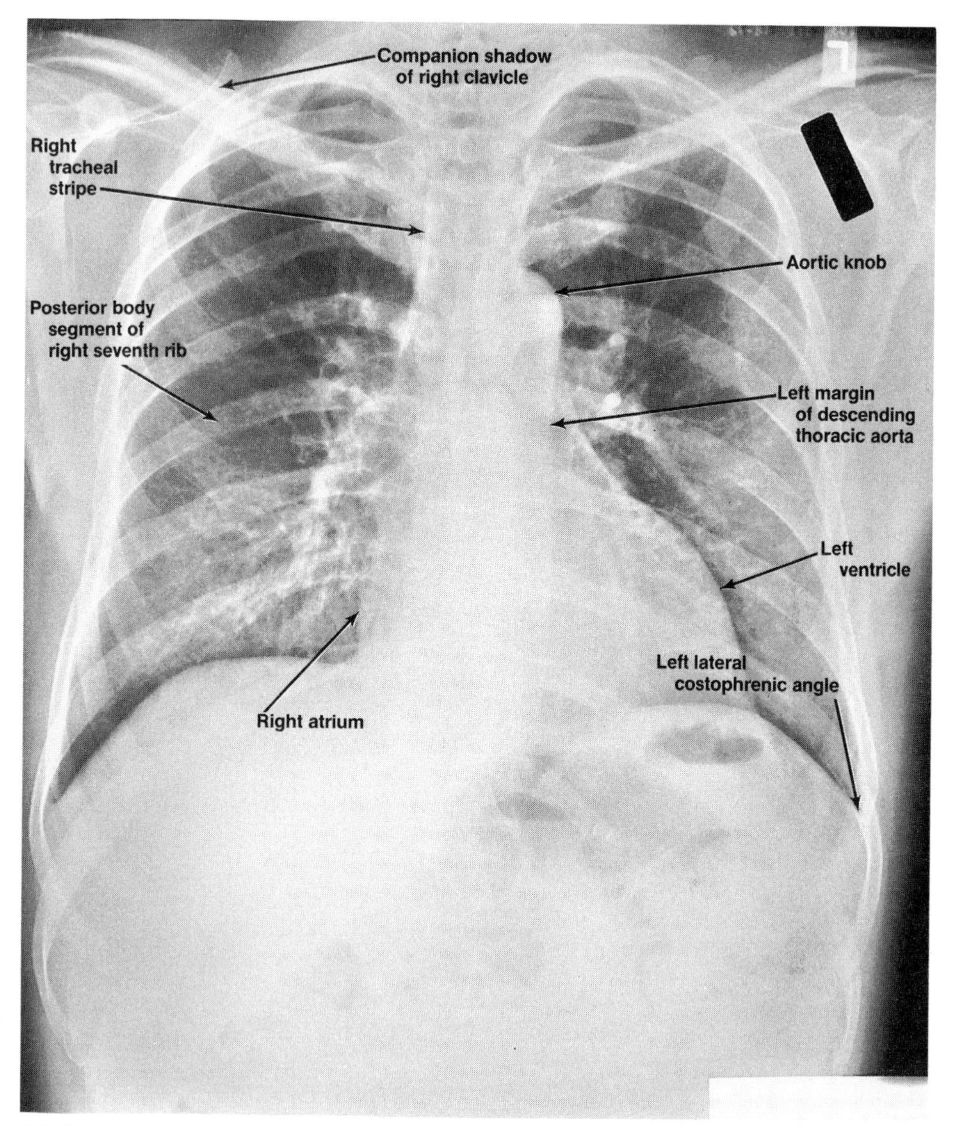

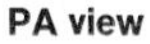
PA view

Case 12 discussion. [*Chapter 3 II A, B*] The chest films appear normal. The PA chest film was properly taken: it is adequately penetrated (since the bodies of the thoracic vertebrae are discernible within the central cardiovascular shadow), and the coronal plane of the patient's body was oriented perpendicular to the path of the x-ray beam (since the medial ends of the clavicles are equidistant from the midlines of the bodies of the thoracic vertebrae). The clavicles, the bodies and pedicles of the vertebrae, and the ribs do not show any notable abnormalities (such as lytic or sclerotic lesions). Each clavicle is accompanied by its companion shadow. There is no evidence of generalized cardiomegaly, as the cardiothoracic ratio is about 0.5 (which is the maximum magnitude within the normal range of the ratio). The left and right borders of the central cardiovascular shadow are well delineated; the left margin of the descending thoracic aorta is also well defined. The lumina of the trachea and its main stem bronchi are visible; the width of the right tracheal stripe is normal and the size of the subcarinal angle is normal. The left hilum is higher than the right hilum. The lung fields and their vascularity appear normal. The lateral costophrenic angles appear normal. The right dome of the diaphragm is higher than the left dome; although this relationship is the most common one, its reversal would not by itself have any significance. The lateral chest film establishes that the gas bubble underlying the left dome of the diaphragm is located in the fundus of the stomach and that the other collections of gas seen in the PA chest film are colonic gas located in the splenic flexure or the distal part of the transverse colon.

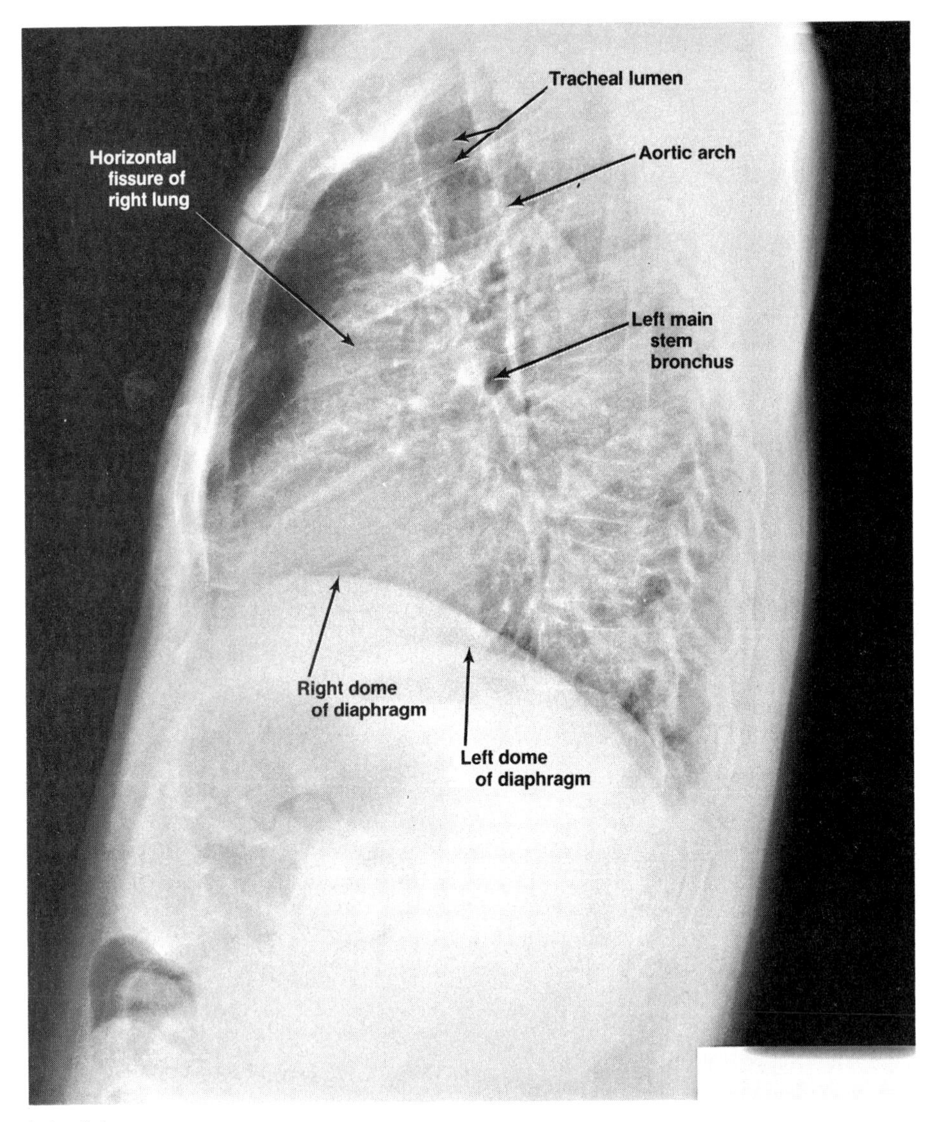

Lateral view

In the lateral chest film, the bodies of the thoracic vertebrae appear, as they should, progressively more radiolucent inferiorly, since the lateral view superimposes the radiodensities of the posterior parts of both lungs on the bodies of the thoracic vertebrae, and the radiolucency of the parenchyma of each lung appears to increase inferiorly as the chest widens. The ascending aorta, aortic arch, and upper part of the descending thoracic aorta are visible. As the tracheal lumen descends obliquely through the superior mediastinum, it crosses the highest part of the aortic arch. The water-density stripe representing the posterior tracheal wall and collapsed esophagus together is normal in width and appearance. The small, almost circular air-density area in the upper part of the retrocardiac area most likely represents the left main stem bronchus; the fine, water-density line that arcs anteriorly from just above this air-density circle represents the horizontal fissure of the right lung. The oblique fissures of the lungs are not clearly visible; however, their failure to project as fine water-density lines can be encountered under both normal and abnormal conditions. The retrosternal area, which principally represents the superimposed radiolucencies of the anterior bronchopulmonary segments of the upper lobes of both lungs, appears normal. Vascular markings in the retrocardiac area obscure the posterior wall of the cardiac shadow; the retrocardiac area represents the superimposed radiodensities of the basal bronchopulmonary segments of the lower lobes of both lungs. The posterior costophrenic angles, which show the lowest region of the costodiaphragmatic recess in each pleural cavity, appear normal. The domed water-density shadow directly over the fundic gas bubble represents the left dome of the diaphragm and the wall of the cardiac region of the stomach.

Case 13

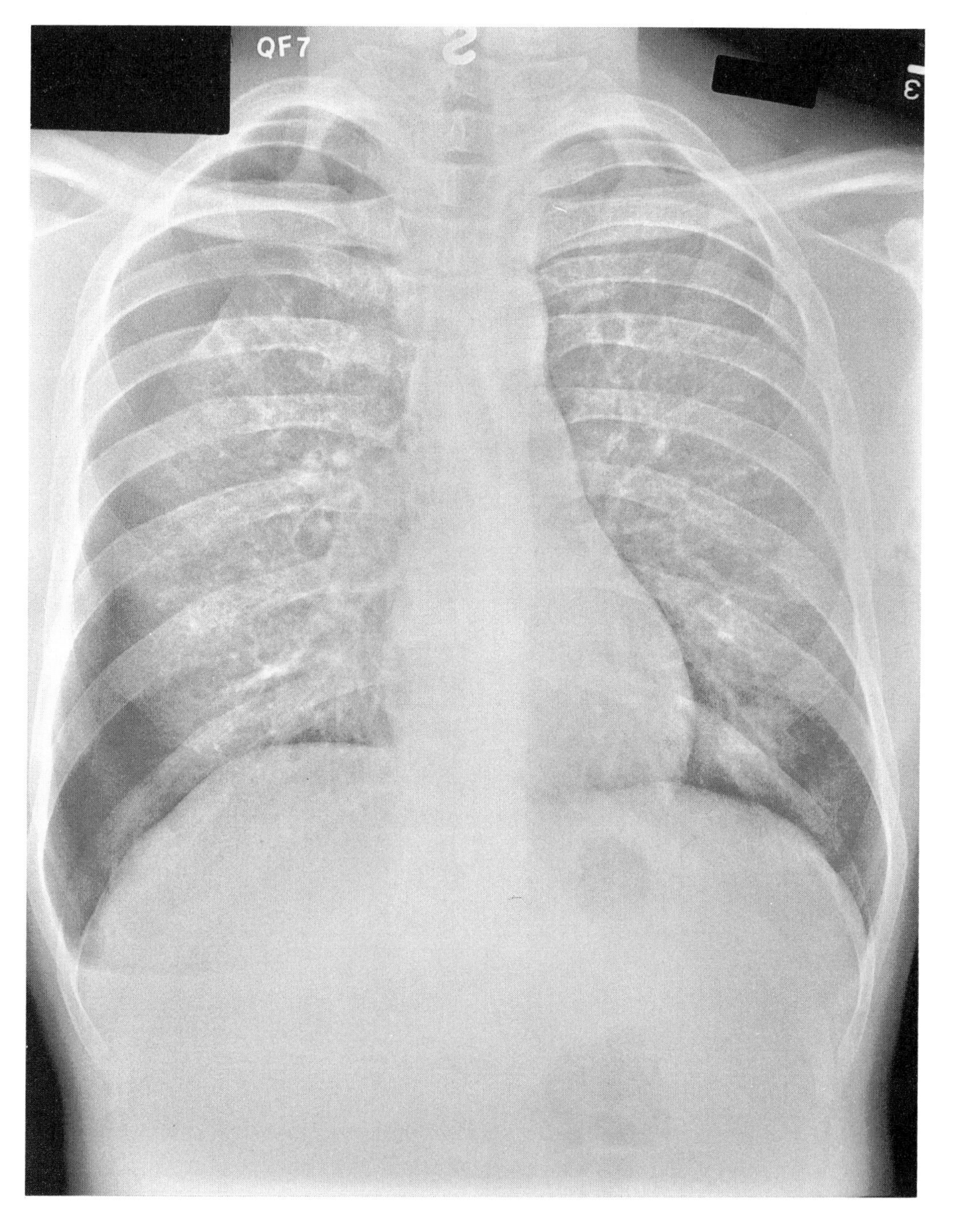

PA chest film of a 28-year-old man with dyspnea (i.e., shortness of breath).

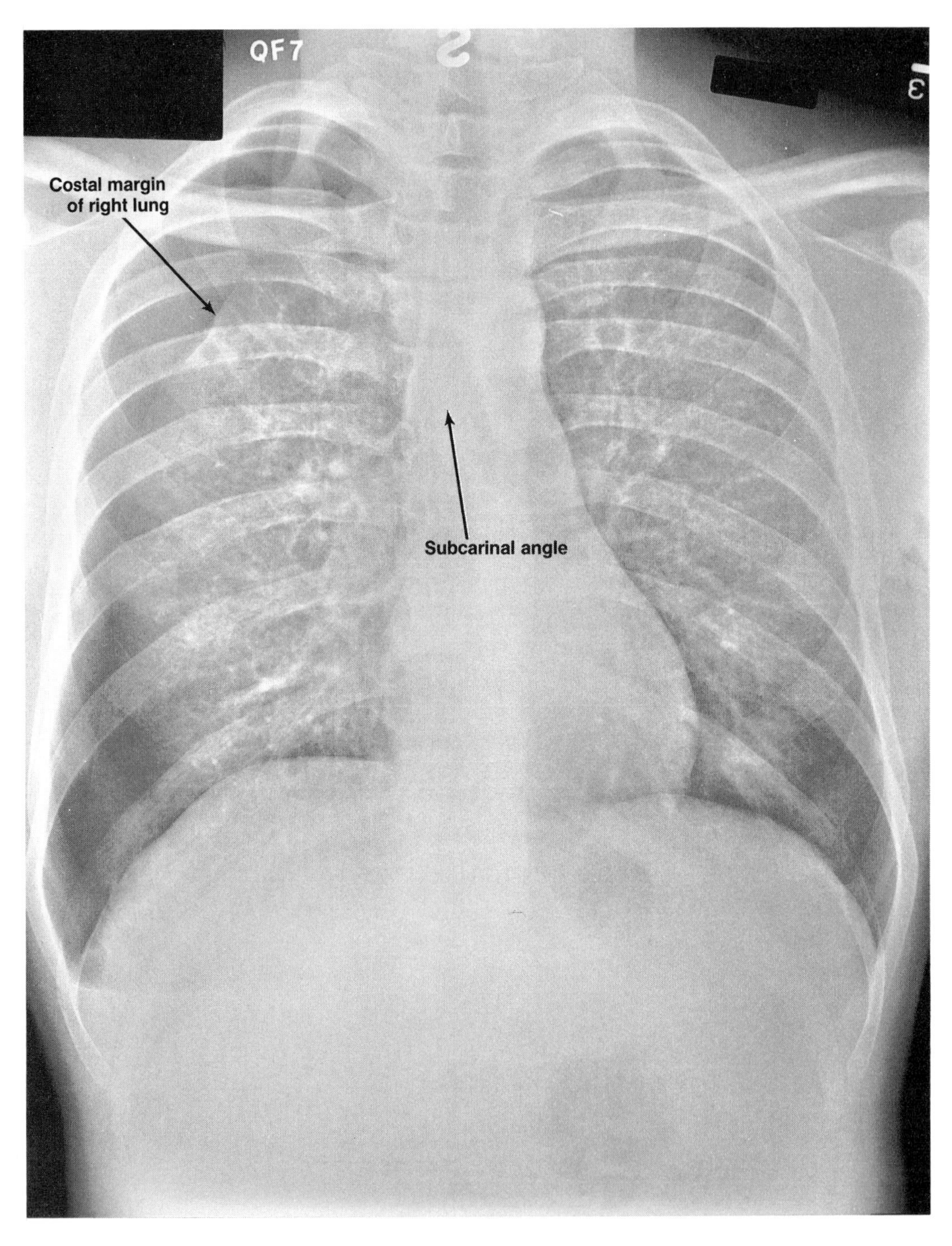

Case 13 discussion. [*Chapter 3 IV D 6*] The chest film shows a pneumothorax of the right lung. The apex of the right lung is seen near the medial end of the right fourth posterior interspace; the costal margin of the right lung curves inferolaterally from the apex toward the lateral end of the right dome of the diaphragm. The right pneumothorax has produced a slight mediastinal shift to the left; this is evidenced in two ways: (1) the right lower border of the cardiovascular shadow is superimposed on the right lateral border of the vertebral column, and (2) the mediastinal shift to the left has diminished the subcarinal angle.

Case 14

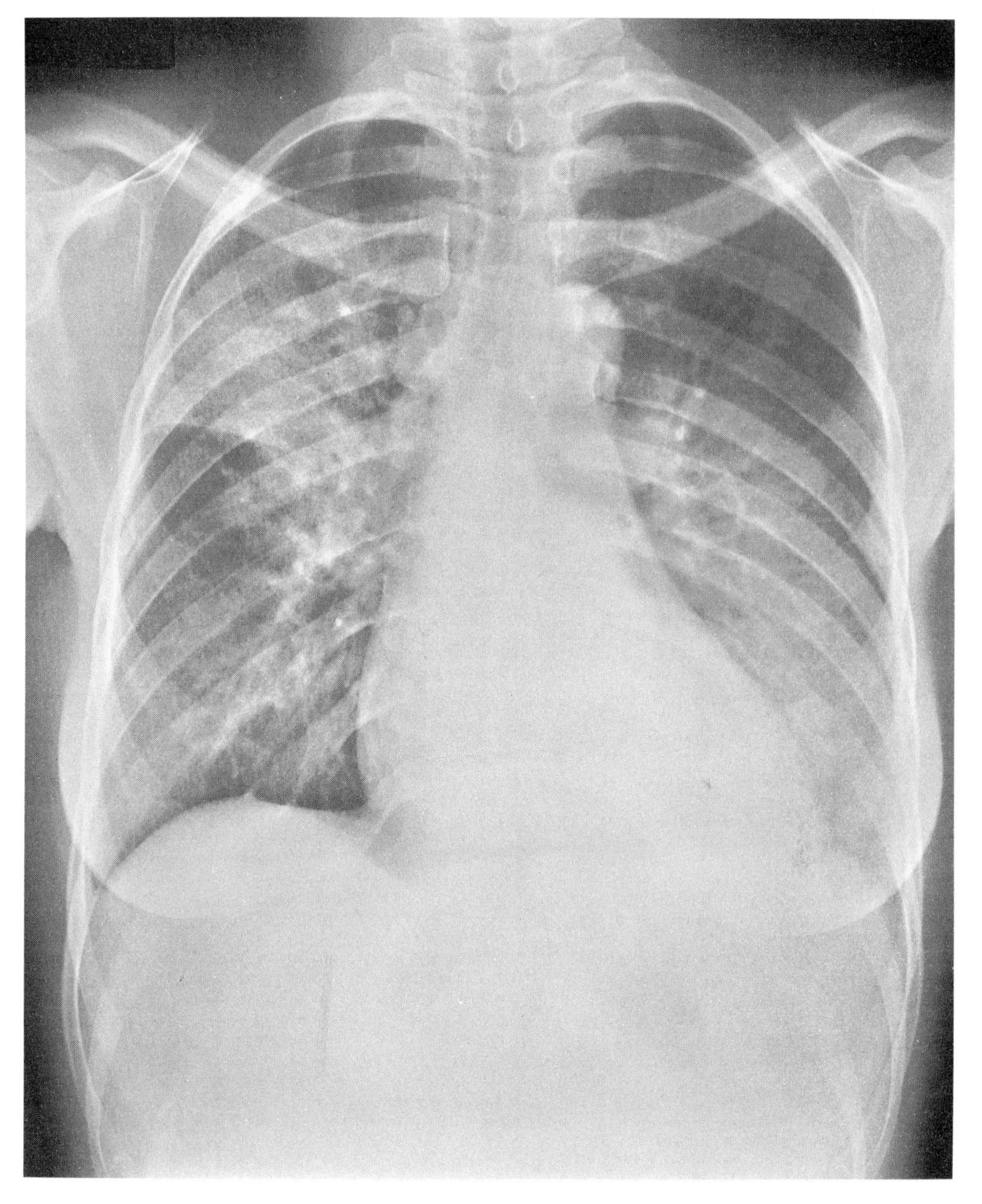

PA and lateral chest films of a 44-year-old woman with fever, cough, and dyspnea.

continued on next page

Case 14 *continued*

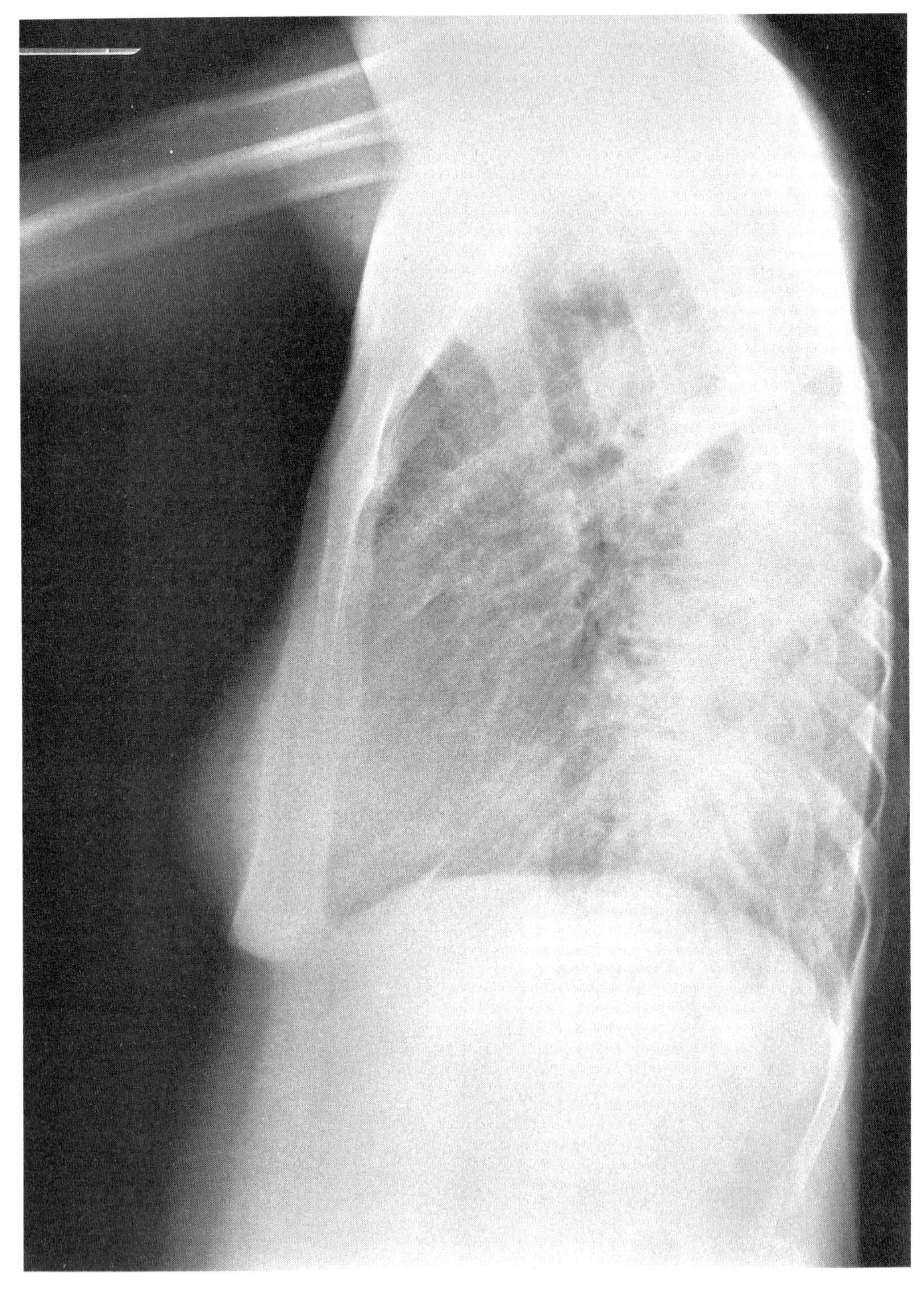

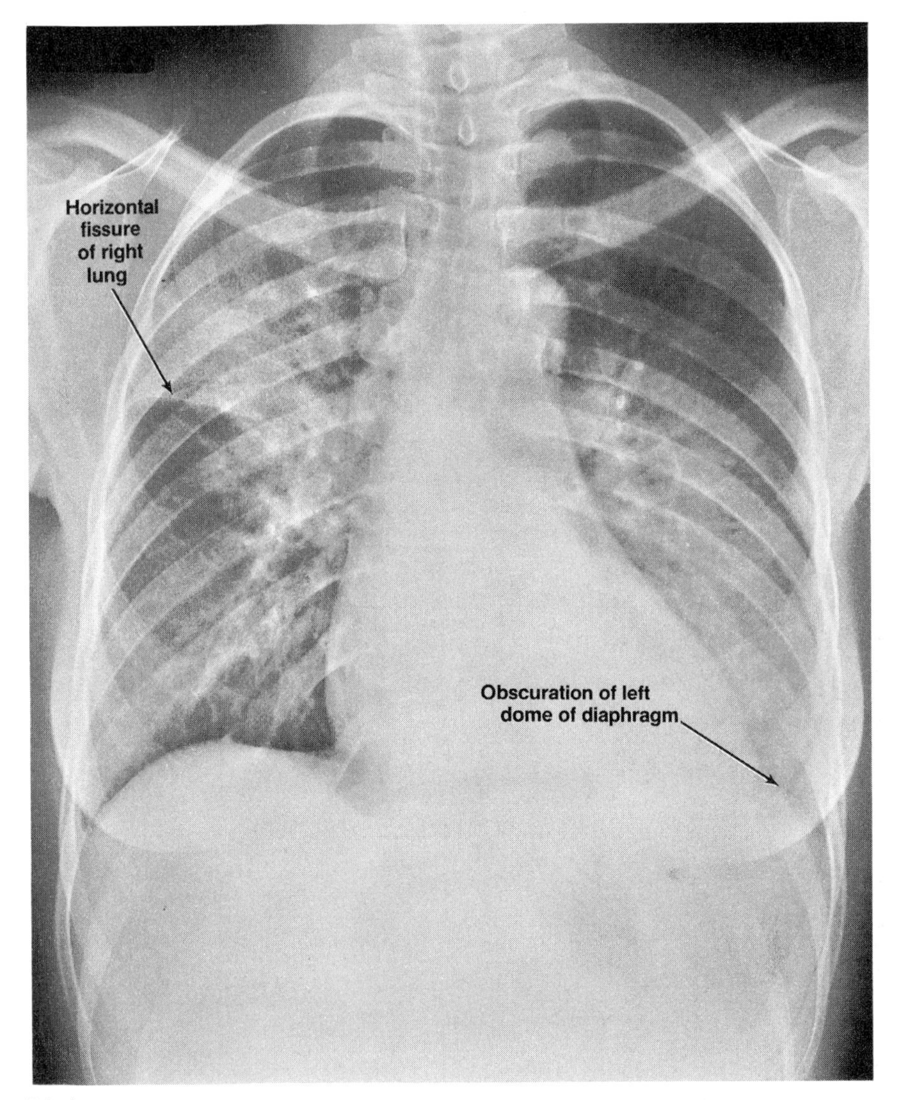

PA view

Case 14 discussion. [*Chapter 3 IV D 2*] The PA chest film shows consolidation of the upper part of the right lung and the lower part of the left lung.

Three findings indicate that the consolidation process in the right lung involves its upper lobe:

(1) The PA chest film shows that the area of consolidation is bordered inferiorly by the horizontal fissure and thus is located, at least in part, in the upper lobe.

(2) The PA chest film shows that the consolidation has produced a silhouette sign; specifically, it has obscured the upper part of the right border of the cardiovascular shadow. This particular silhouette sign indicates that the consolidation process in the upper lobe involves at a minimum the anterior bronchopulmonary segment.

(3) The lateral chest film shows consolidation of both the retrosternal area and an area directly posterior to the lower end of the tracheal lumen. The consolidation of the retrosternal area is due to the consolidation of the anterior segment of the right lung's upper lobe; this is because the retrosternal area shows the superimposed radiolucencies of principally the anterior bronchopulmonary segments of the upper lobes of both lungs. The area directly posterior to the tracheal lumen shows the radiolucencies of the apical and posterior segments of the upper lobe of the right lung superimposed upon those of the apical posterior segment of the upper lobe of the left lung. Therefore, consolidation of this area indicates that the consolidation process also involves one or both of the apical and posterior segments in the upper lobe of the right lung.

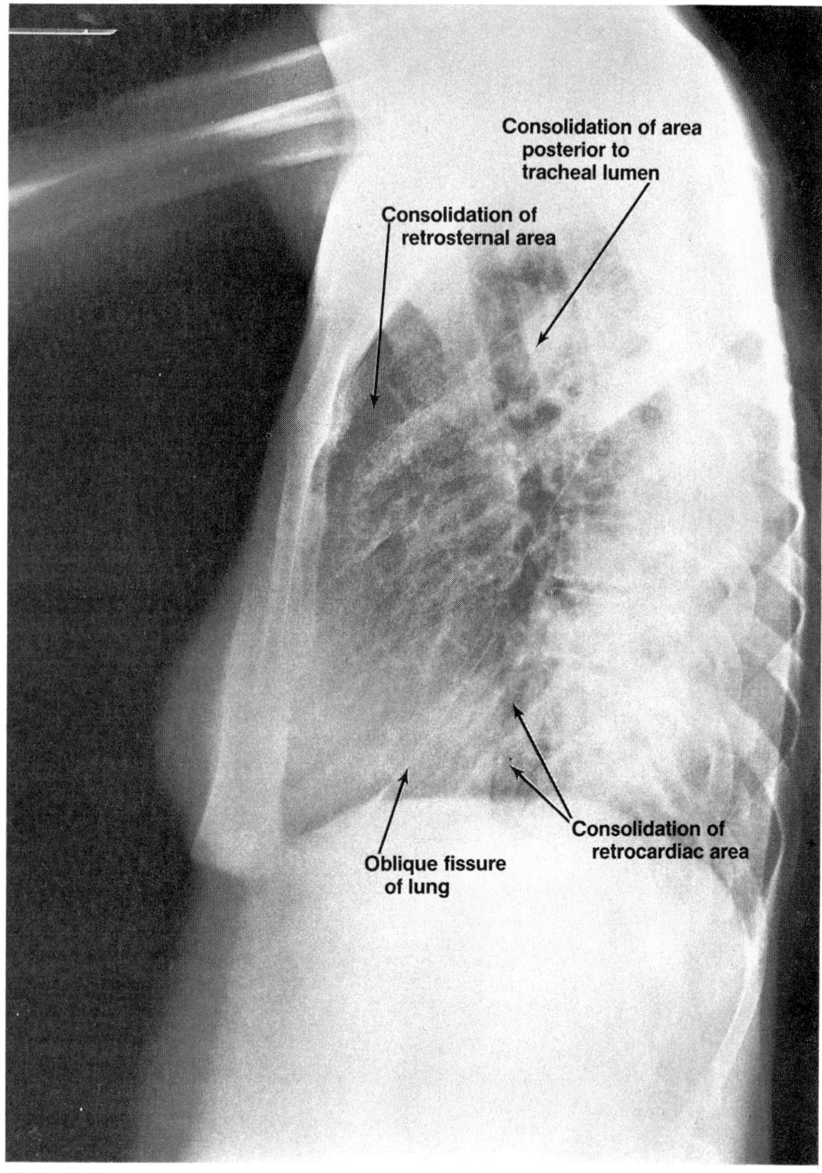

Lateral view

Two findings indicate that the consolidation process in the left lung involves its lower lobe:

(1) The PA chest film shows that the consolidation has produced a second silhouette sign; specifically, it has obscured the lateral margin of the left dome of the diaphragm. This particular silhouette sign indicates that the consolidation process is located, at least in part, in the lower lobe and involves one or more of its basal bronchopulmonary segments.

(2) The lateral chest film shows consolidation of the retrocardiac area; the retrocardiac area shows the superimposed radiodensities of principally the basal bronchopulmonary segments of the lower lobes of both lungs. The consolidation in the retrocardiac area has obscured the left dome of the diaphragm, is superimposed in part upon the bodies of the lower thoracic vertebrae, and lies posterior to the fine water-density lines representing the oblique, or major, fissures of the lungs. All these findings are consistent with the conclusion that the consolidation in the lower part of the left lung involves one or more of the basal segments of its lower lobe.

Pneumonia was responsible for this patient's respiratory symptoms and radiographic findings.

Case 15

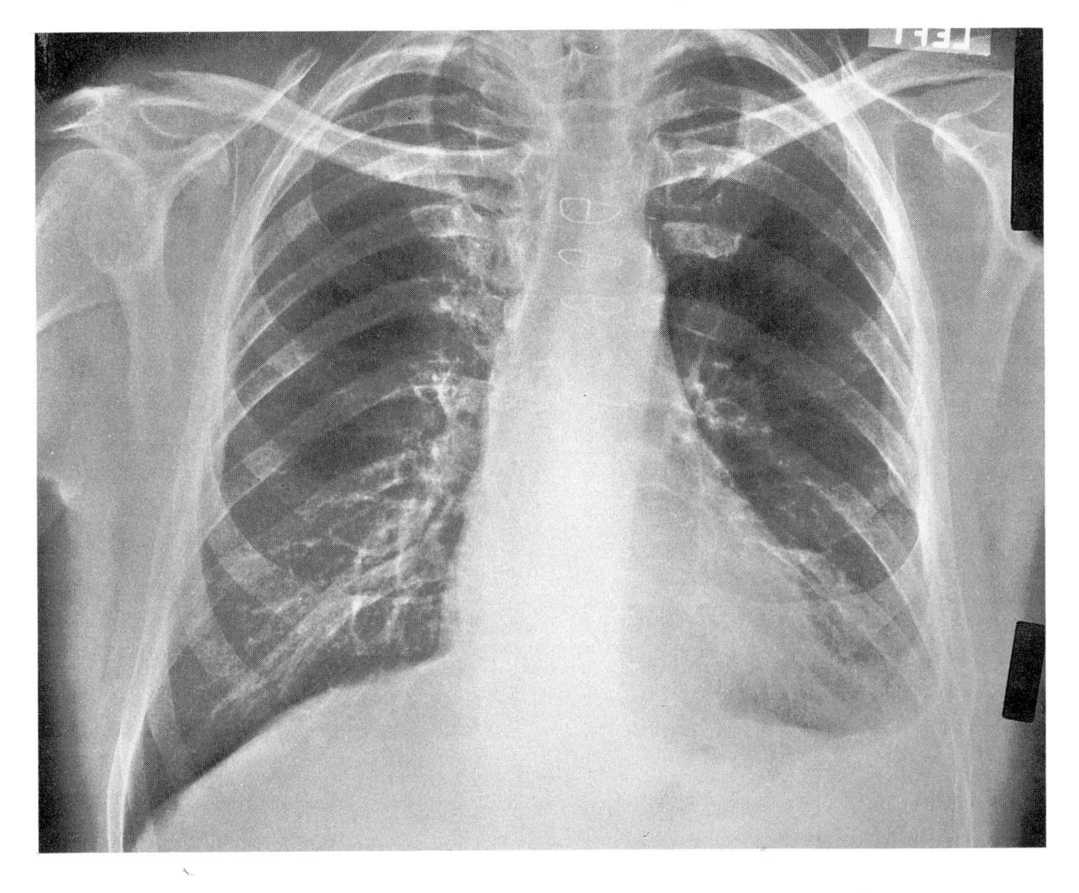

PA and lateral chest films of a 64-year-old man who has recently undergone coronary artery bypass surgery.

continued on next page

Case 15 *continued*

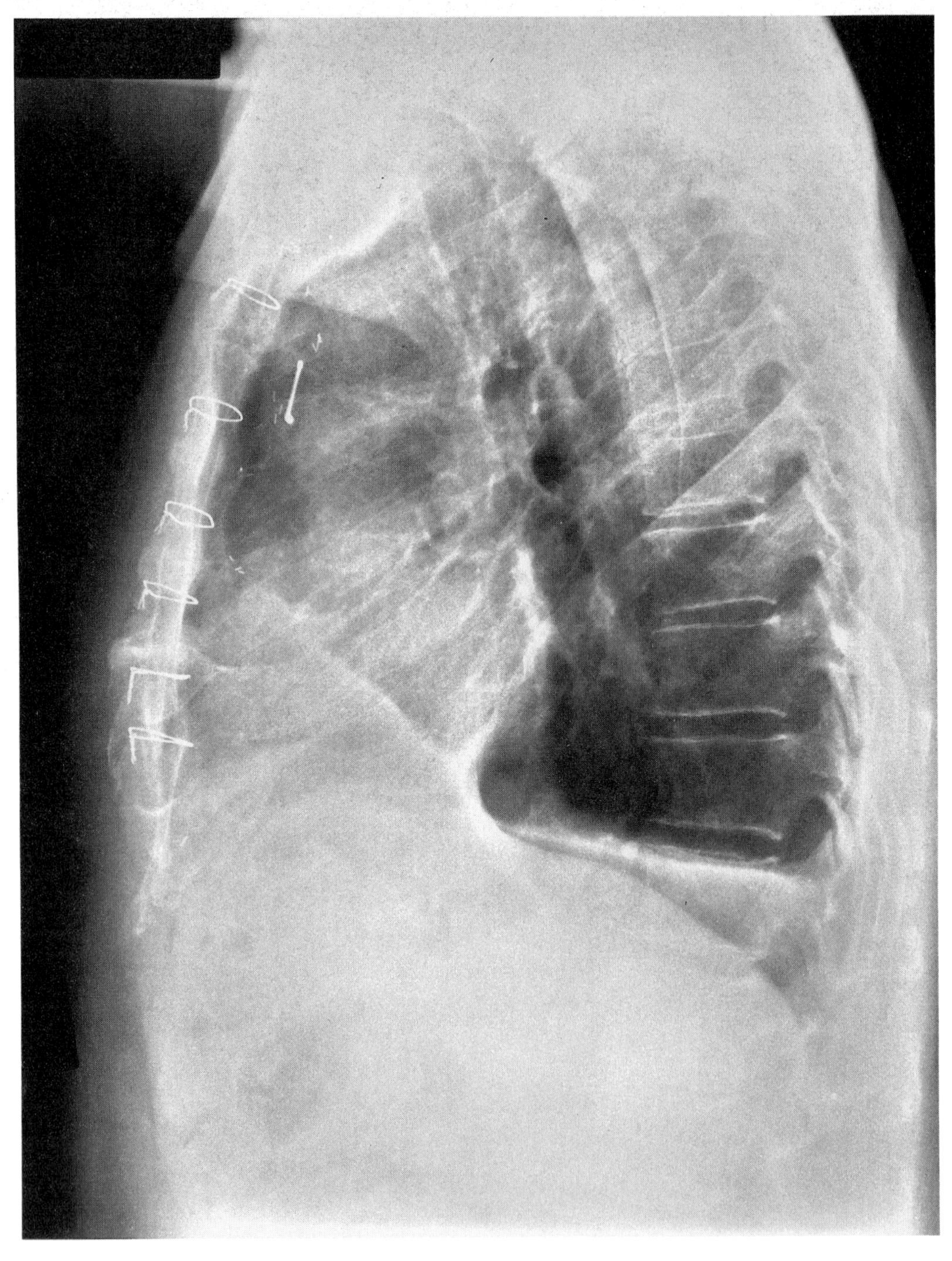

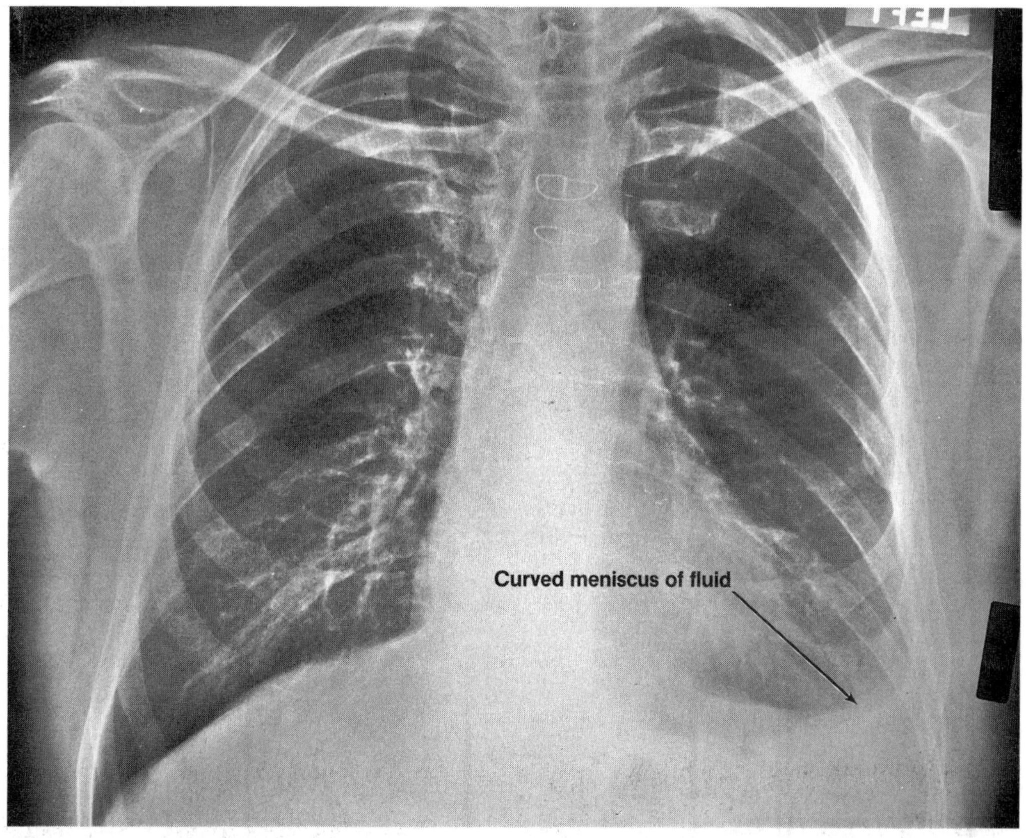

PA view

Case 15 discussion. [*Chapter 3 IV D 5*] The PA chest film shows a curved meniscus of fluid in the lower portion of the left pleural cavity and obscuration of the lower part of the heart's left border. The pleural effusion in the left pleural cavity already exceeds 500 ml in volume, as it has completely filled the lateral and anterior margins of the costodiaphragmatic recess. The lateral chest film shows that the pleural effusion in the posterior part of the left pleural cavity has risen to the level of the upper border of the body of the tenth thoracic vertebra.

continued on next page

Case 15 discussion *continued*

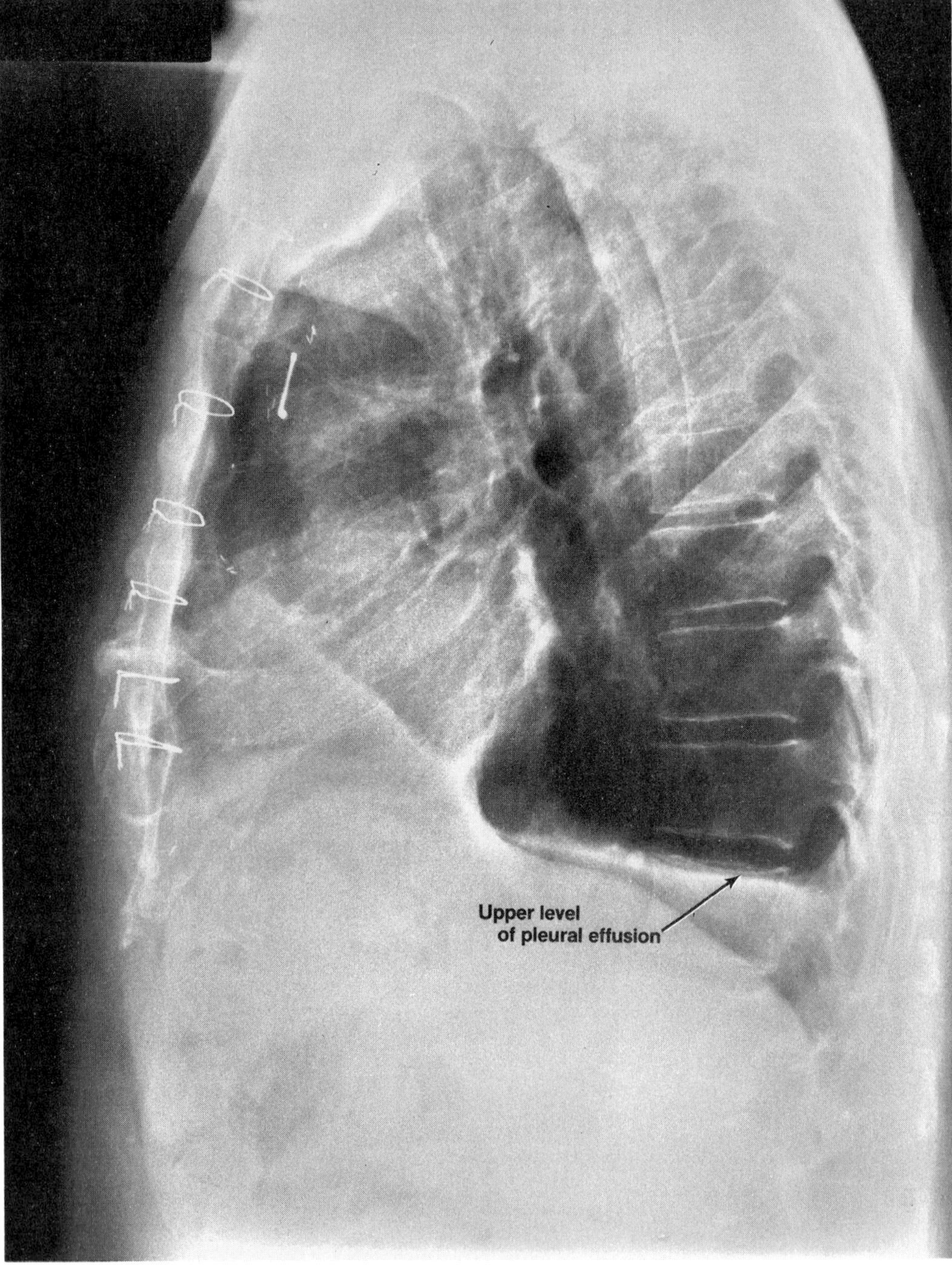

Lateral view

Case 16

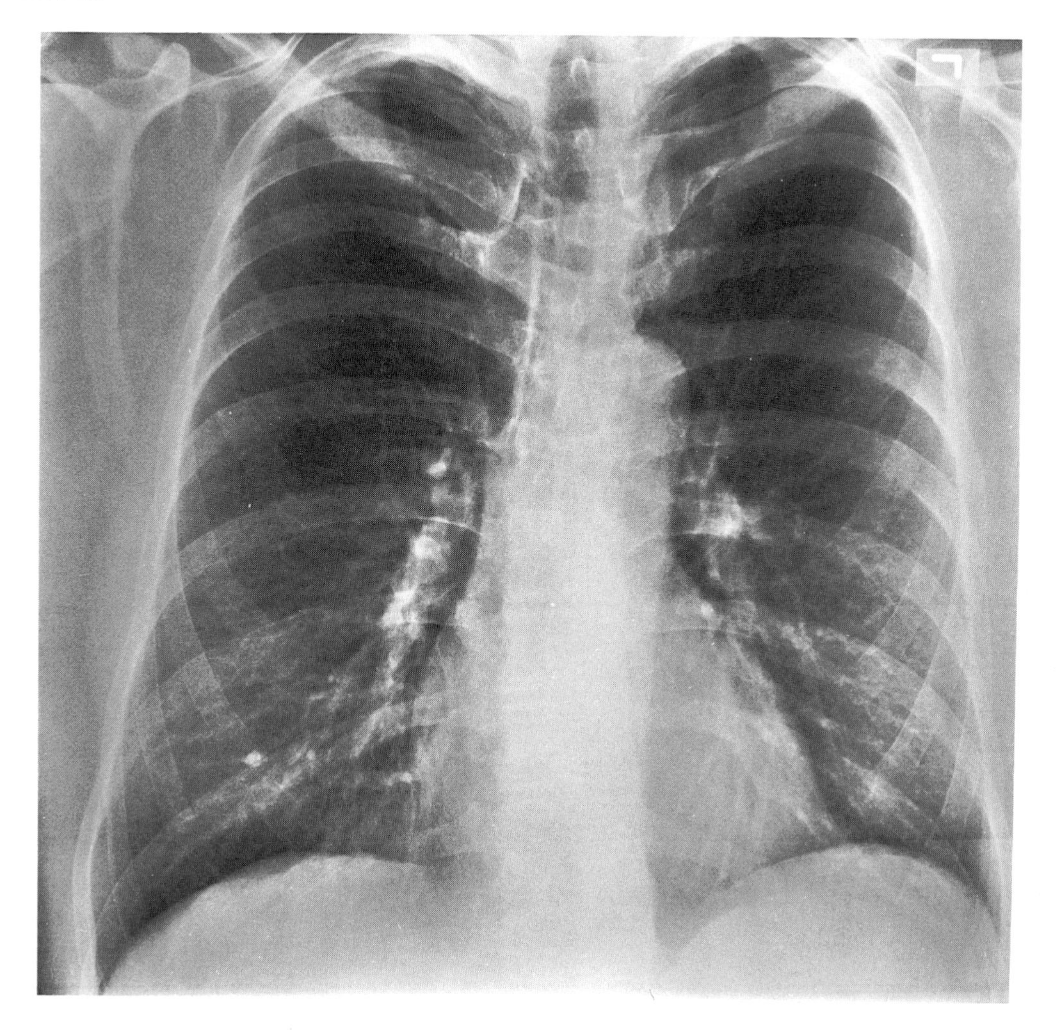

PA and lateral chest films taken during the annual physical examination of a 47-year-old man.

continued on next page

Case 16 *continued*

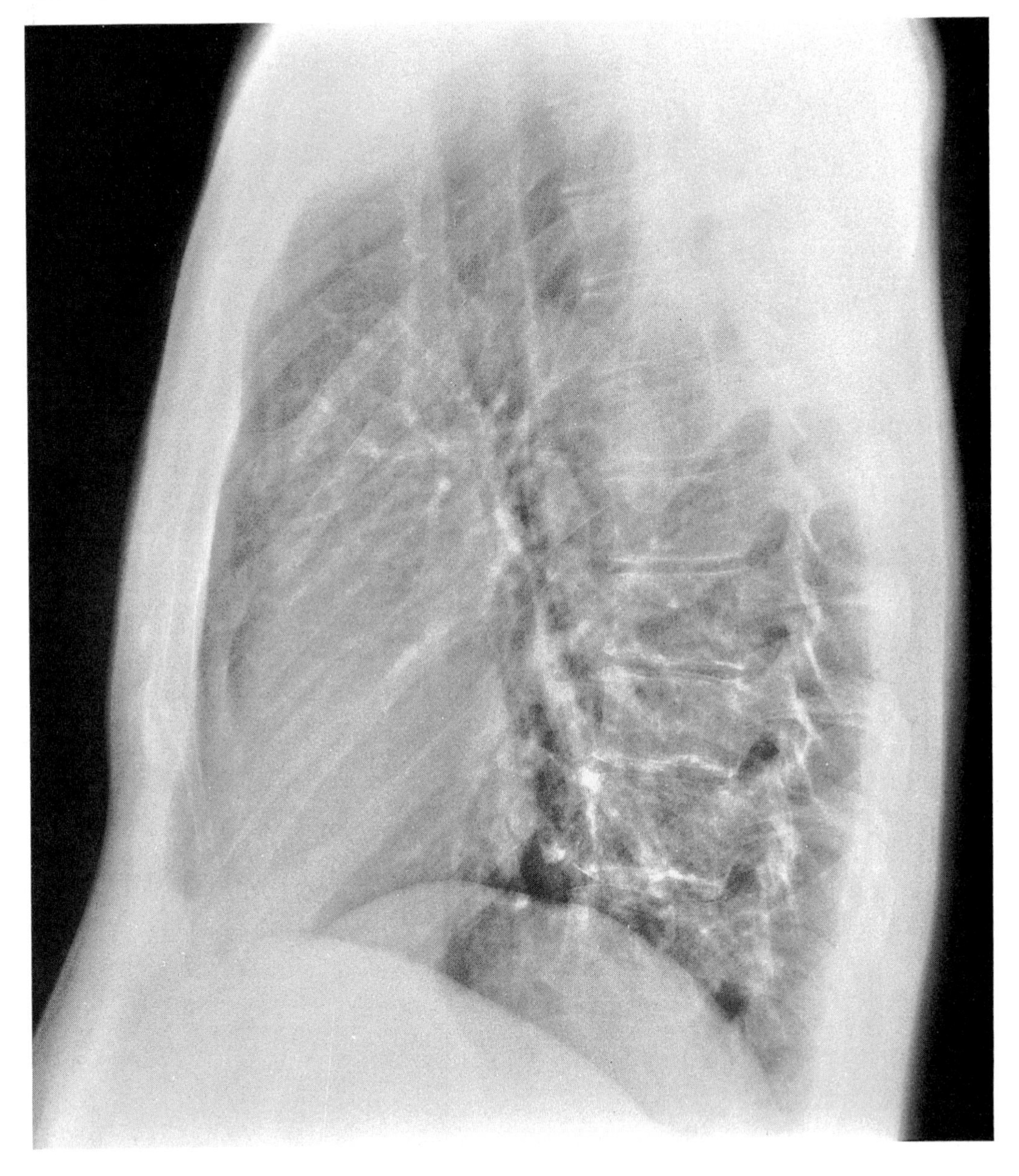

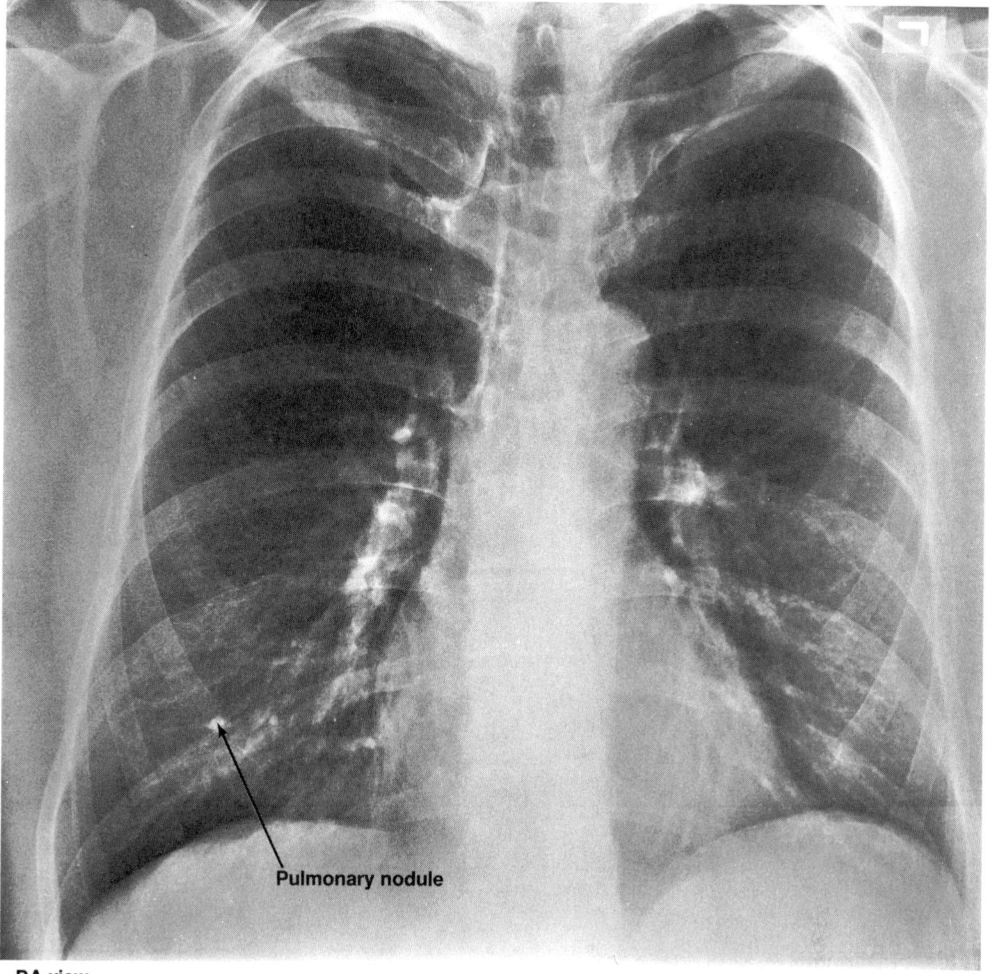

PA view

Case 16 discussion. [*Chapter 3 IV D 1*] The PA chest film shows a pulmonary nodule in the midregion of the right ninth posterior interspace; the lower margin of the nodule is superimposed upon the superior margin of the posterior segment of the right tenth rib. The lateral chest film shows the nodule, which has a stellate-shaped upper border and a smoothly curved lower border, in the retrocardiac area, and thus within the lower lobe of the right lung. Since the nodule lies at some distance inferolateral to the right hilum, it does not represent the superimposed images of two or more pulmonary vessels. Its size, relative radiopacity, and distinct border (especially when viewed in the lateral chest film) strongly suggest that it is calcified (the nodule measures 5 mm in diameter, and solitary nodules 1 to 5 mm in diameter are distinctly visible only if calcified). The nodule may be classified as a benign calcified granuloma if its appearance and size are determined to be the same as in chest films taken during the past 2 years or remain the same in chest films taken after the next 6 months.

continued on next page

Case 16 discussion *continued*

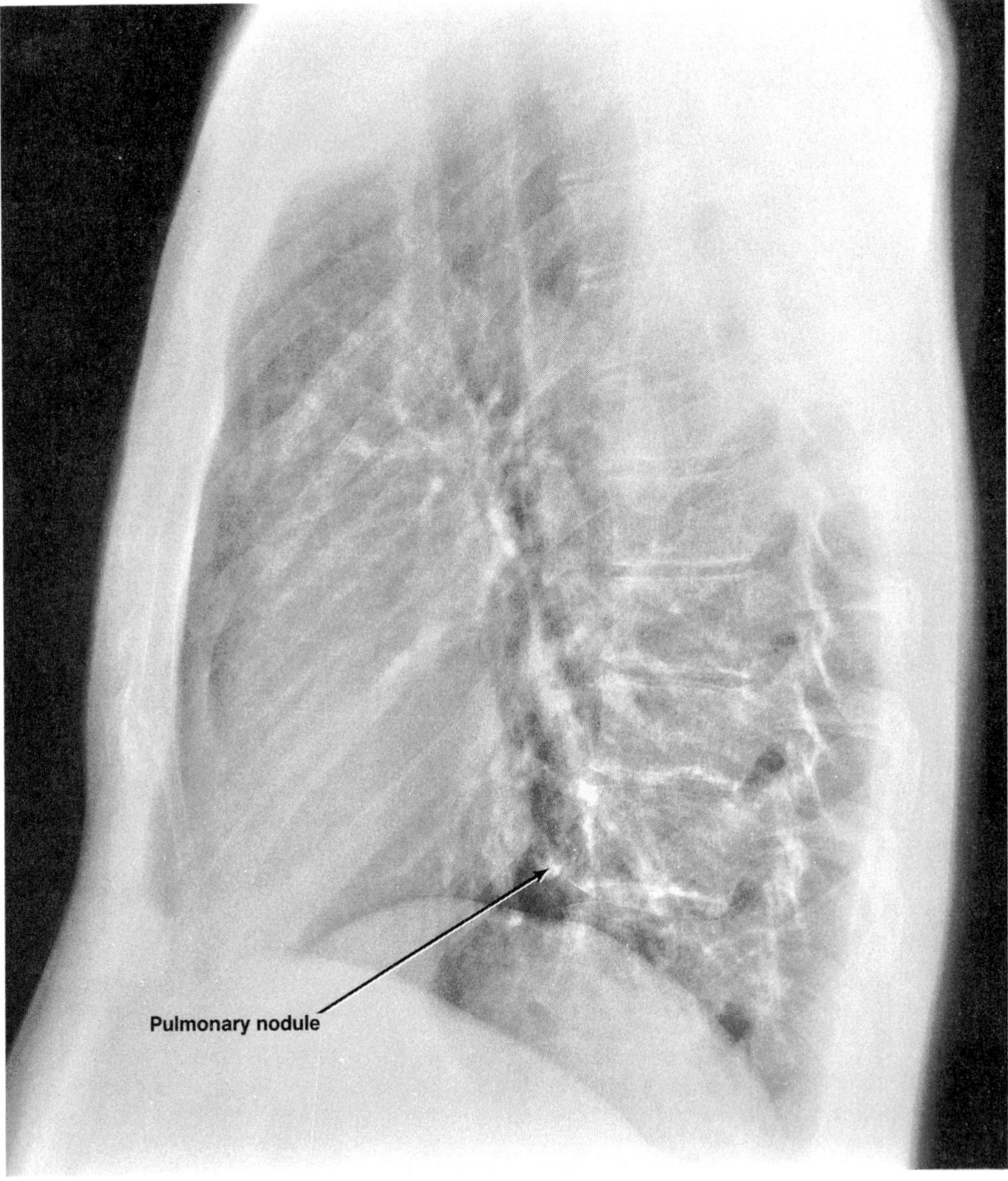

Lateral view

Case 17

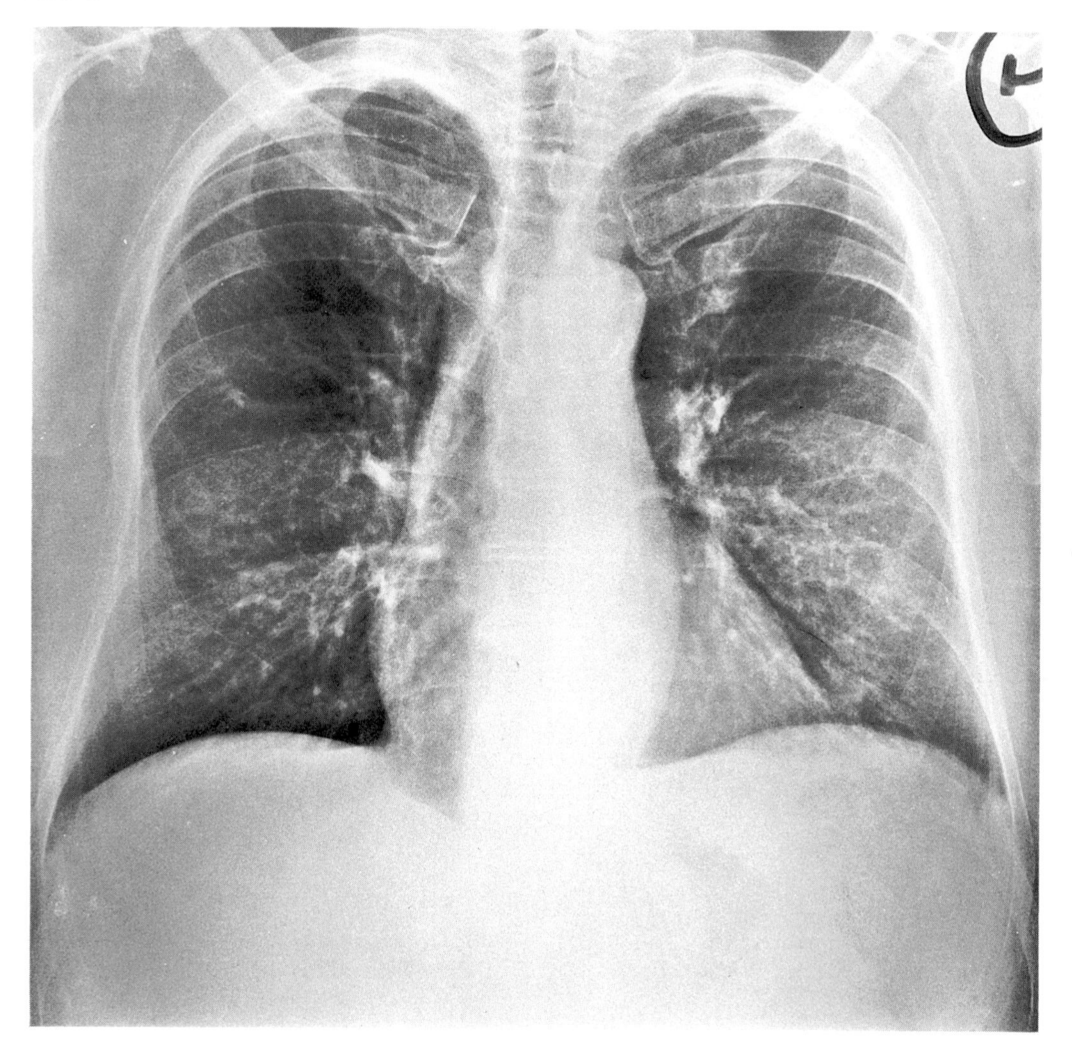

PA and lateral chest films taken during the annual physical examination of a 55-year-old man.

continued on next page

Case 17 *continued*

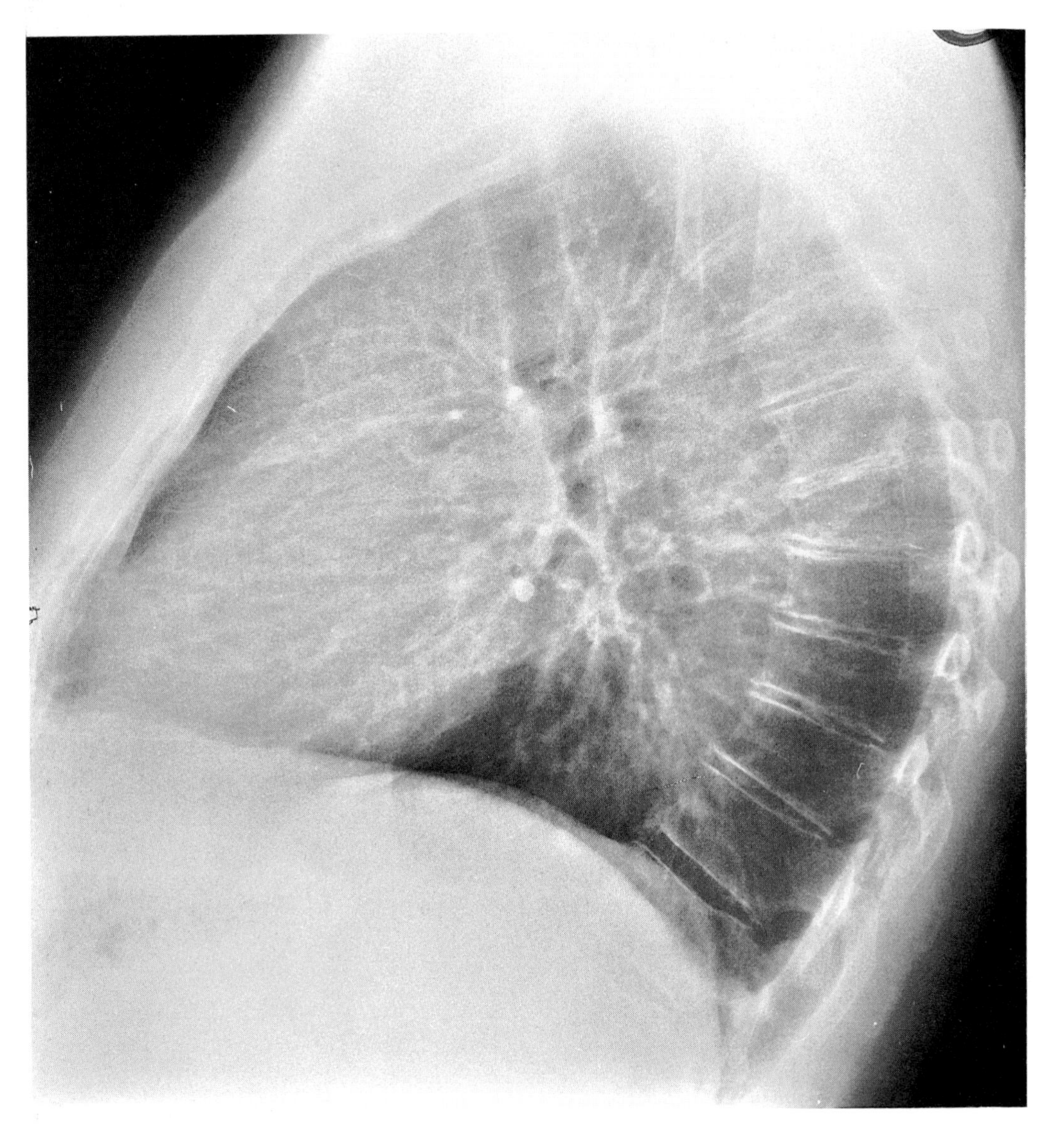

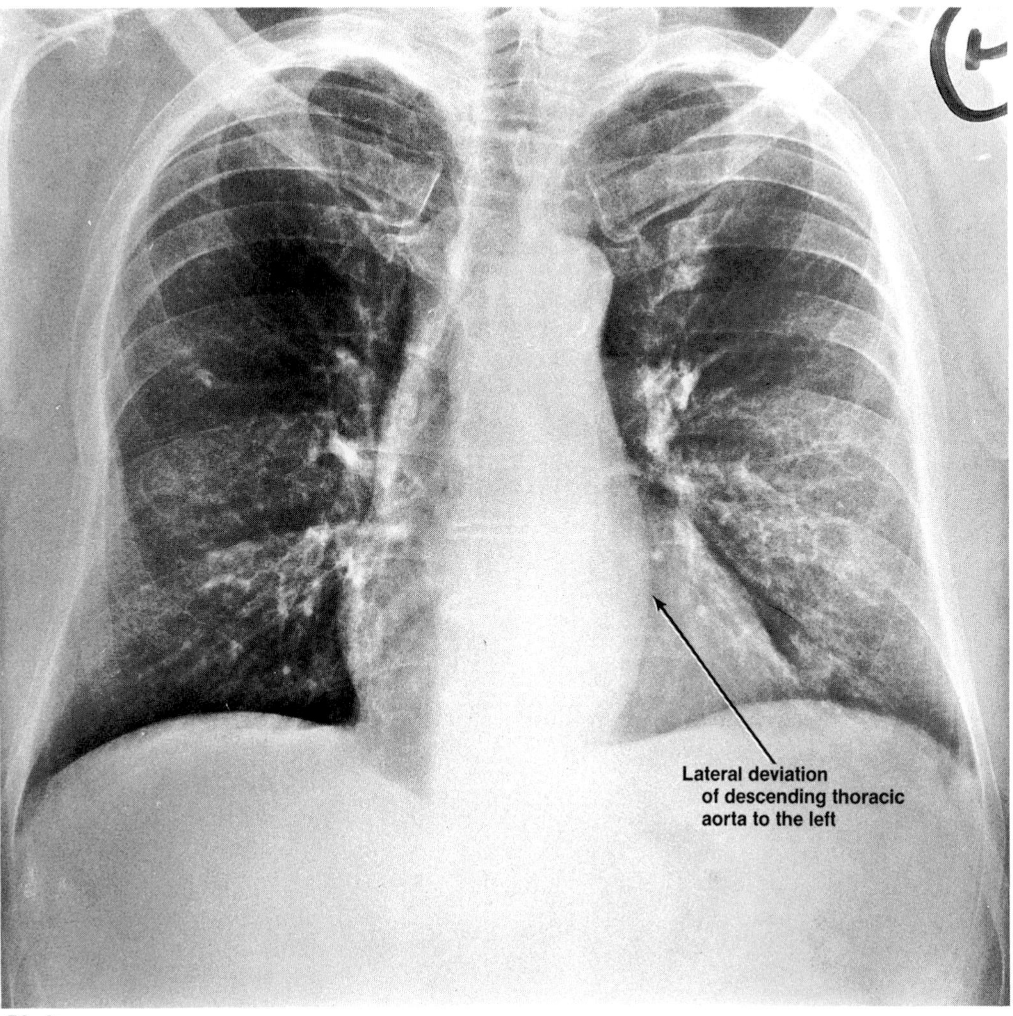

PA view

Case 17 discussion. [*Chapter 3 II A 3 d, B 2 b*] The lateral chest film shows marked kyphosis (i.e., exaggerated anterior curvature) of the thoracic part of the vertebral column. The T6–T7 intervertebral disk and the body of the seventh thoracic vertebra are noticeably compressed, most likely due to an old compression fracture of the body of the seventh thoracic vertebra and resultant loss of anterior stature. The thoracic kyphosis accounts for the bell-shaped outline of the chest wall in the PA chest film. The PA chest film also shows a lateral deviation of the descending thoracic aorta to the left, due to tortuosity secondary to arteriosclerotic change.

continued on next page

Case 17 discussion *continued*

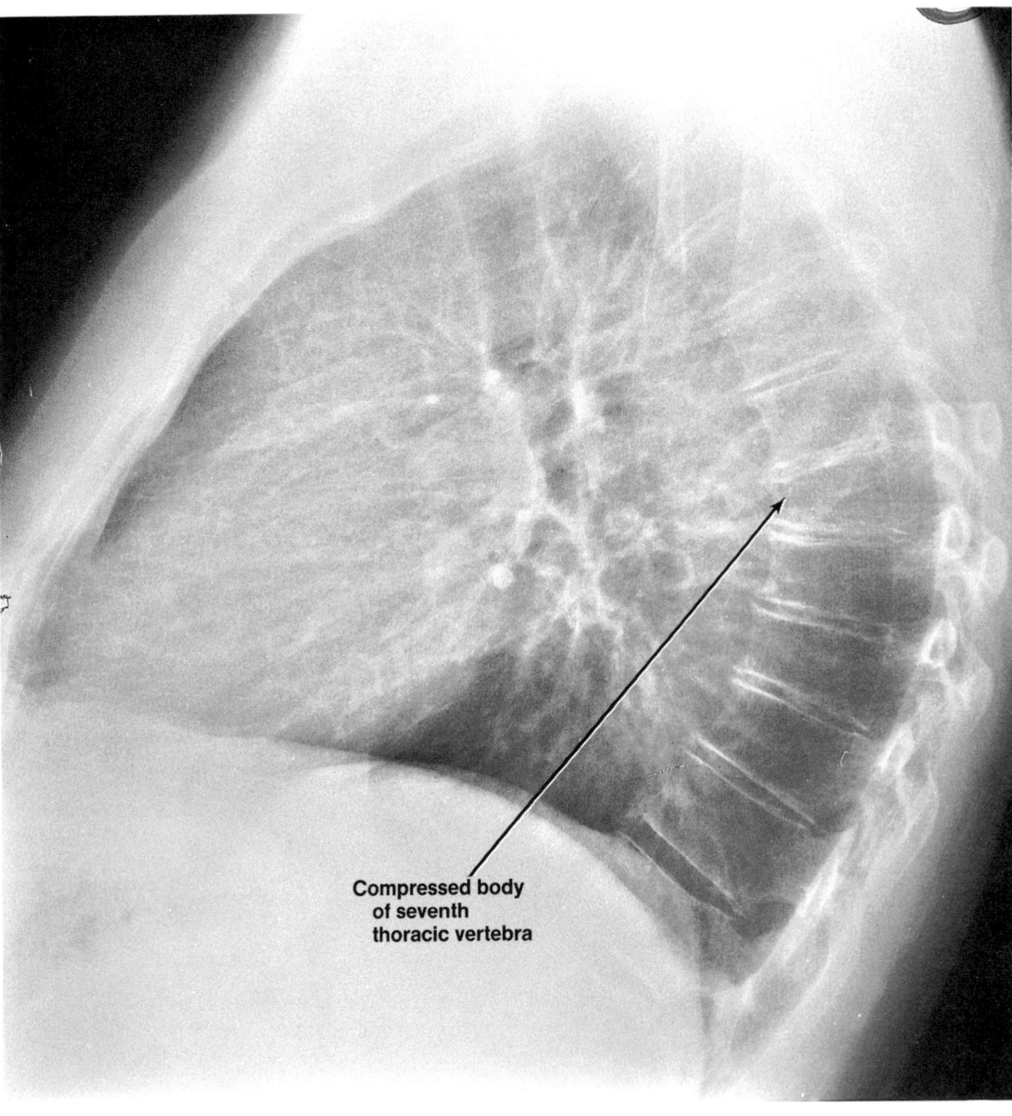

Lateral view

Case 18

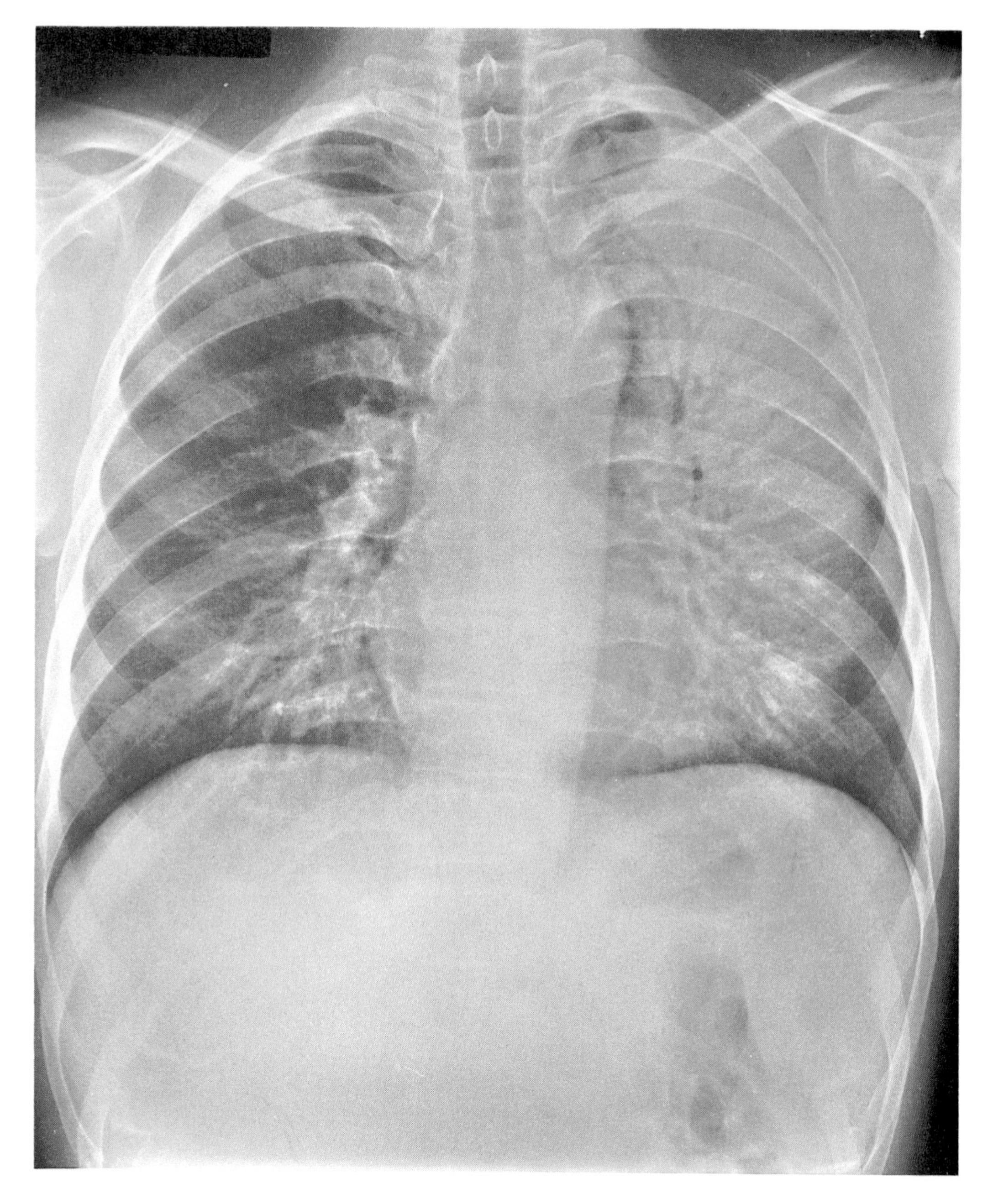

PA and lateral chest films of a 41-year-old man with fever, sputum-productive cough, and dyspnea.

continued on next page

Case 18 *continued*

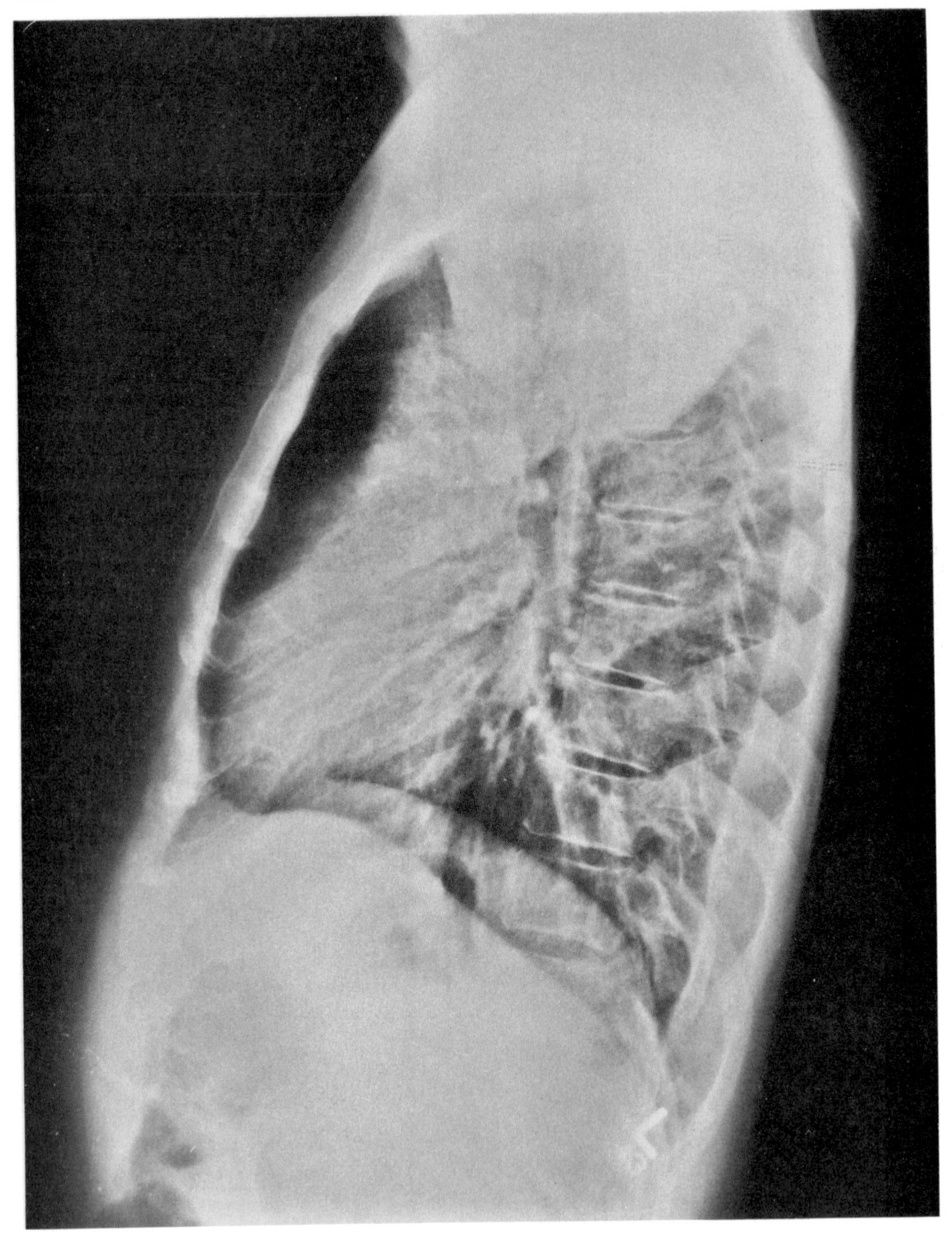

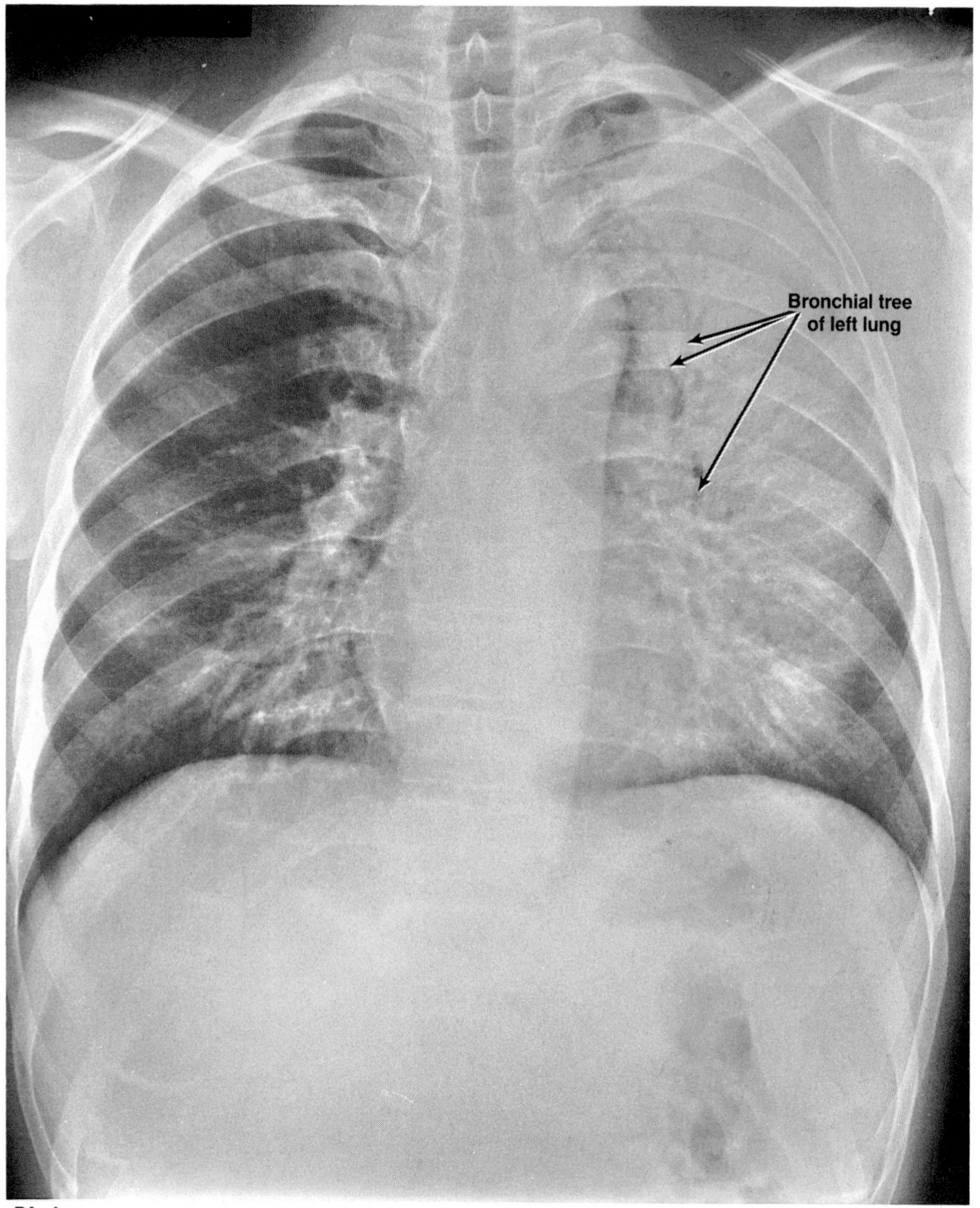

PA view

Case 18 discussion. [*Chapter 3 IV D 2*] The PA chest film shows an air bronchogram and consolidation in the upper and middle regions of the left lung. The bronchial tree of the left lung can be seen because the air density of its airways contrasts with the water density of the surrounding opacified alveoli. Three findings indicate that the consolidation process involves all of the bronchopulmonary segments of the left lung's upper lobe:

(1) The lateral chest film shows a uniformly radiopaque wedge-shaped area of consolidation in the upper part of the left lung. The location of the anterior and posterior borders of this wedge-shaped area indicate that the consolidation has occurred in the apical posterior segment of the upper lobe. However, the mediastinal borders of these segments are not significantly consolidated, since there is no obscuration of the aortic knob in the PA chest film.

(2) The PA chest film shows that a consolidated part of the left lung has obscured the silhouette of the pulmonary trunk and the upper part of the left ventricle along the left border of the cardiovascular

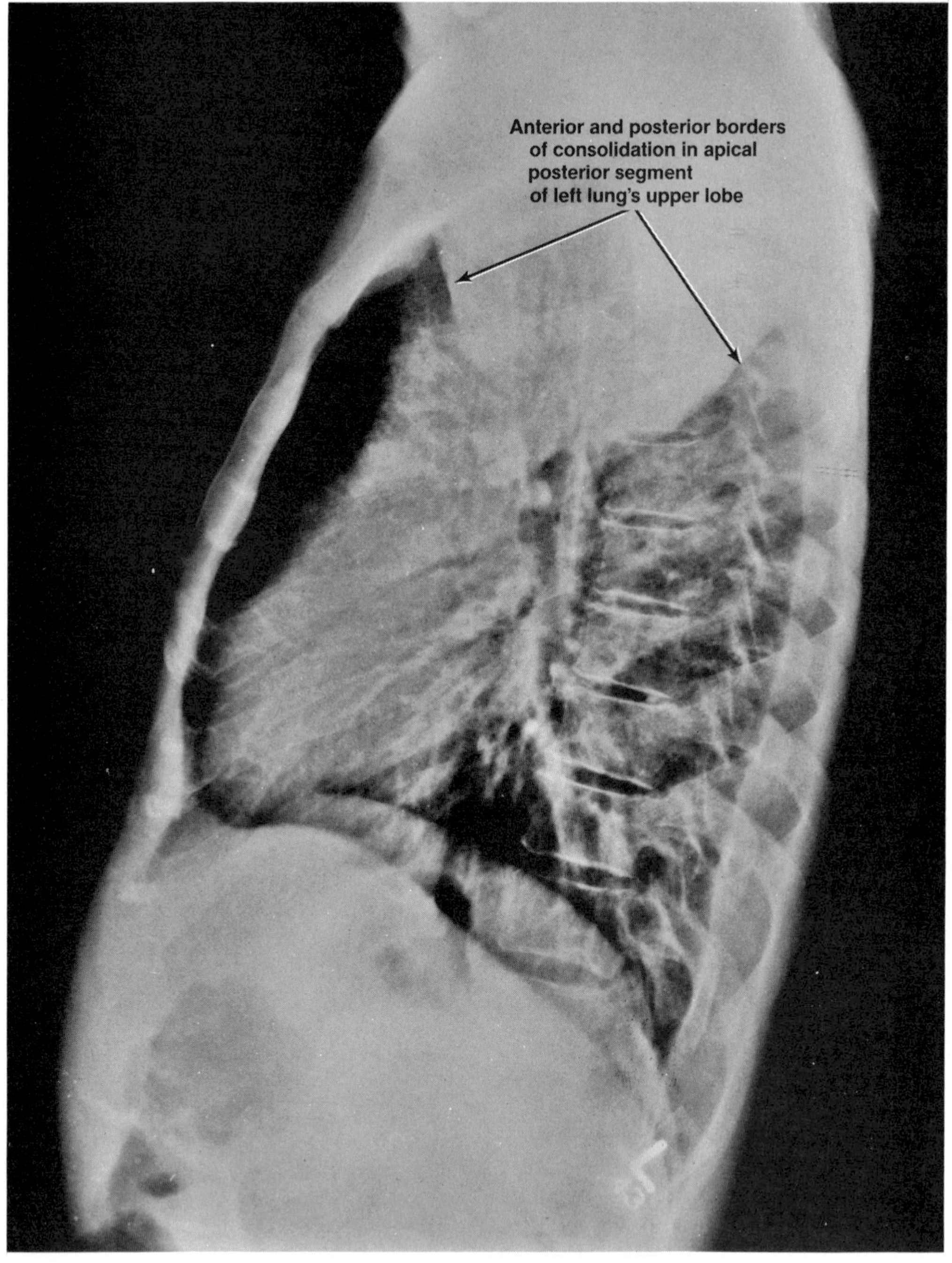

Lateral view

shadow. This silhouette sign indicates that the consolidation process involves the anterior bronchopulmonary segment of the upper lobe.

(3) The PA chest film shows that a consolidated part of the left lung has obscured the silhouette of most of the left ventricle along the left border of the cardiovascular shadow. This silhouette sign indicates that the consolidation process involves one or both of the left lung's lingular segments.

Pneumonia was responsible for this patient's respiratory symptoms and radiographic findings.

Case 19

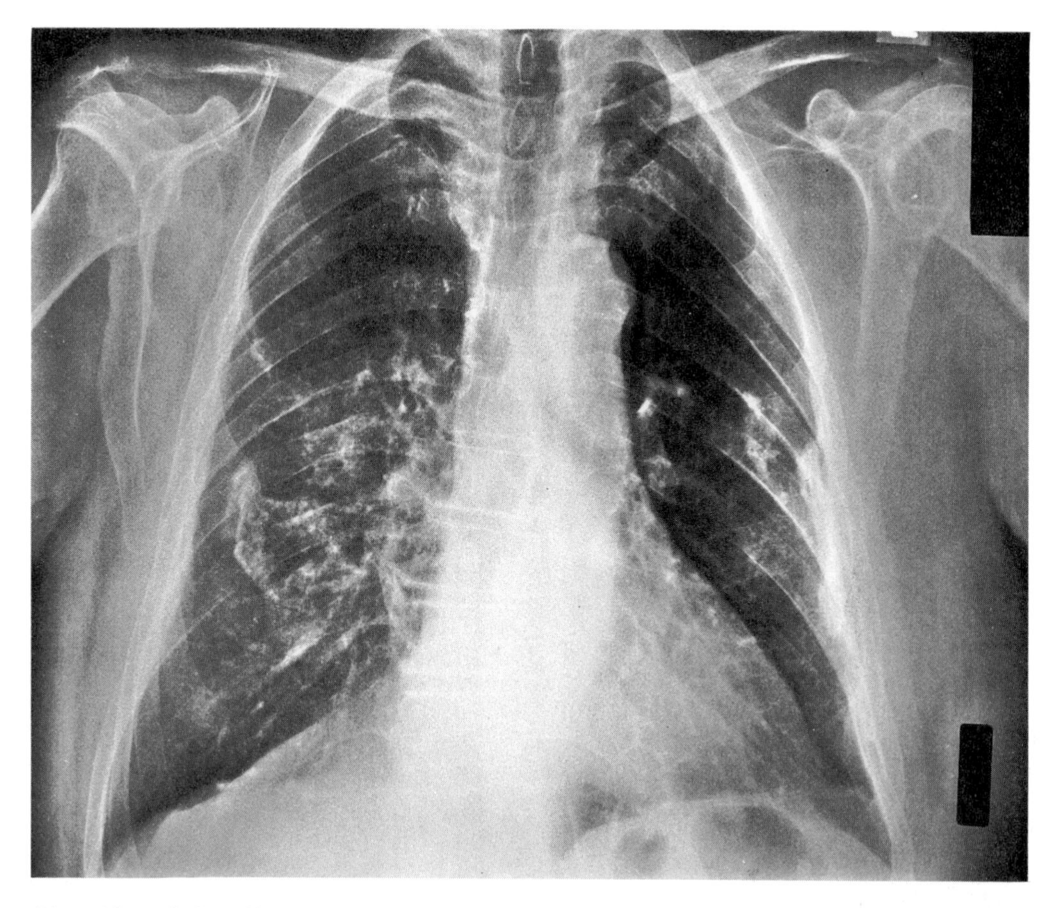

PA and lateral chest films taken during the annual physical examination of a 77-year-old man.

continued on next page

Case 19 *continued*

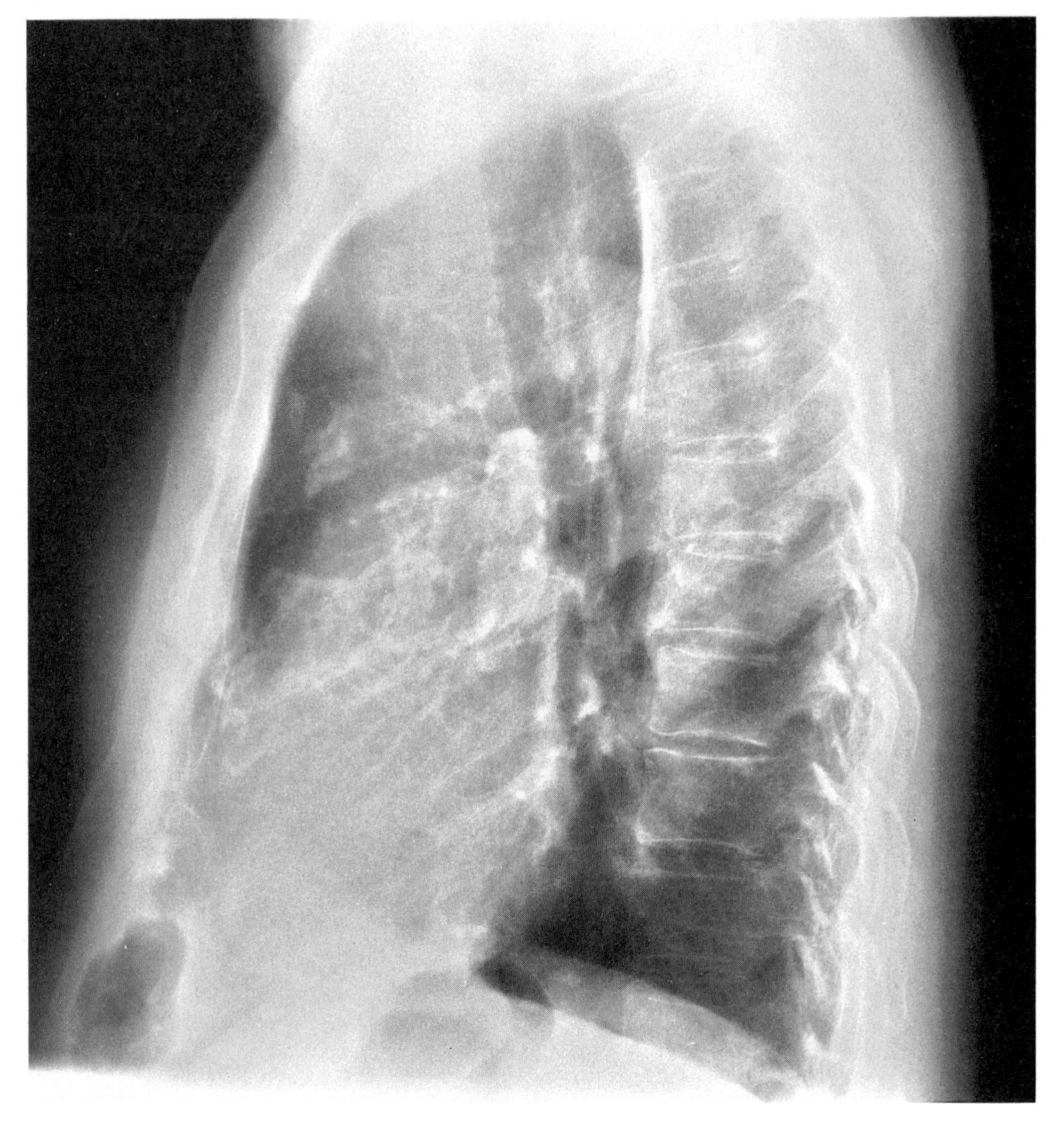

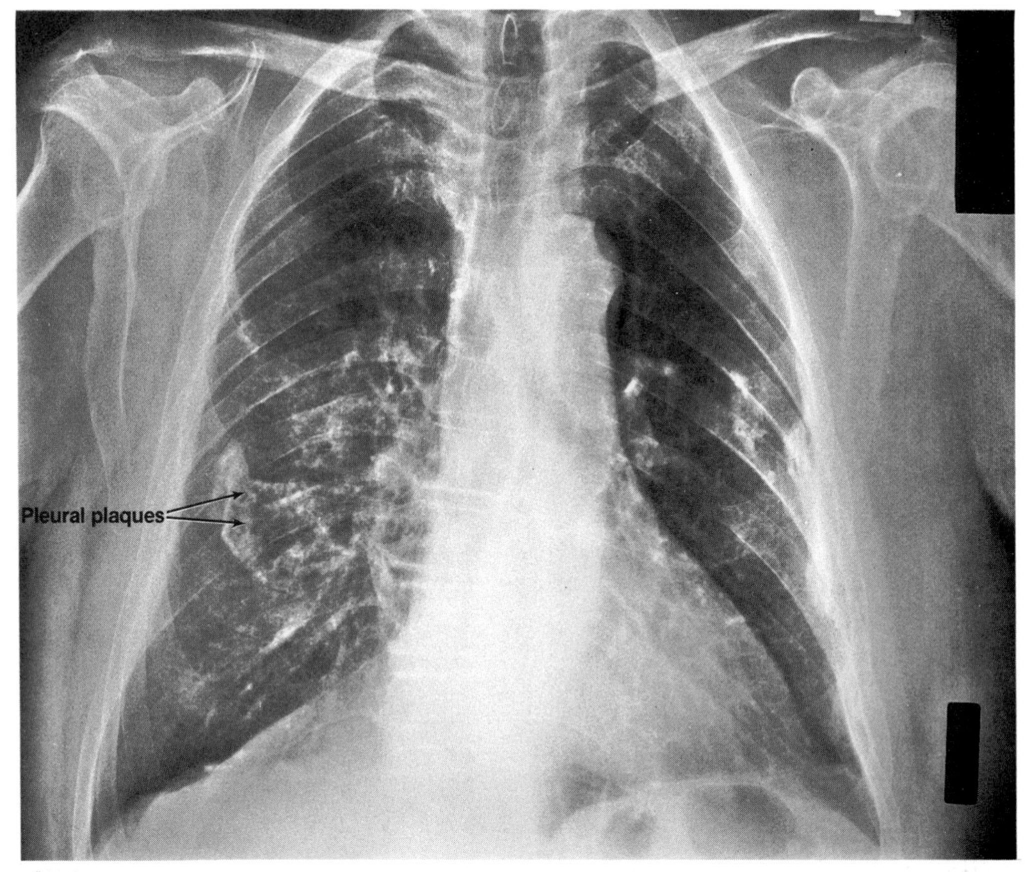

PA view

Case 19 discussion. The PA chest film shows radiodense lesions with irregular borders in mainly the midregions of the lung fields; the densest cluster of lesions is located in the midregion of the right lung field, superimposed upon the tenth and eleventh posterior rib segments and the intervening tenth interspace. The lateral chest film shows some of the larger lesions superimposed upon the upper half of the cardiac shadow. The PA chest film also shows diffuse interstitial fibrosis (i.e., diffuse thickening of pulmonary interstitial tissues) in the basal regions of the lung fields.

The radiodense lesions represent pleural plaques. Their distribution in the lung fields suggests the patient's previous exposure to asbestos fibers. Asbestos-induced pleural plaques develop on the parietal pleura, occurring in greatest density in the midregions of the lung fields and in least density in the apical and basal regions. Although exposure to asbestos fibers for only a few months can suffice to induce pleural plaques, the plaques do not appear until after a latency period of 10 to 20 years. It is common for the plaques to calcify with increasing age. The diffuse interstitial fibrosis in the basal regions of the lung fields is another pathologic change characteristic of asbestos exposure.

continued on next page

Case 19 discussion *continued*

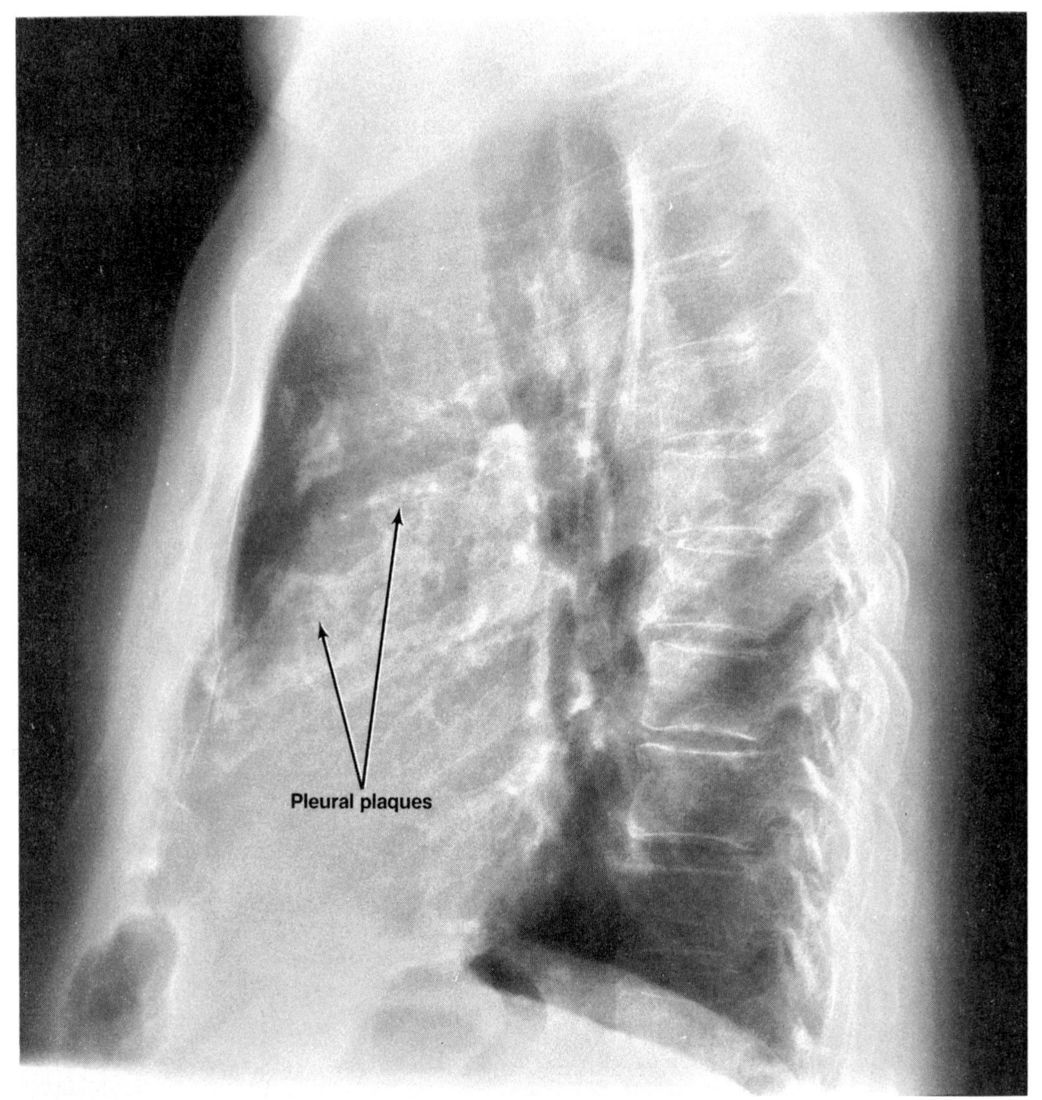

Lateral view

Case 20

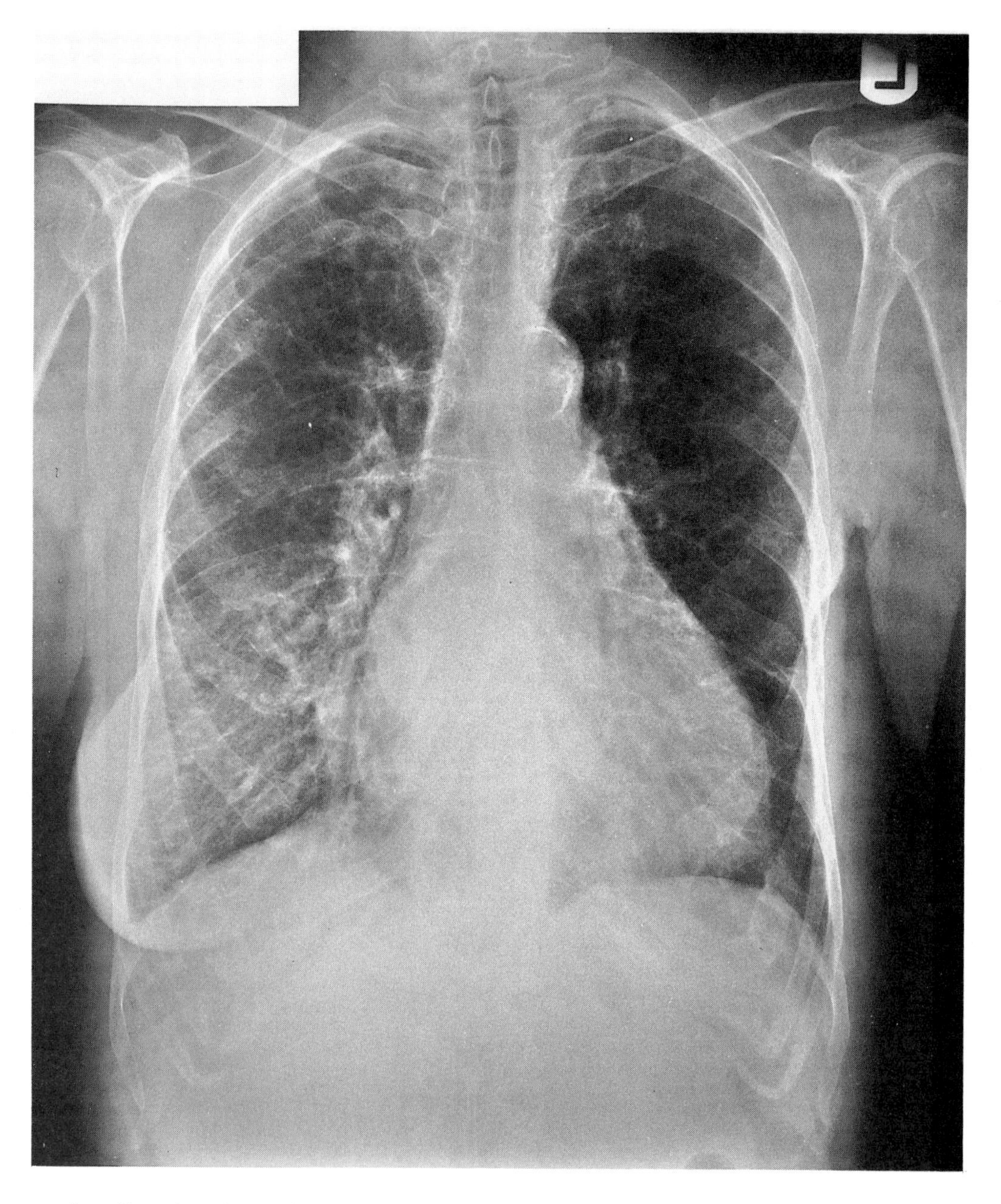

PA chest film taken during the annual physical examination of an 80-year-old woman.

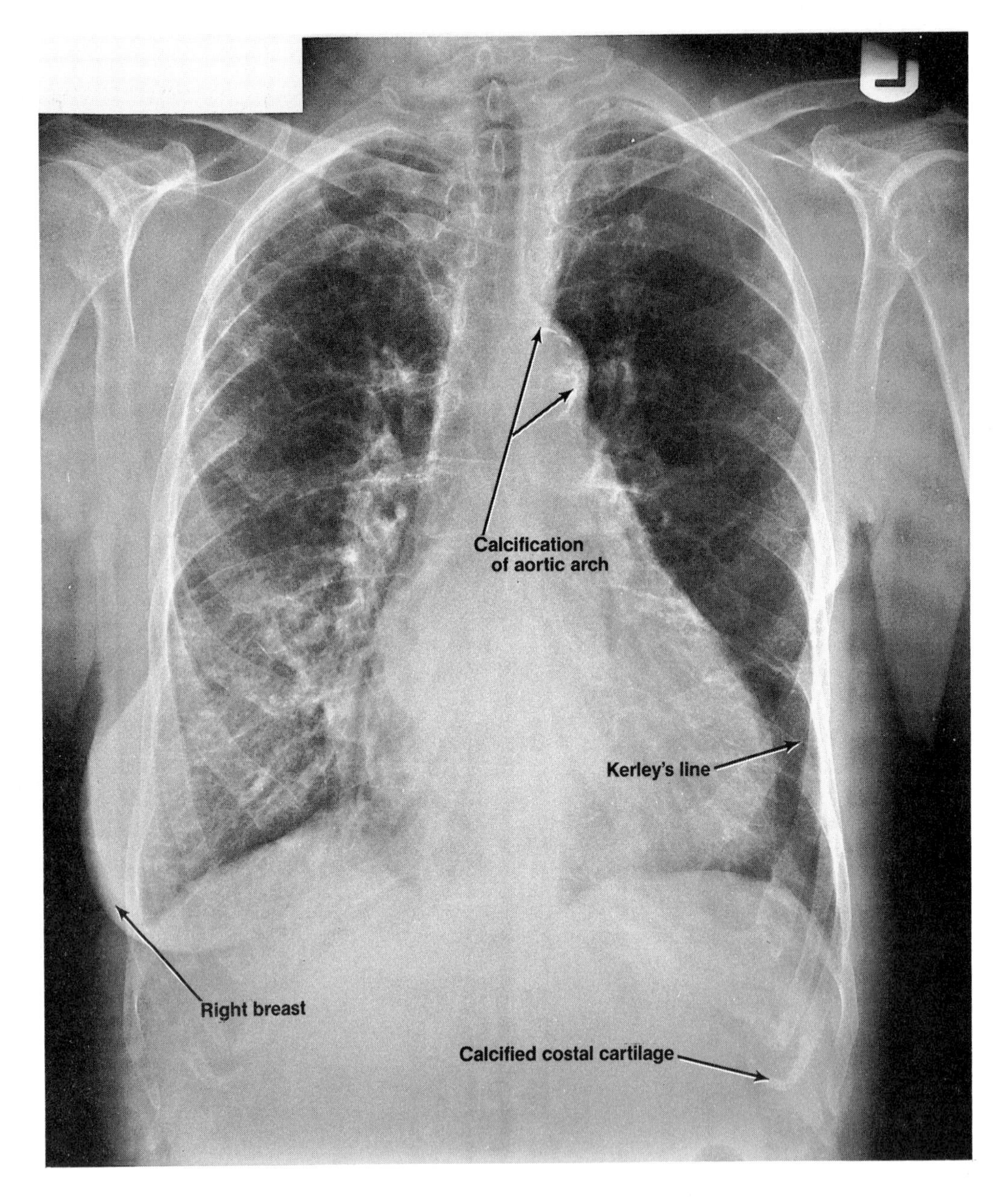

Case 20 discussion. [*Chapter 3 IV D 3*] The PA chest film shows an absence of the soft tissue shadows of the left breast, Kerley's lines bilaterally in the basal regions of the lung fields, calcification of the aortic arch, and partial calcification of the costal cartilages along the costal margins. The soft tissue shadows of the left breast are absent because the woman has undergone a mastectomy for cancer of the left breast. Kerley's lines represent thickened interlobular connective tissue septa or distended interlobular lymphatics.

Case 21

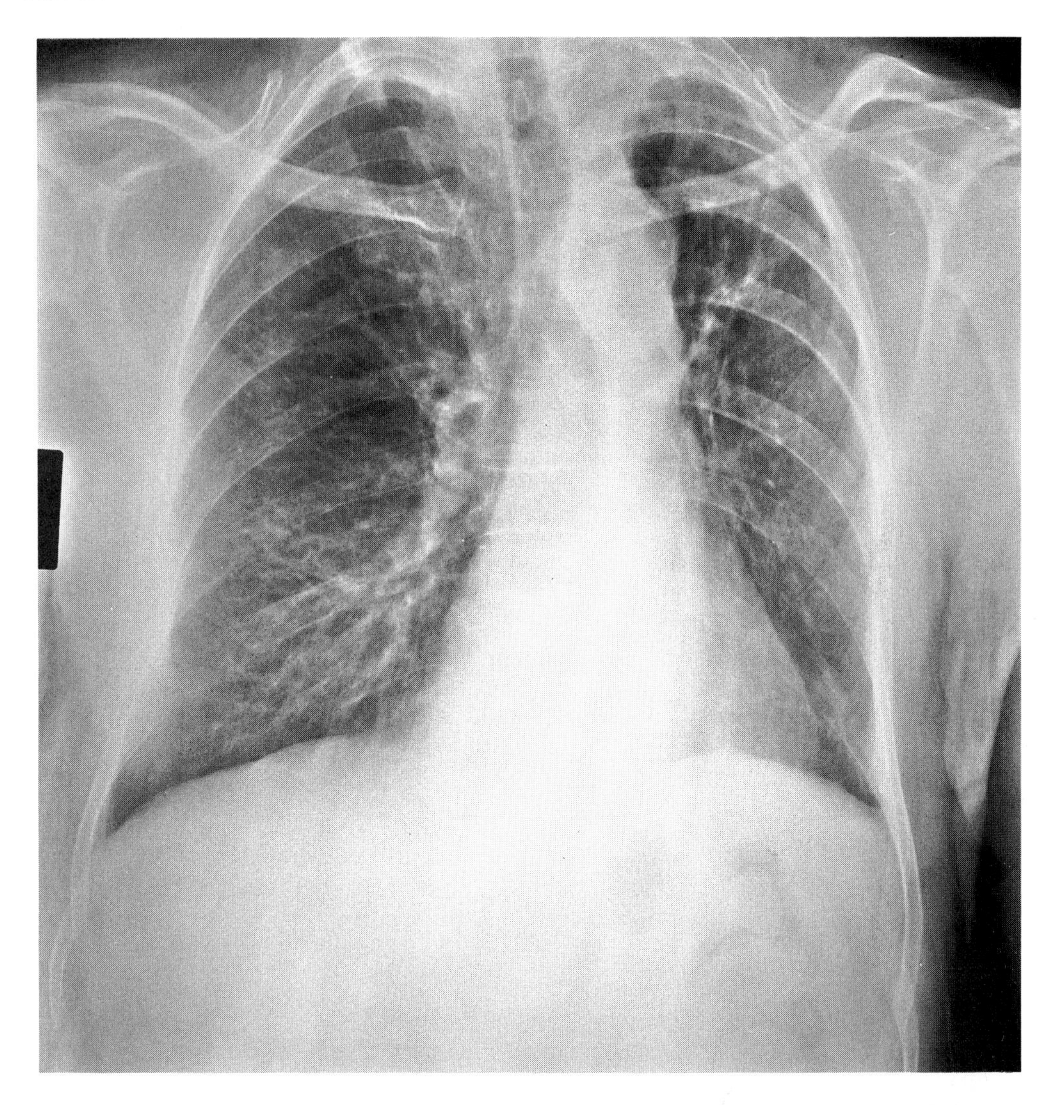

PA and lateral chest films taken during the annual physical examination of a 61-year-old man.

continued on next page

Case 21 *continued*

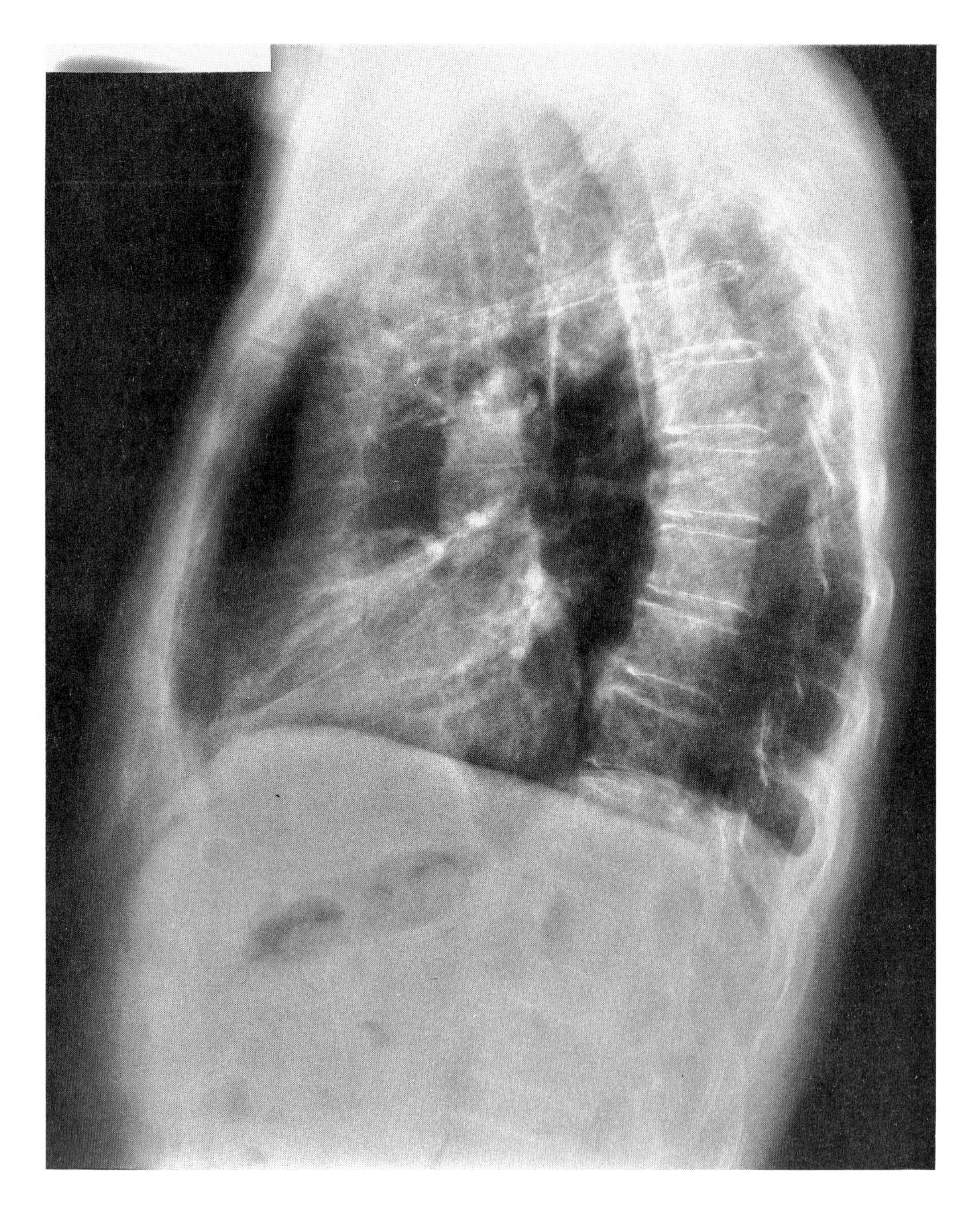

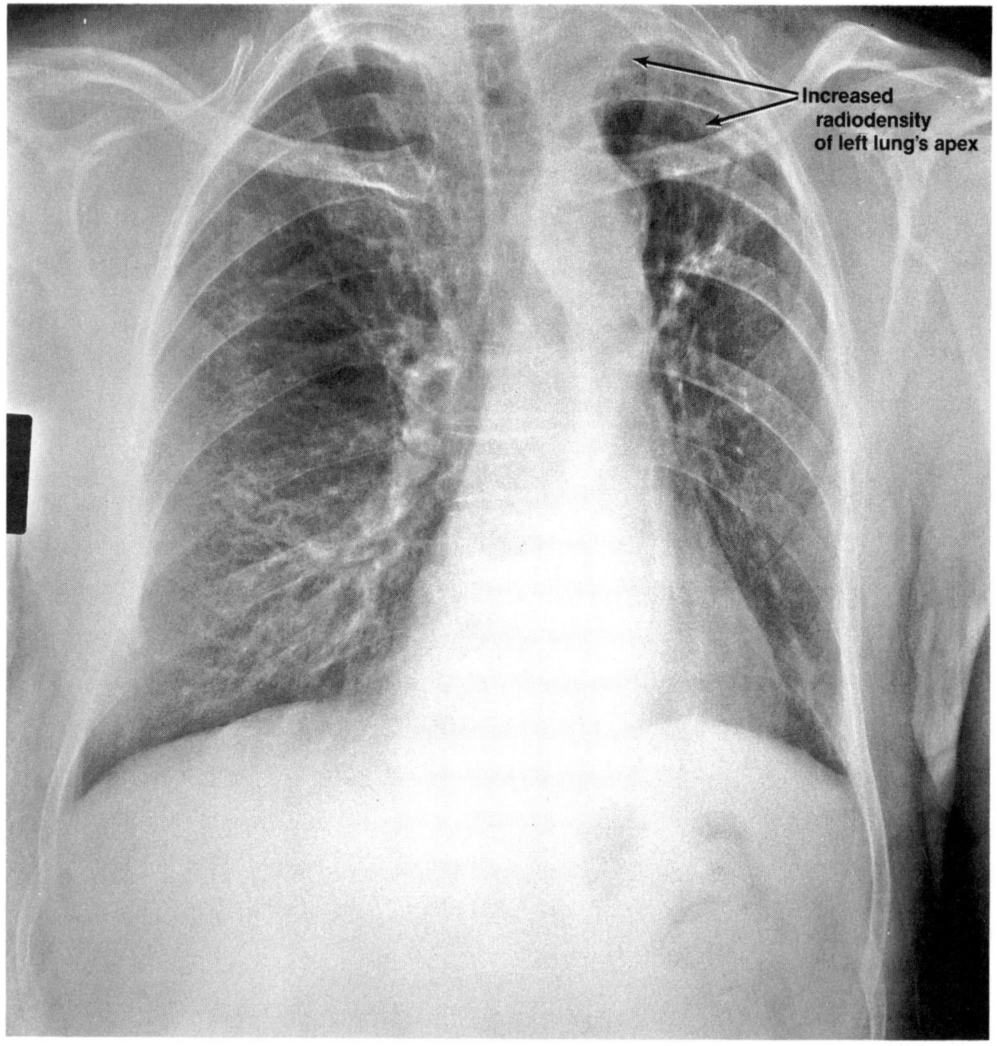

PA view

Case 21 discussion. The PA chest film shows increased radiodensity of the apex of the left lung field (especially evident in the second and third interspaces). The lateral chest film shows that the left lung region of increased radiodensity appears in the area directly posterior to the lower end of the tracheal lumen. The area directly posterior to the tracheal lumen shows the radiolucencies of the apical posterior segment of the left lung's upper lobe superimposed upon the radiolucencies of the apical and posterior segments of the right lung's upper lobe. In this instance, the increased radiodensity of the apical posterior segment of the left lung's upper lobe represents fibrotic scarring that is a sequela of prior episodes of pneumonia.

continued on next page

Case 21 discussion *continued*

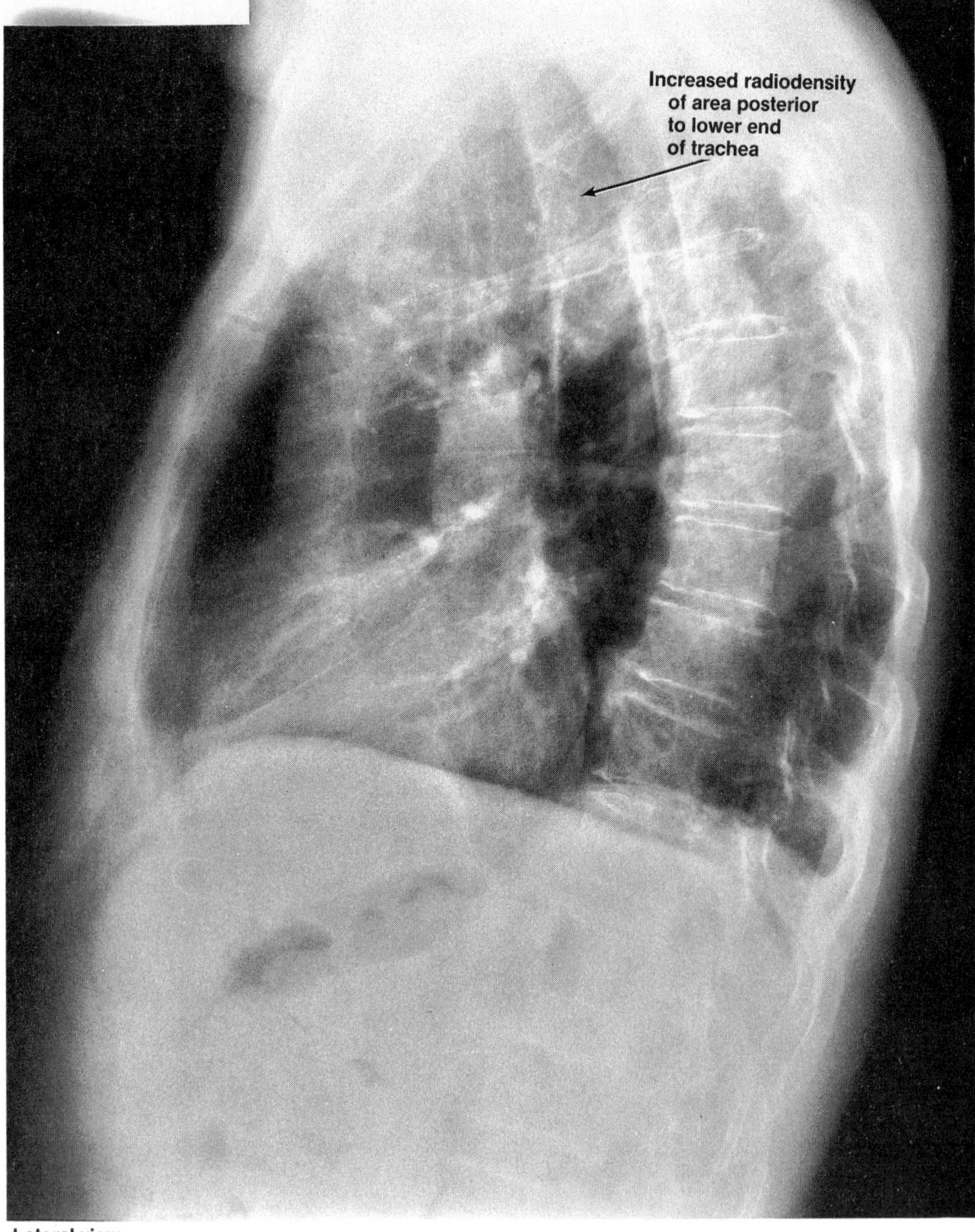

Lateral view

Case 22

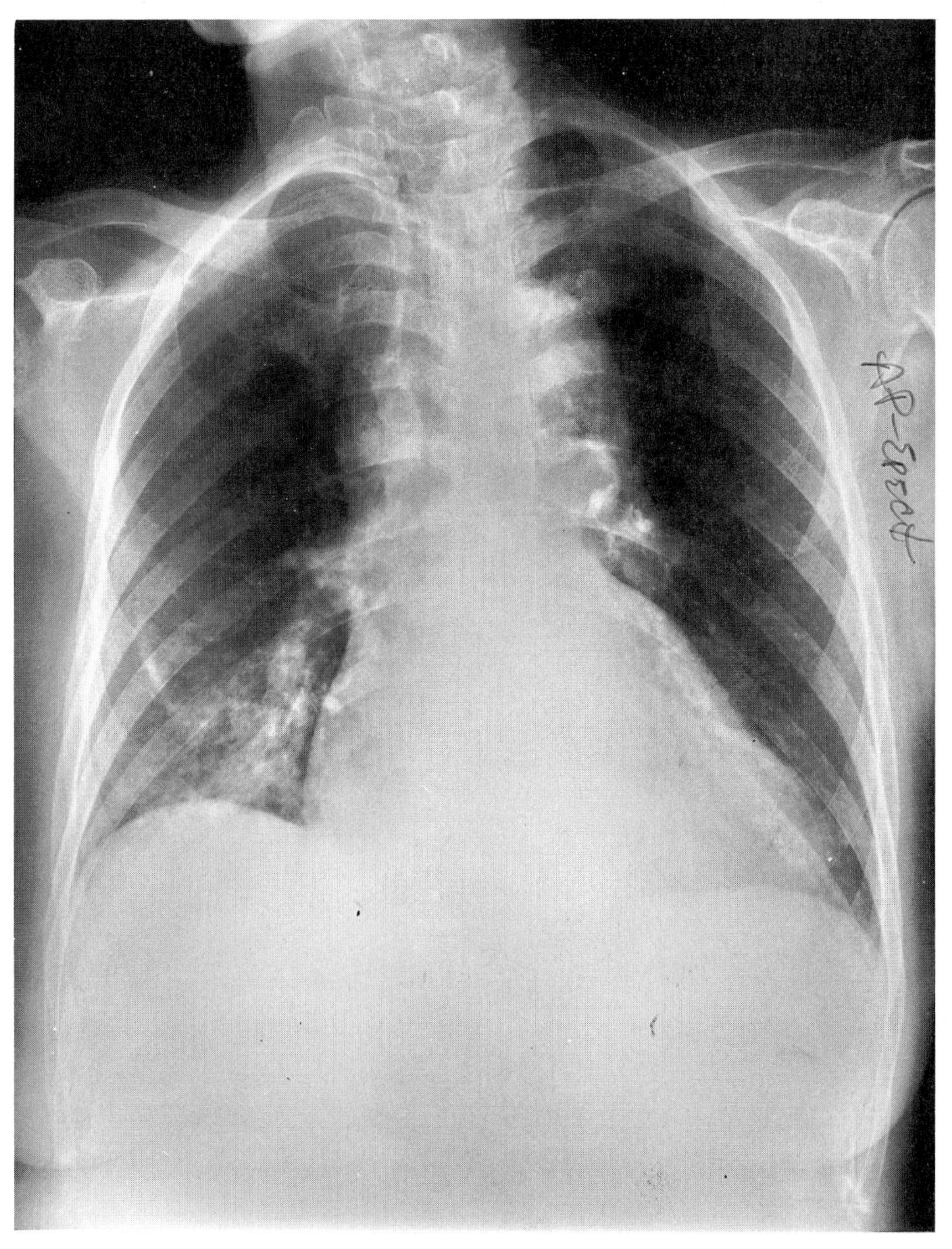

AP erect chest film of an 82-year-old woman with chest pain.

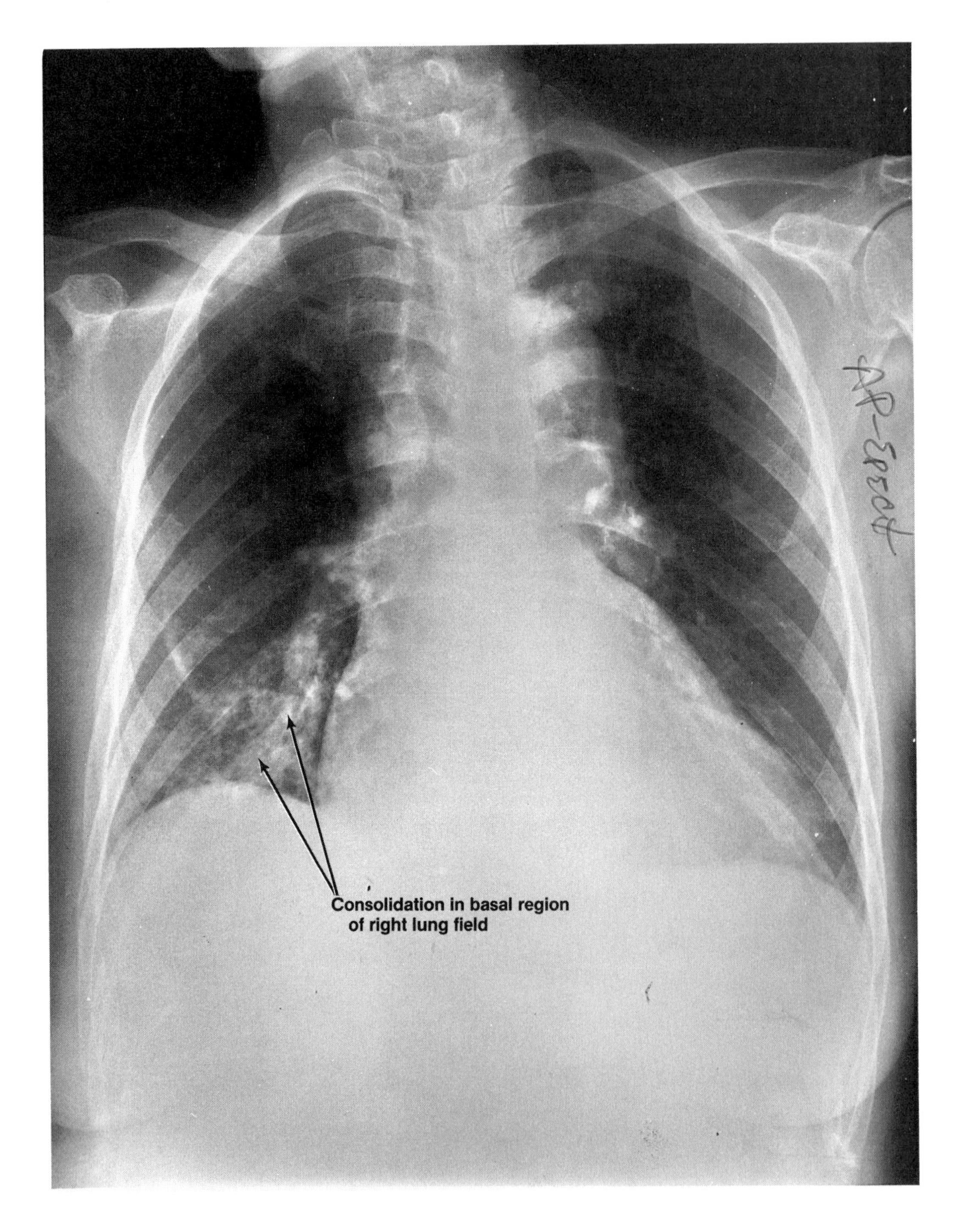

Case 22 discussion. [*Chapter 3 IV D 2 c (2) (b) (vi)*] The AP chest film shows areas of consolidation in the lower half of the right lung field. Some of the areas of consolidation are located in one or more of the basal segments of the right lung's lower lobe since these areas are superimposed upon the silhouette of the right dome of the diaphragm; the consolidated areas have not, however, obscured the silhouette of the right dome of the diaphragm. In this case, further examination showed the patient to be suffering from pneumonia of the right lung's lower lobe.

Case 23

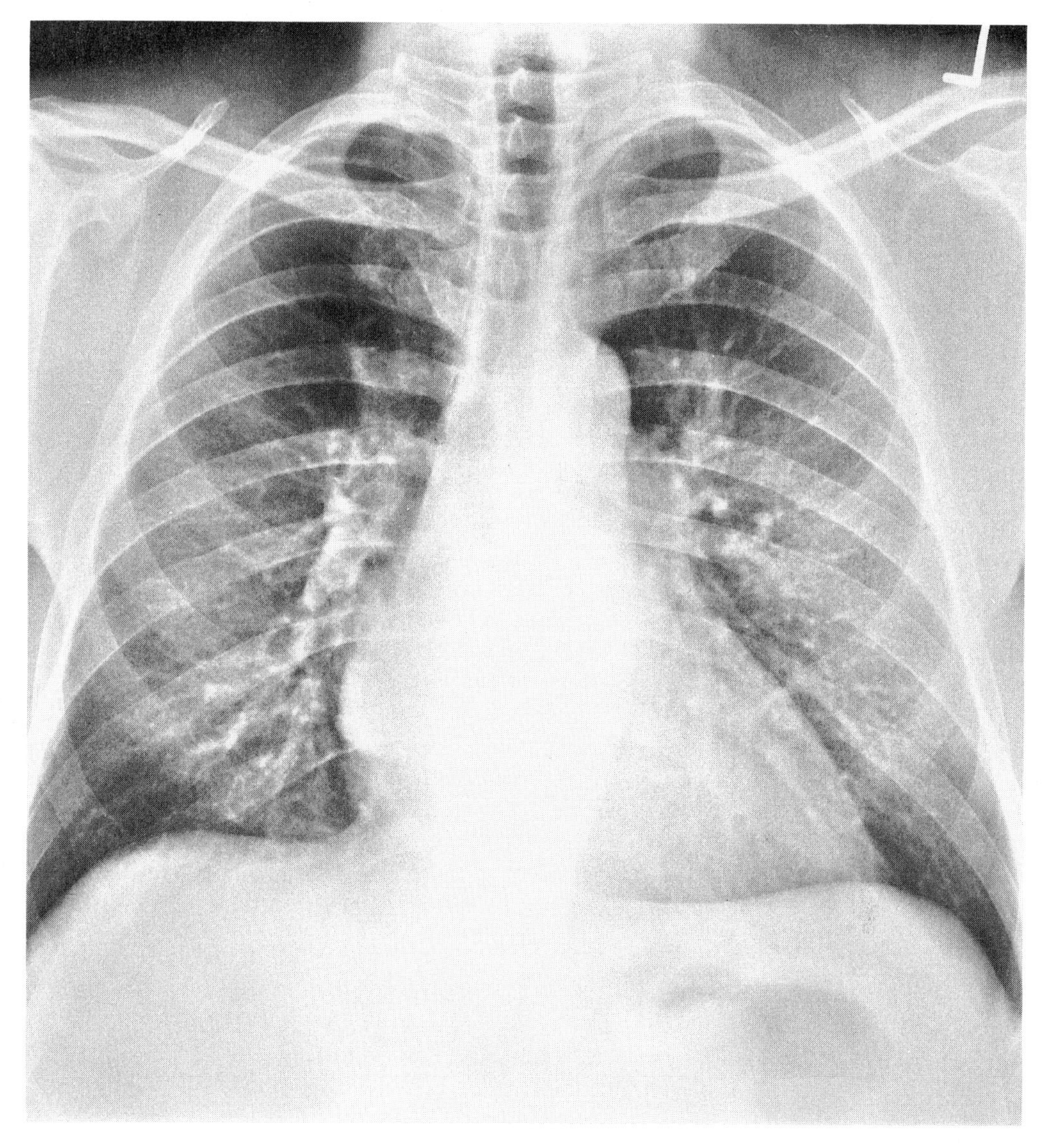

PA and lateral chest films taken during the annual physical examination of a 49-year-old man.

continued on next page

Case 23 *continued*

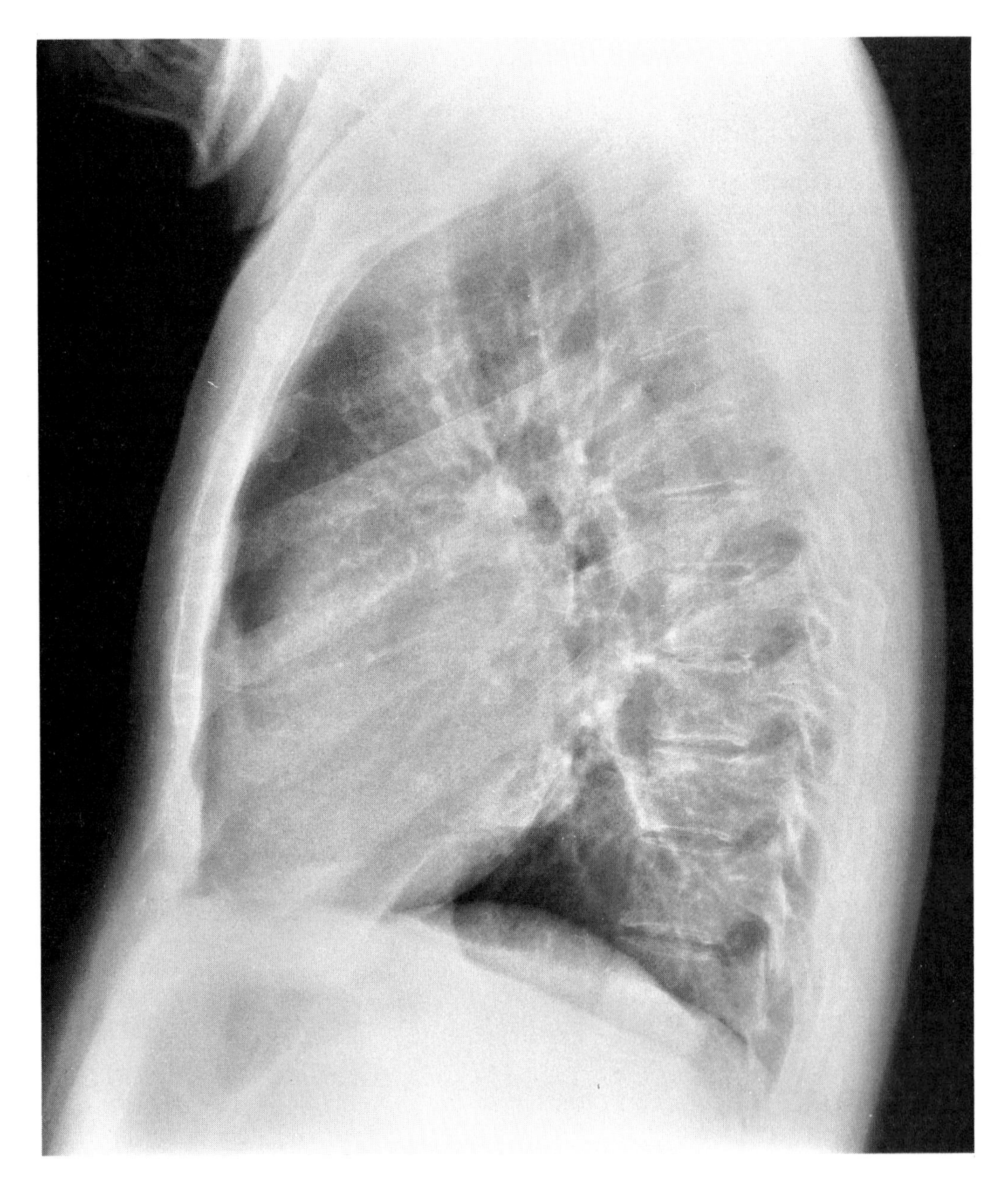

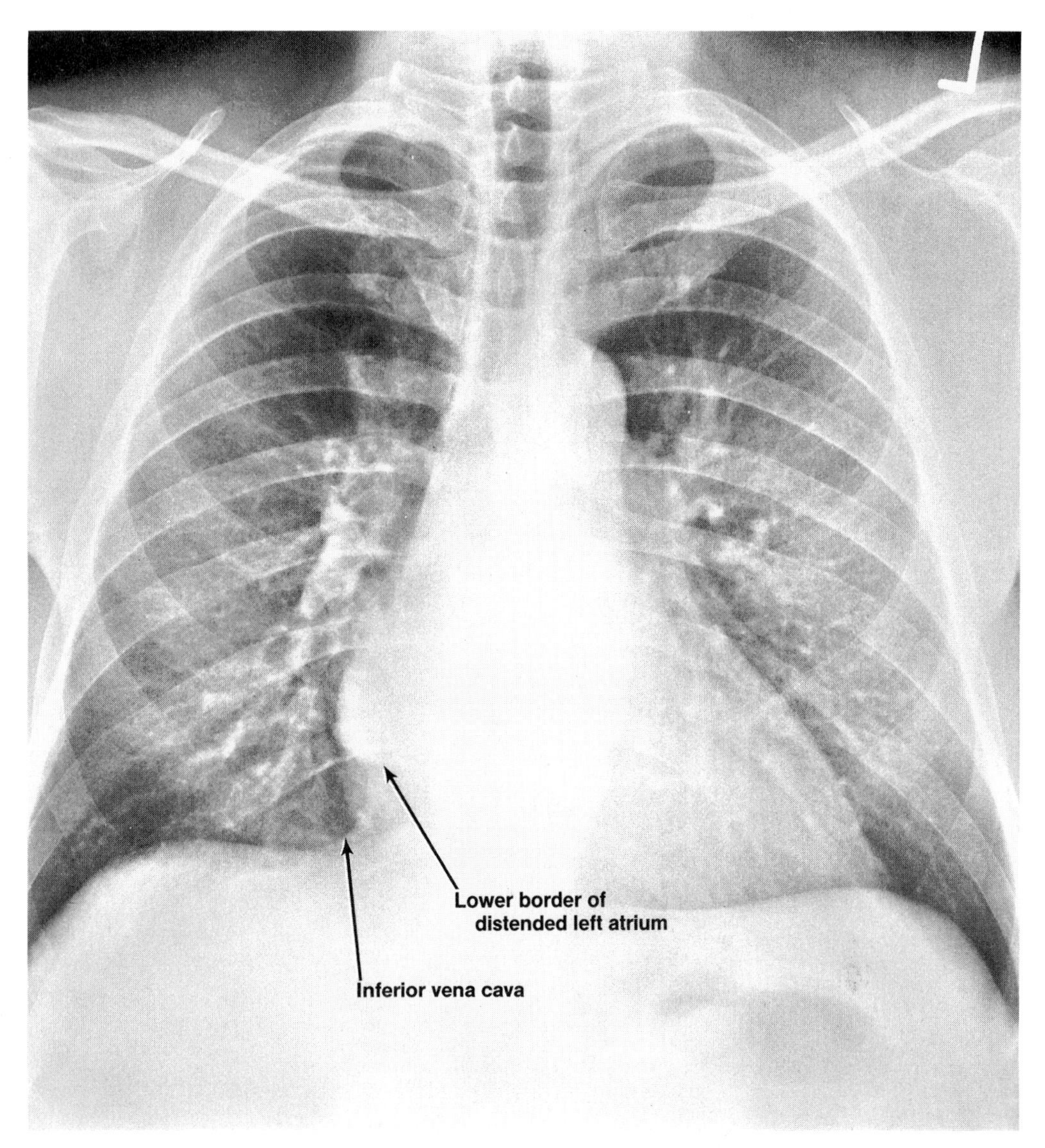

PA view

Case 23 discussion. [*Chapter 3 IV C 1 b*] The lower right corner of the cardiovascular shadow in the PA chest film shows the area of the union of the inferior vena cava with the right atrium bordered superiorly by an area of greater radiodensity; the areas of different radiodensity are separated by a horizontal boundary. The lateral chest film shows a moderate posterior bulge in the midregion of the posterior border of the cardiac shadow. In this case, an enlarged left atrium accounts for both of these abnormal findings. The horizontal boundary between the areas of different radiodensity in the lower right corner of the cardiovascular shadow of the PA chest film represents the lower border of the distended left atrium. There is not a similar vertical boundary between areas of different radiodensity along the right side of the cardiovascular shadow because the right border of the distended left atrium is superimposed upon the right border of the right atrium. In the lateral chest film, the midregion of the cardiac shadow's posterior border bulges posteriorly because the middle third of the shadow's posterior border is outlined by the left atrium.

continued on next page

Case 23 discussion *continued*

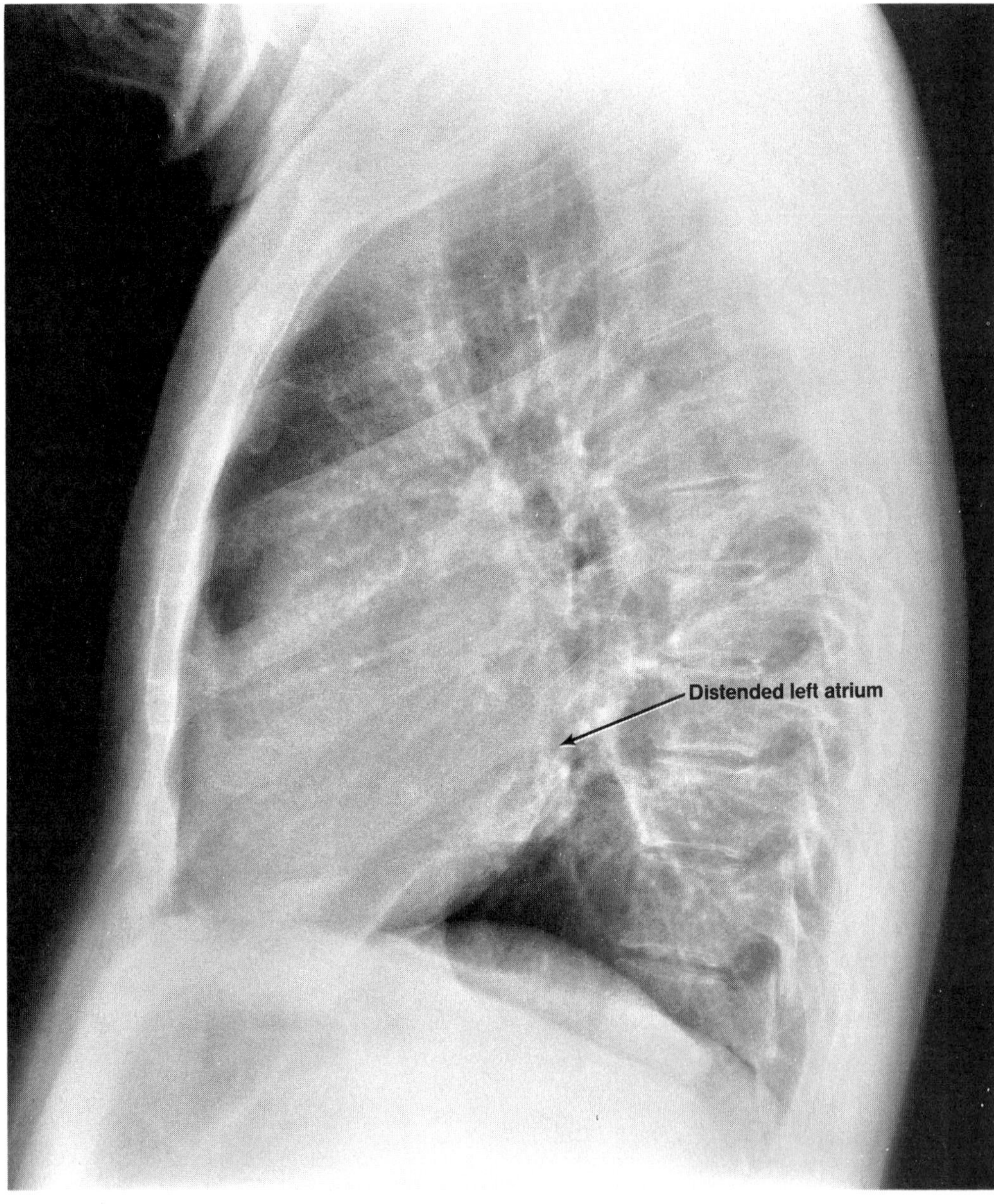

Lateral view

Case 24

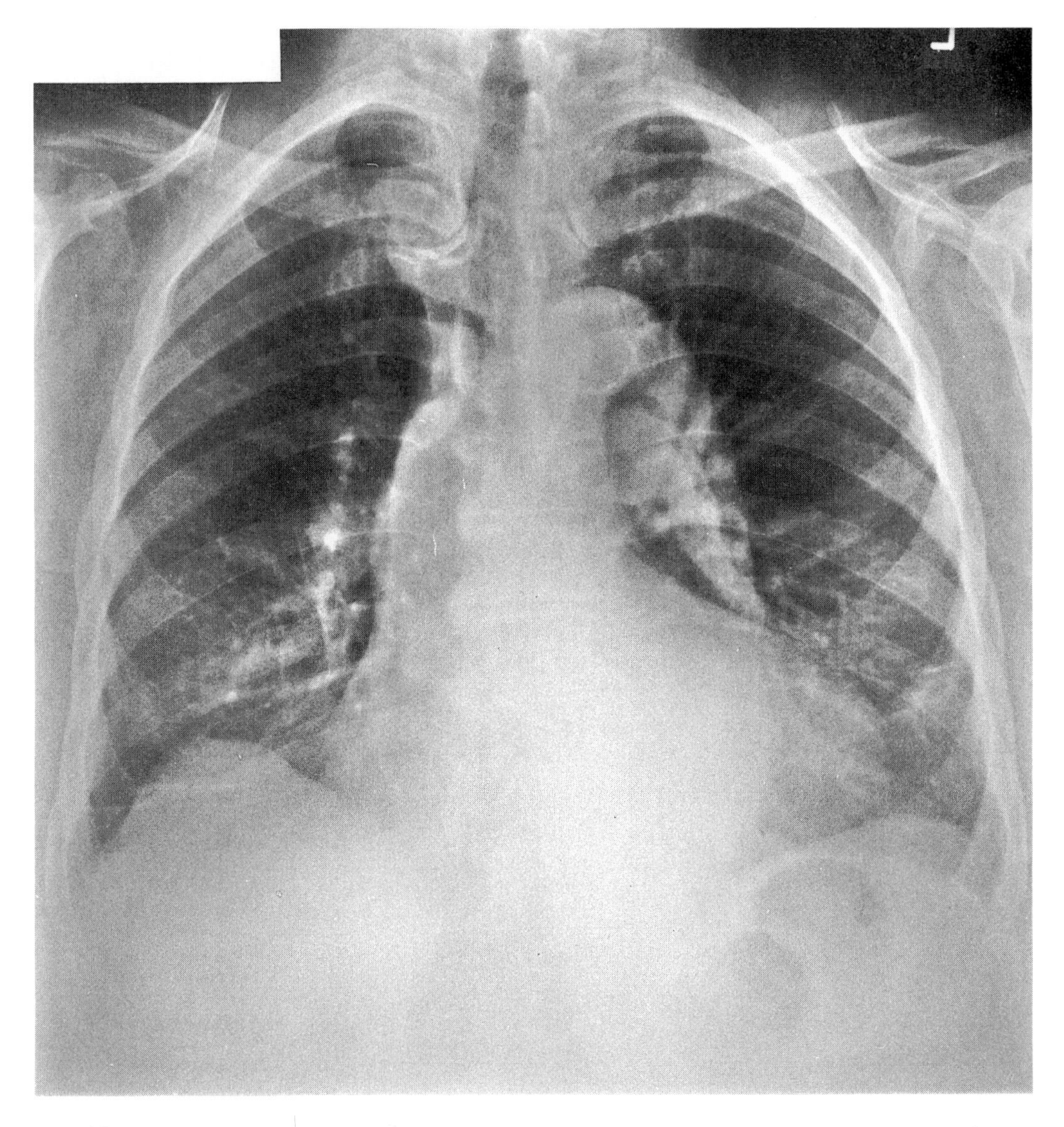

PA and lateral chest films taken during the annual physical examination of an 86-year-old man.

continued on next page

Case 24 *continued*

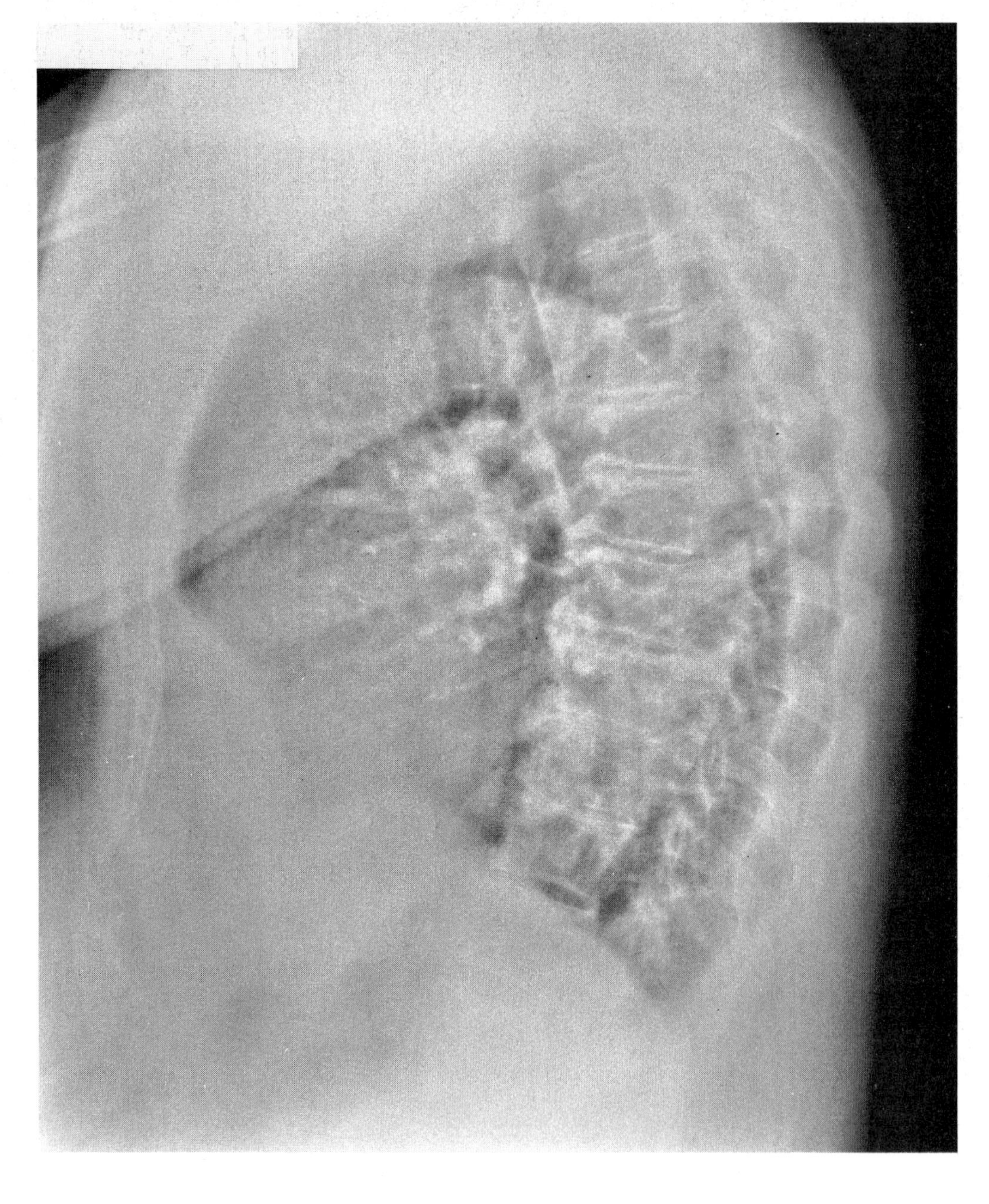

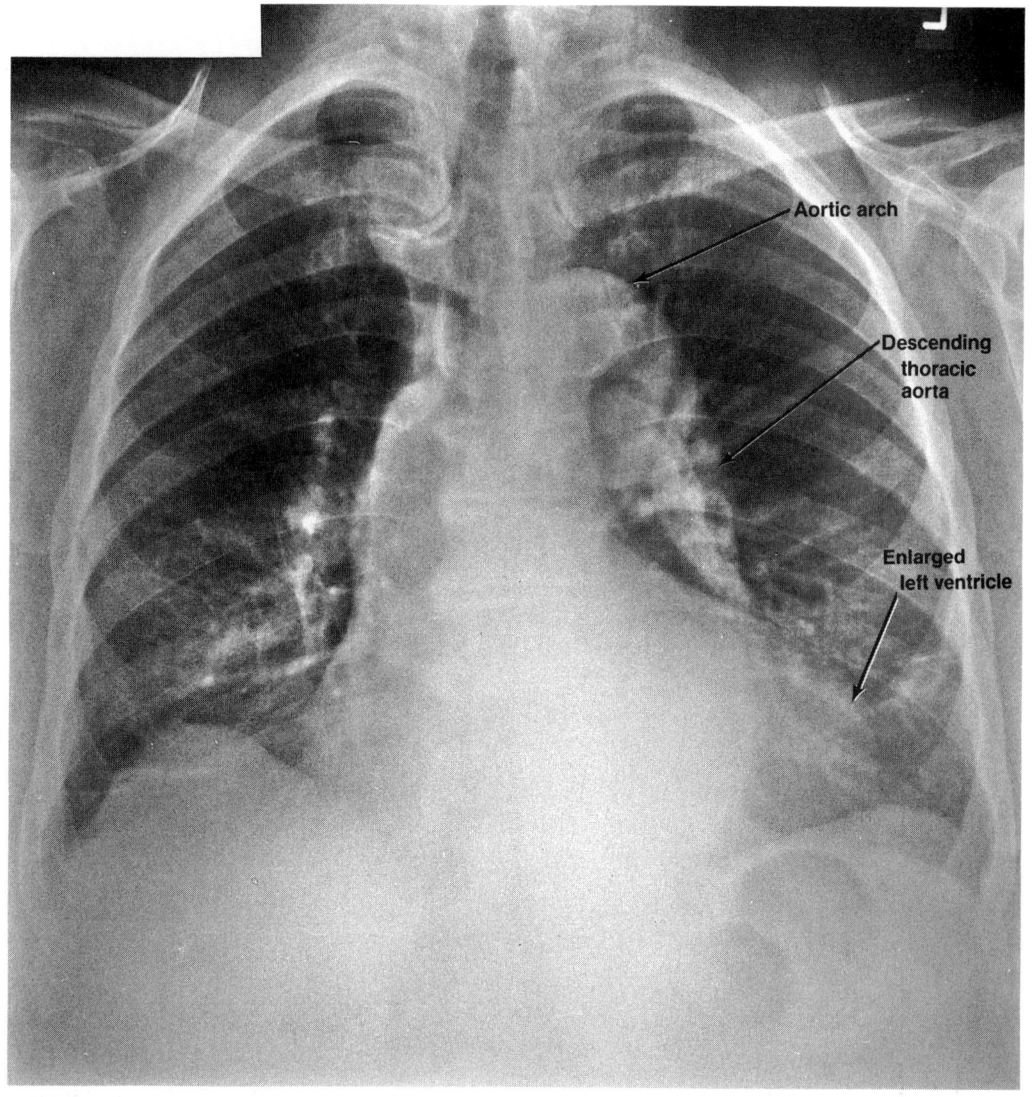

PA view

Case 24 discussion. [*Chapter 3 IV C 1 d, D 5*] The PA chest film shows a moderately enlarged heart and a cardiovascular shadow whose left border is significantly altered by a tortuous aortic arch and descending thoracic aorta. The outward lower bulging of the cardiovascular shadow's left border and lowering of the apex suggest enlargement of the left ventricle. The lateral chest film shows blunting of the posterior costophrenic angles; the PA chest film, however, does not show blunting of the lateral costophrenic angles. It therefore appears that each pleural cavity bears an effusion or pleural thickening along only the posterior margin of its costodiaphragmatic recess.

continued on next page

Case 24 discussion *continued*

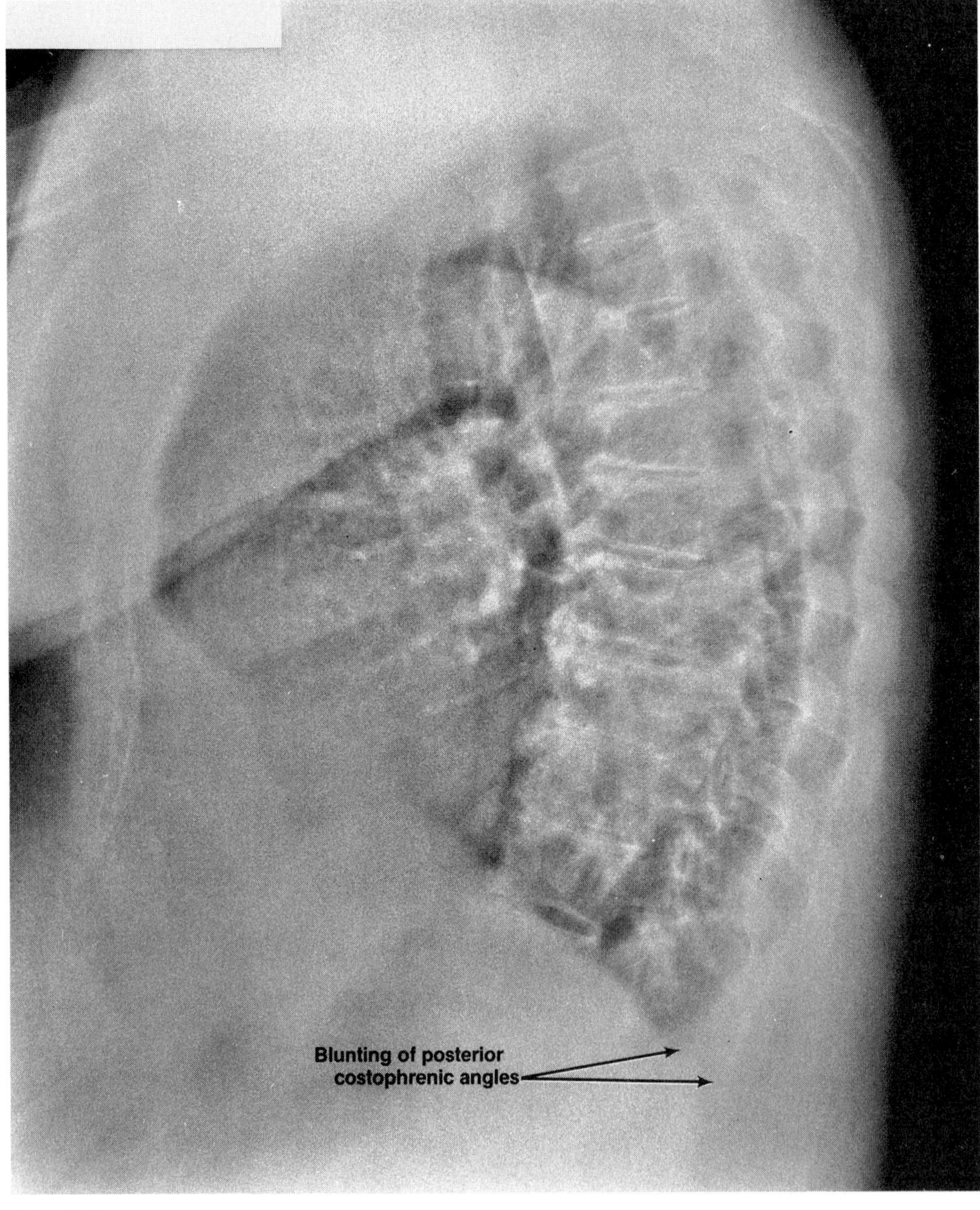

Lateral view

Case 25

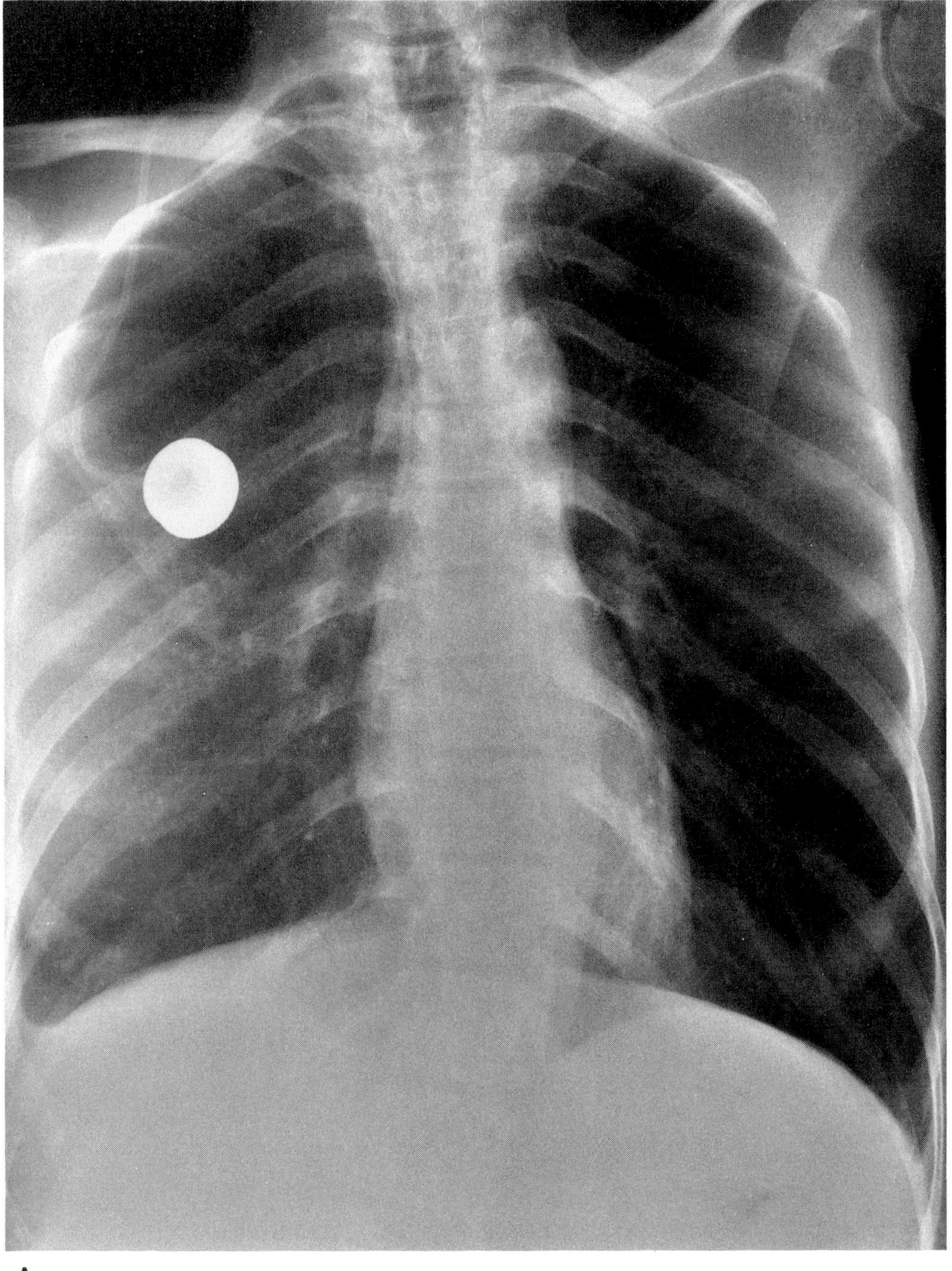

A

(*A*) PA chest film, (*B*) lateral chest film, and (*C*) AP abdominal film of a hospitalized 46-year-old woman.

continued on next page

Case 25 *continued*

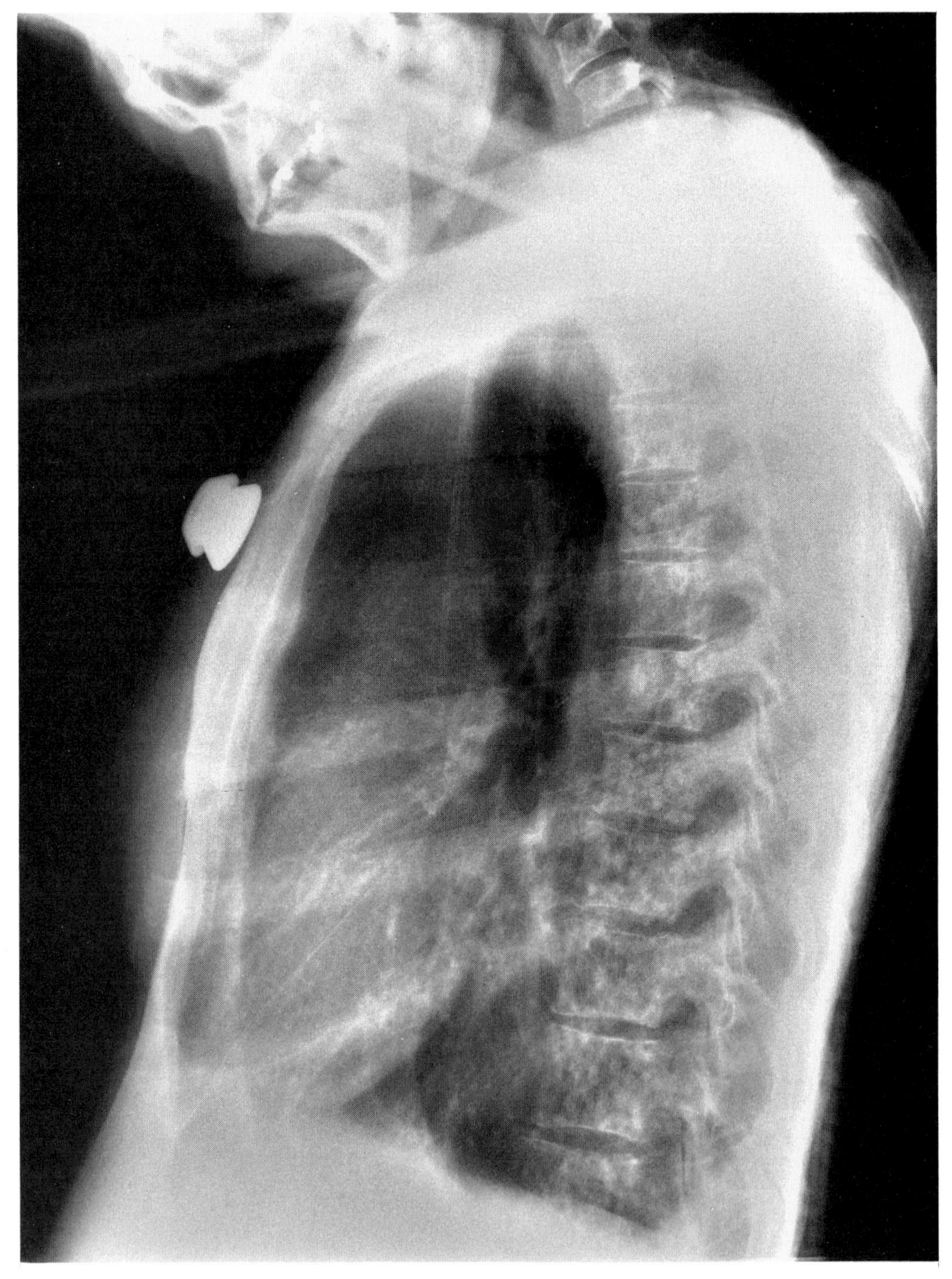

B

Case 25 *continued*

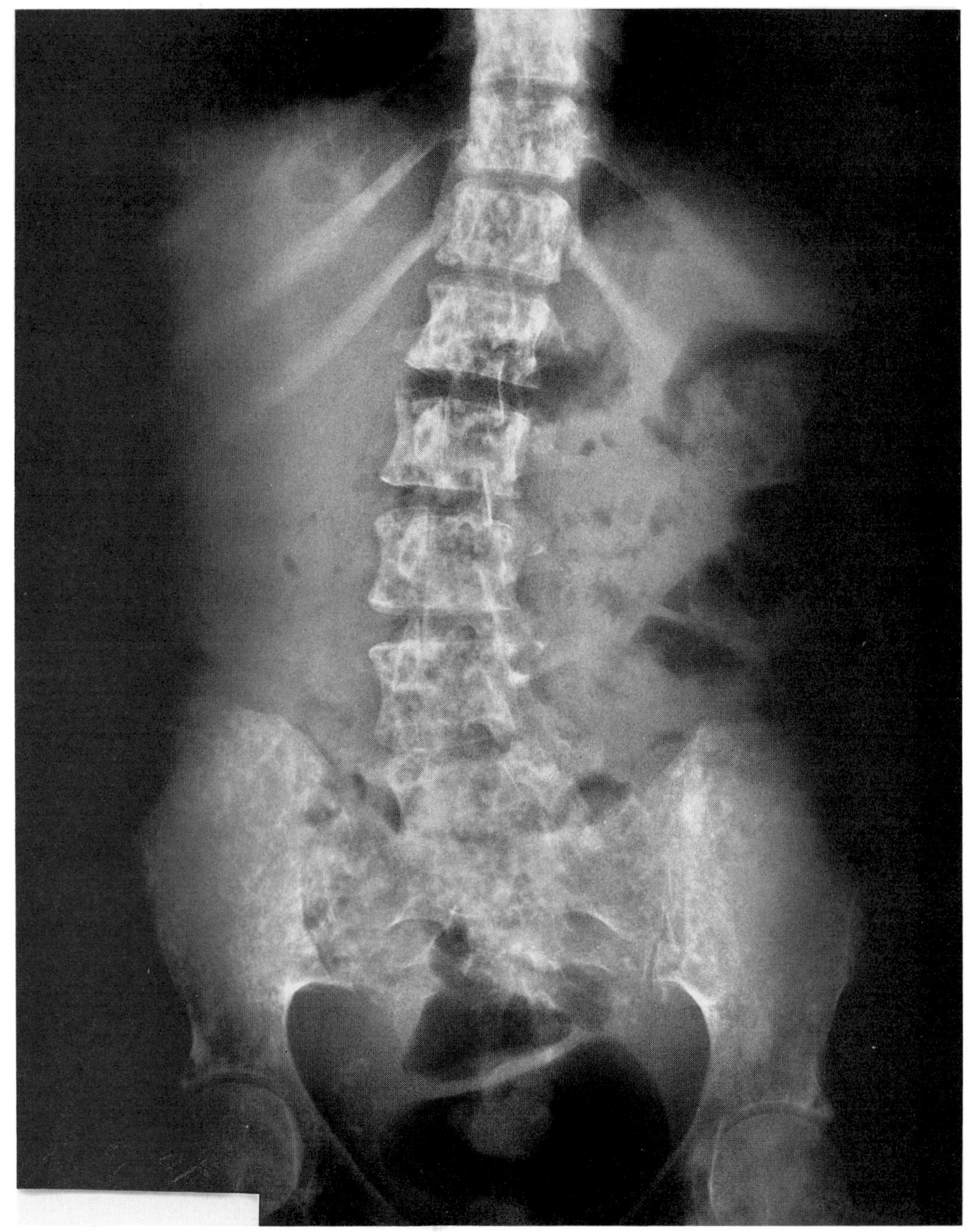

C

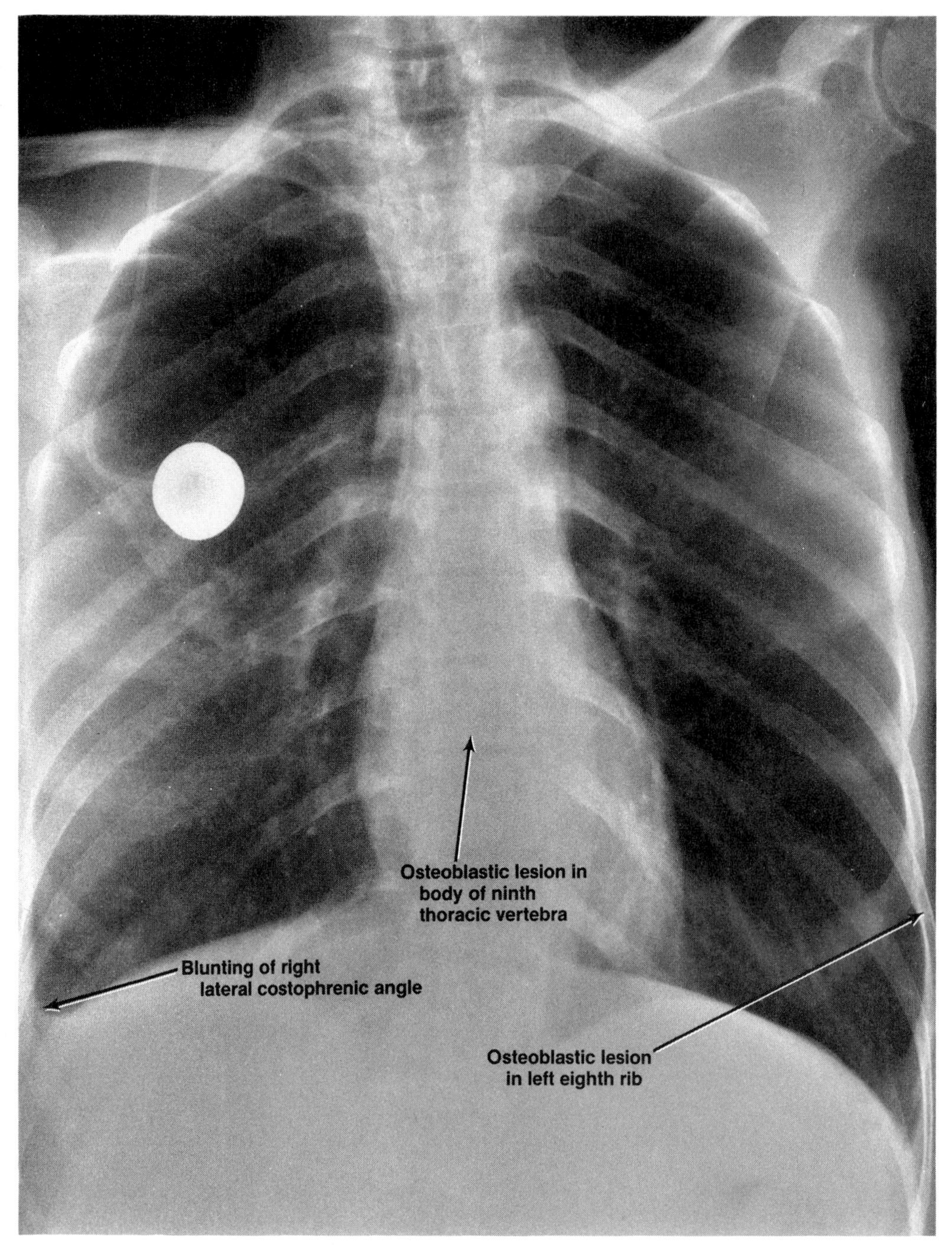

PA view

Case 25 discussion. [*Chapter 3 IV A 2; Chapter 4 IV F*] The PA chest film (radiograph A) shows absence of the soft tissue shadows of the left breast, osteoblastic lesions dispersed throughout the ribs and thoracic vertebrae, and blunting of the right lateral costophrenic angle. The lateral chest film (radiograph B) shows more clearly the dispersion of the osteoblastic lesions throughout the bodies of the thoracic vertebrae; the lateral chest film also shows pleural effusion in the posterior costophrenic angles, or sulci, of the pleural cavities. The AP abdominal film (radiograph C) shows osteoblastic lesions dispersed throughout the bodies of the lumbar vertebrae, the sacrum, and the ileal wings of the innominate bones. The uniformly increased background radiodensity of the abdominal and pelvic

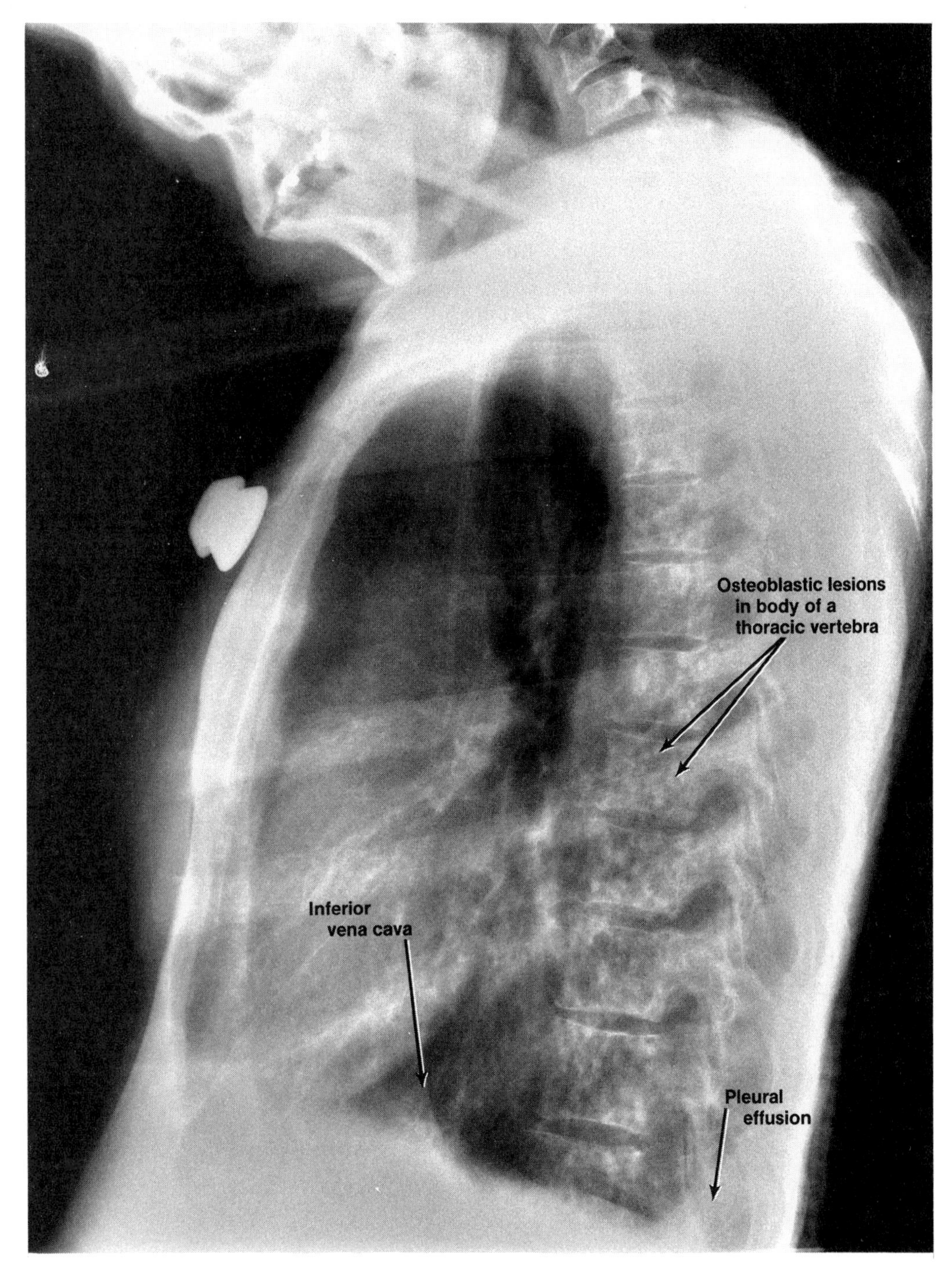

Lateral view

cavities suggests ascites (i.e., excess fluid in the abdominopelvic cavity). The patient had undergone a mastectomy for cancer of the left breast. The osteoblastic lesions displayed in the chest and abdominal films represent advanced skeletal metastases from the primary breast tumor.

continued on next page

Case 25 discussion *continued*

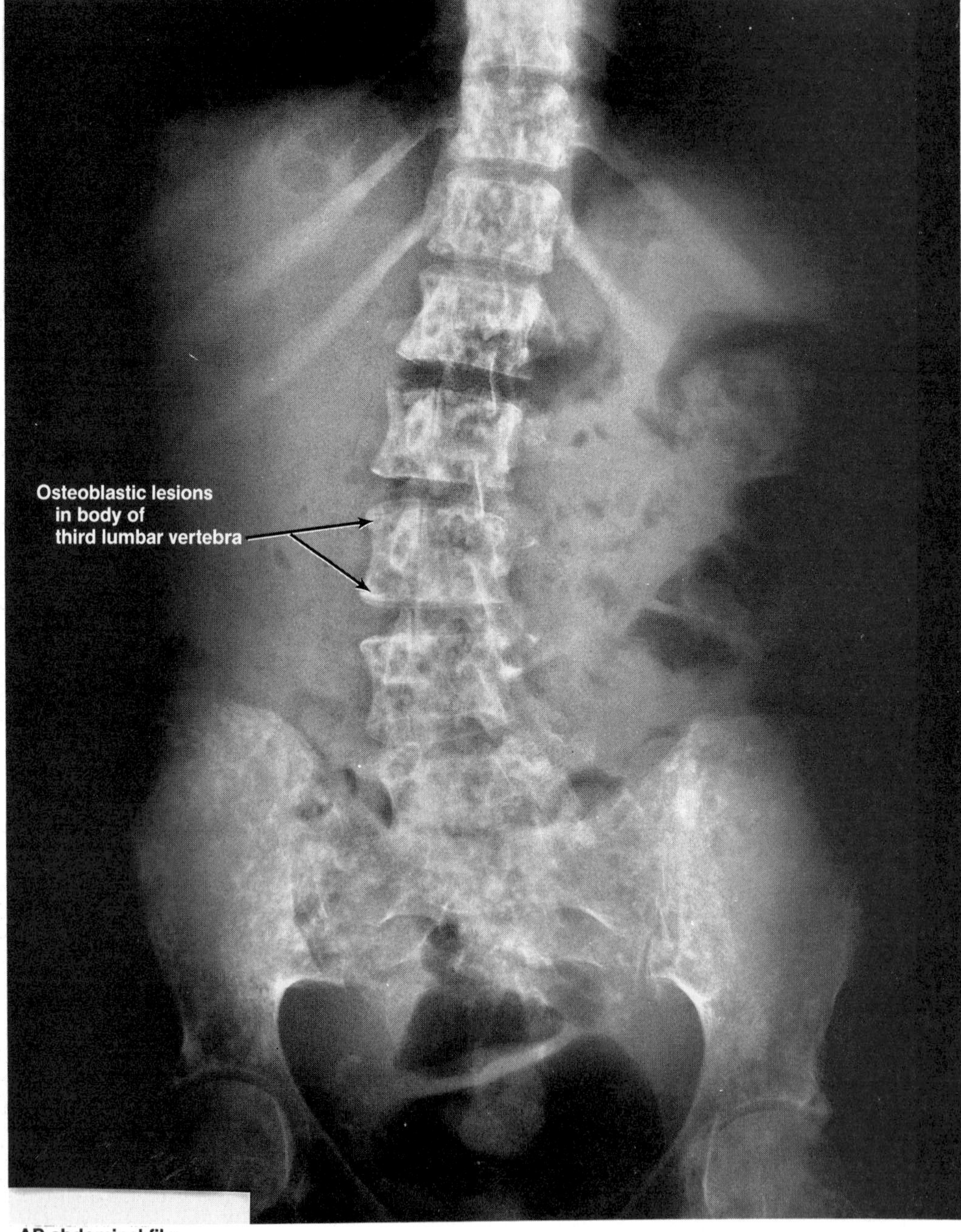

AP abdominal film

Case 26

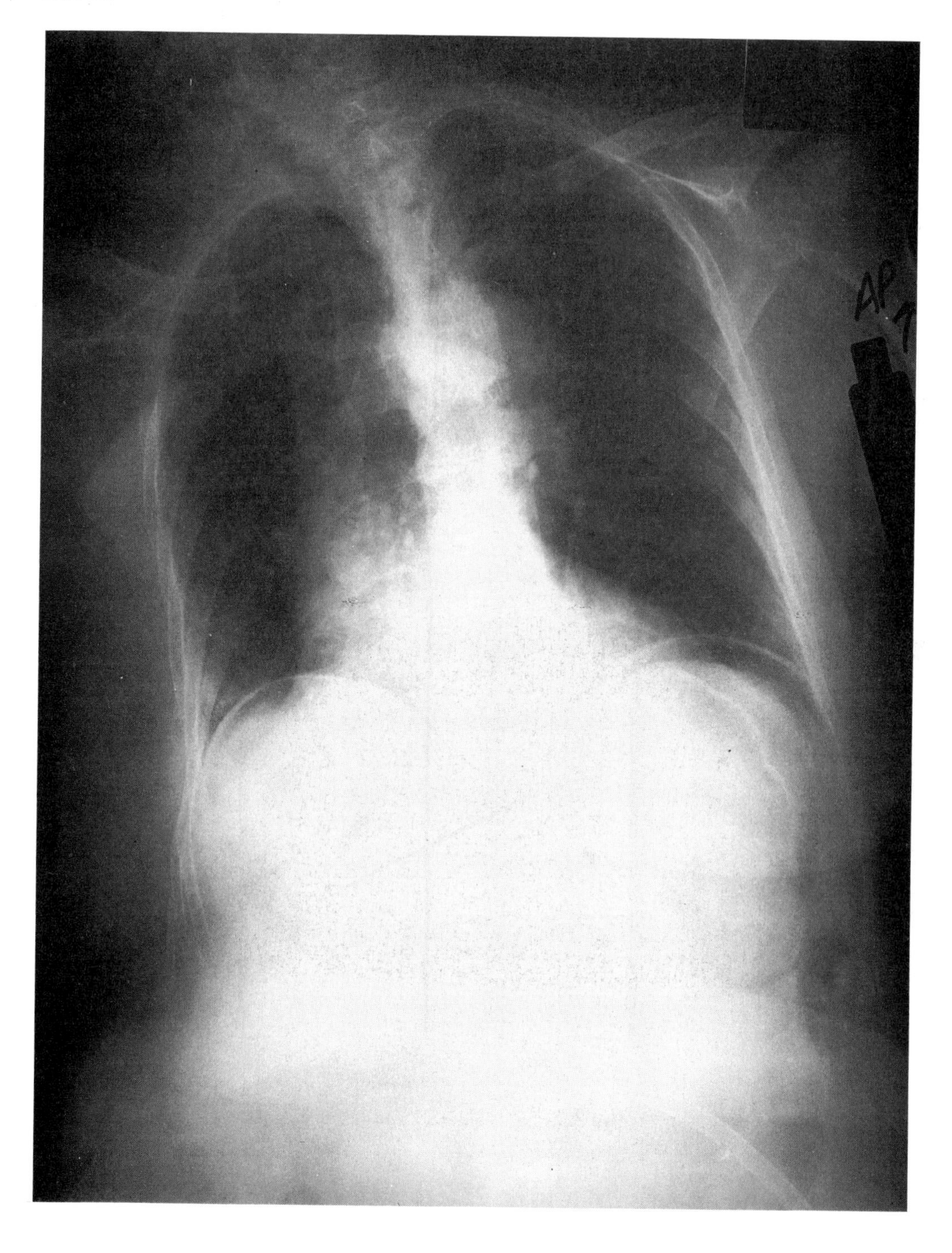

AP erect radiograph of the thorax and upper abdomen of an adult female with acute abdominal and shoulder pain and a history of peptic ulcer disease.

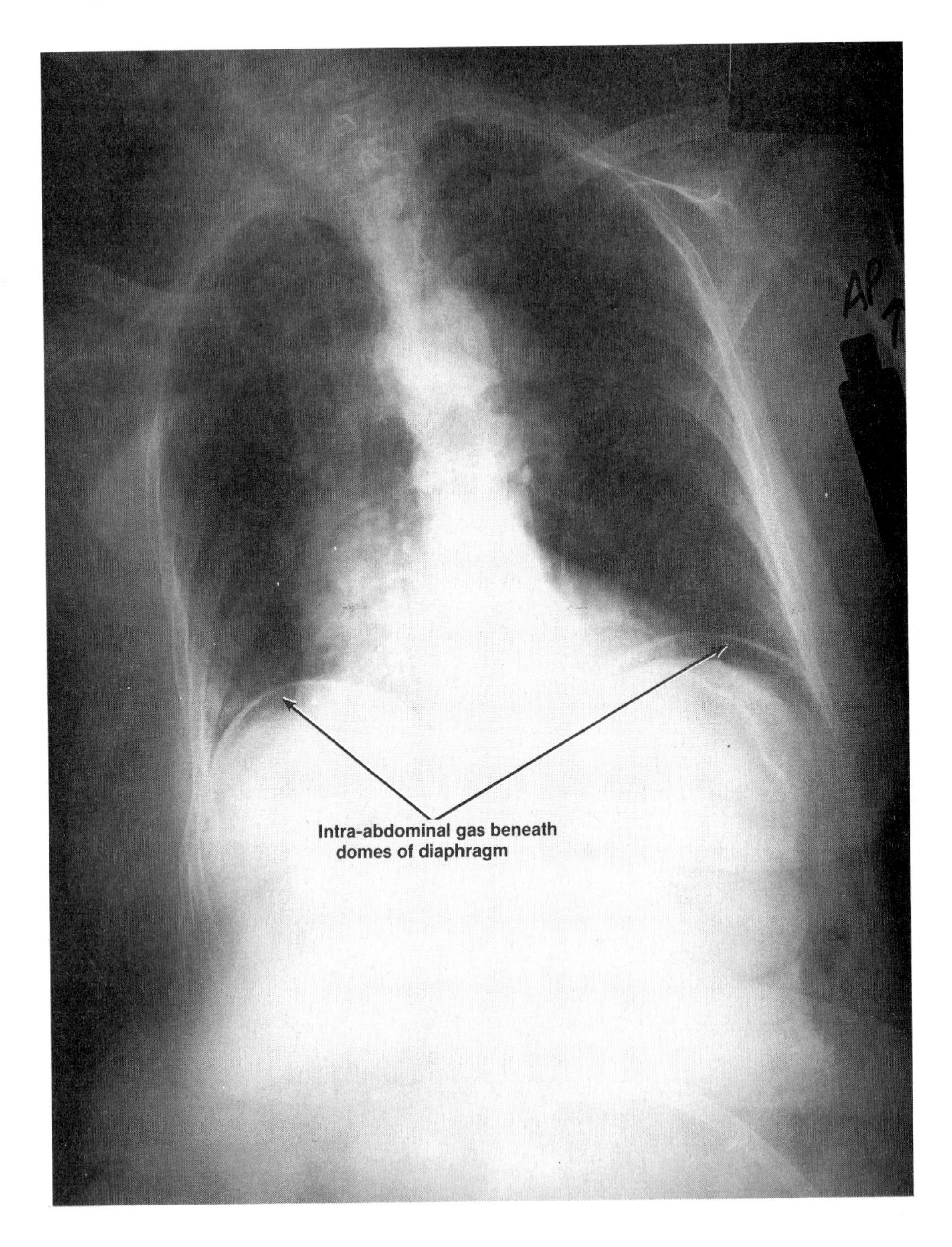

Case 26 discussion. [*Chapter 4 IV C*] The radiograph shows a pneumoperitoneum: both domes of the diaphragm overlie collections of free intra-abdominal gas. The finding of a pneumoperitoneum in association with acute abdominal pain suggests perforation of a hollow abdominal viscus. In this case, the most likely basis of the pneumoperitoneum and acute abdominal pain is perforation of the peptic ulcer. Distension of the diaphragmatic domes by the intra-abdominal gas in association with possible irritation by extravasated gastric or duodenal contents is the basis of referred pain in the shoulders.

Case 27

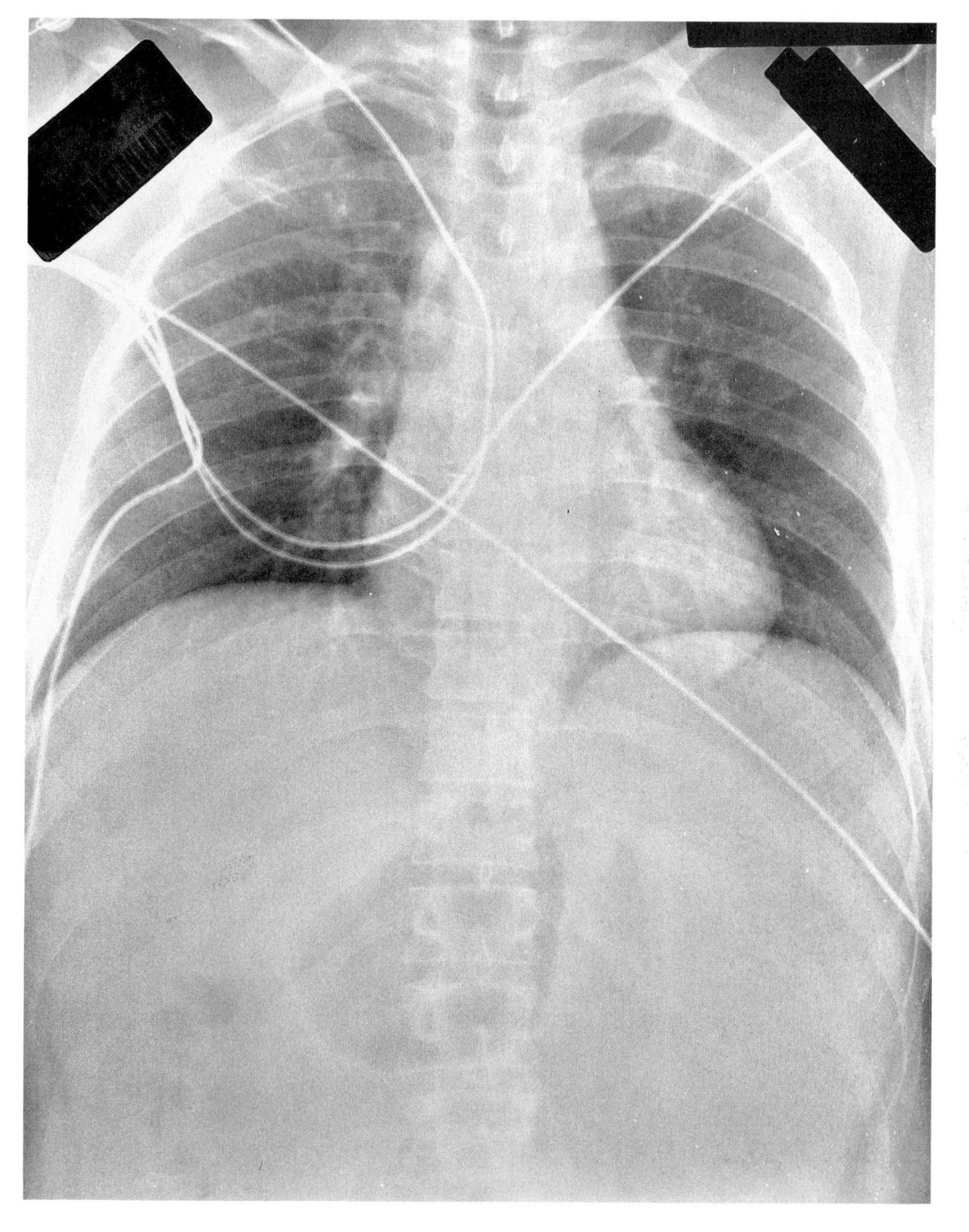

AP supine radiograph of the thorax and upper abdomen of a 39-year-old male brought to the emergency room following blunt abdominal trauma.

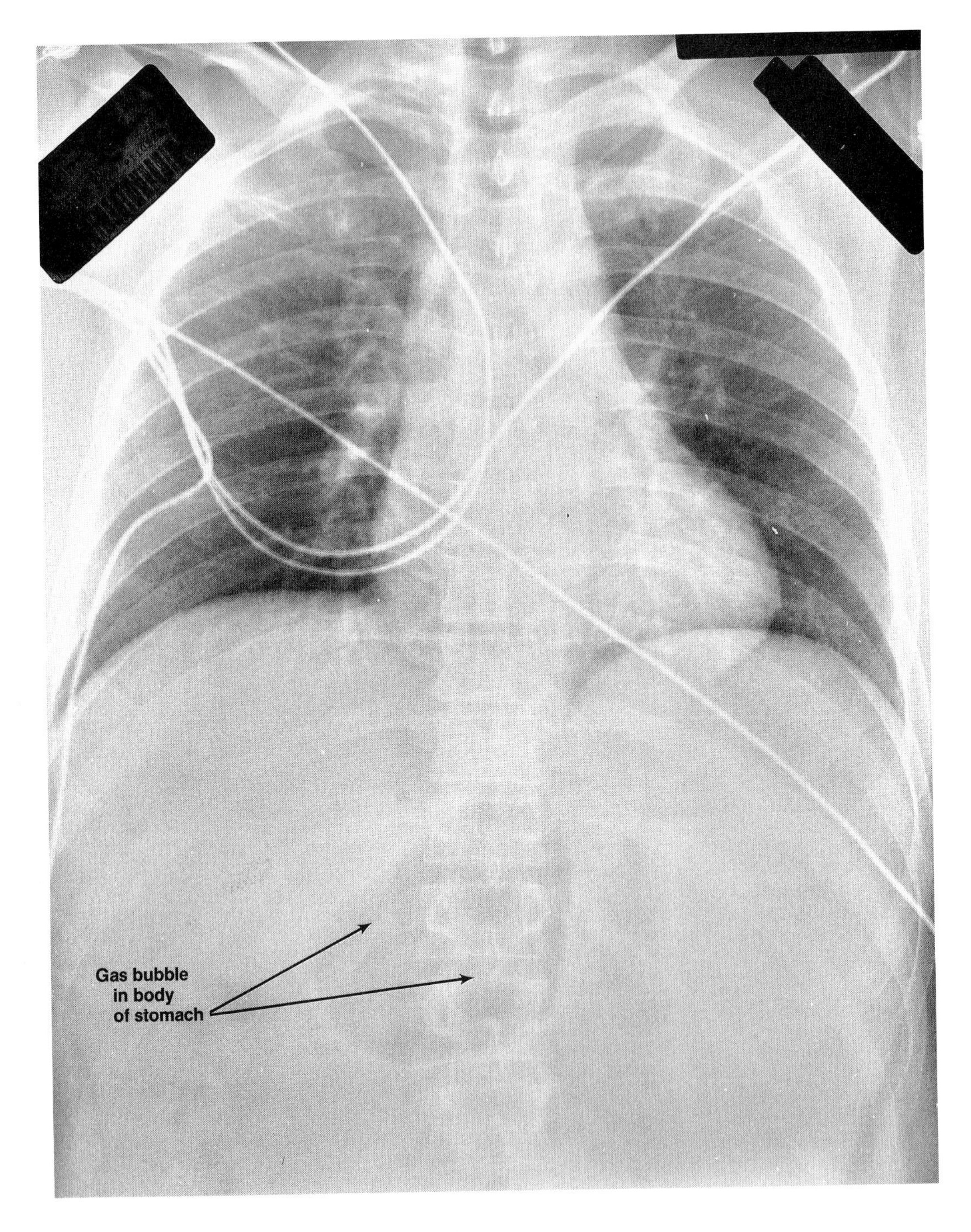

Case 27 discussion. [*Chapter 4 IV D*] The radiograph shows a marked, uniform increase in the background radiodensity of the abdomen; such an increase following trauma to the abdomen generally suggests rupture of an abdominal viscus with marked extravasation of blood into the abdominal cavity. In this case, CT scans of the upper abdomen showed that blood was extravasating from a ruptured spleen and a lacerated liver. The relatively large air-density region in the midline of the upper abdomen represents a large gas bubble in the body of the stomach; the stomach has been inferomedially displaced by the enlarged, ruptured spleen.

Case 28

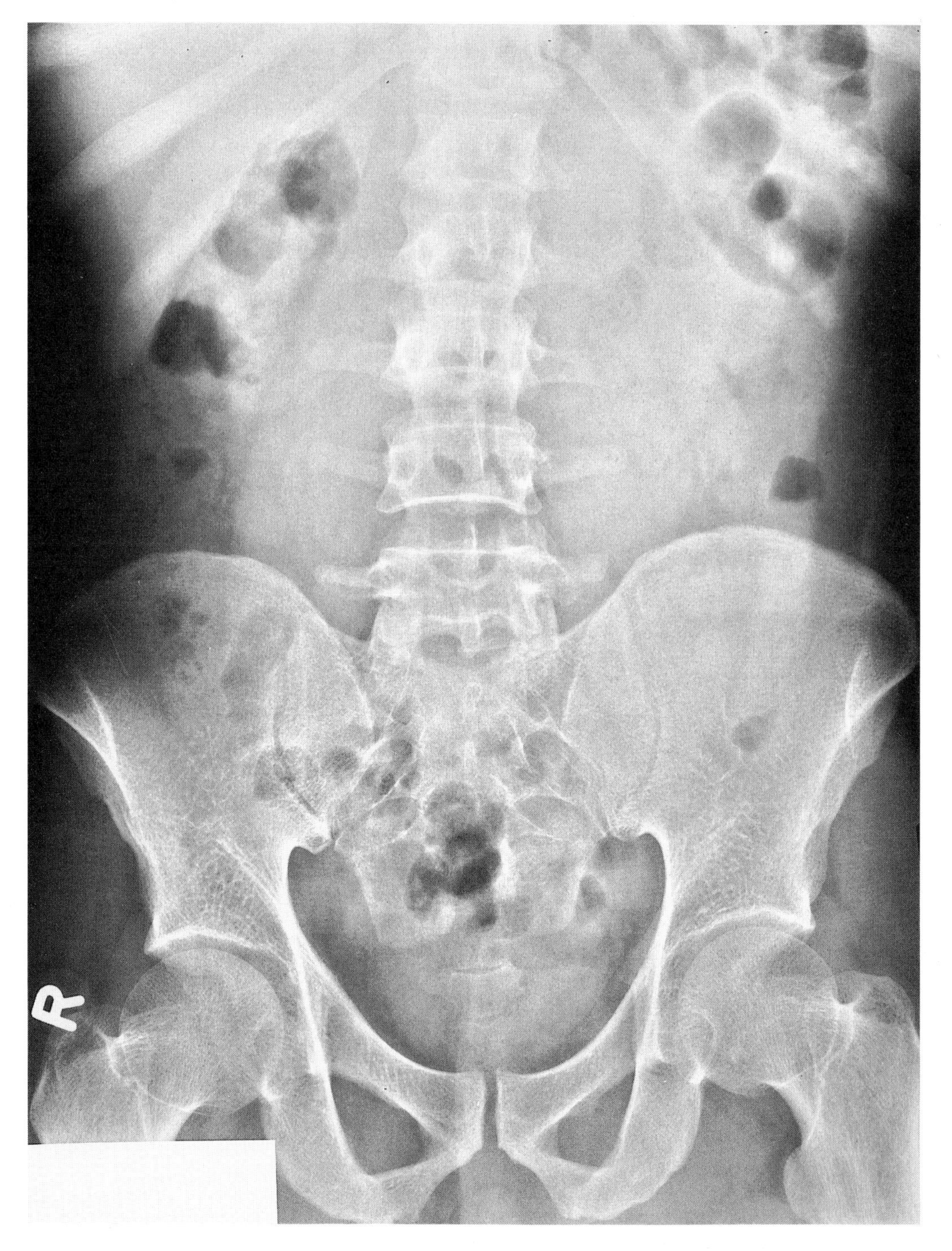

AP supine abdominal radiograph of a 57-year-old man.

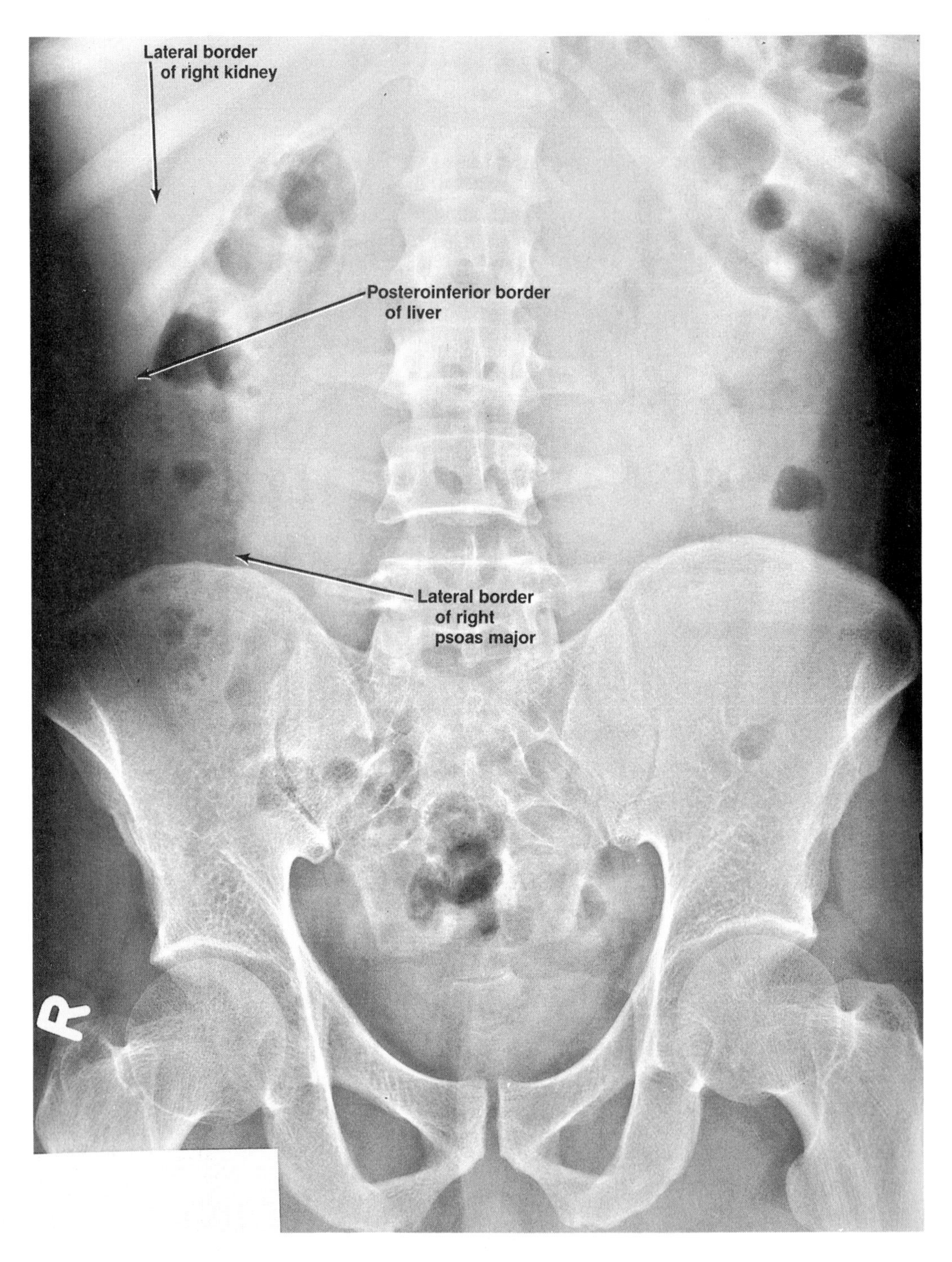

Case 28 discussion. [*Chapter 4 II A, D*] The radiograph shows a nonspecific gas pattern and no abnormalities. Parts of the lateral border of each psoas major muscle are discernible. The posteroinferior border of the liver and the lateral border of the right kidney are also discernible.

Case 29

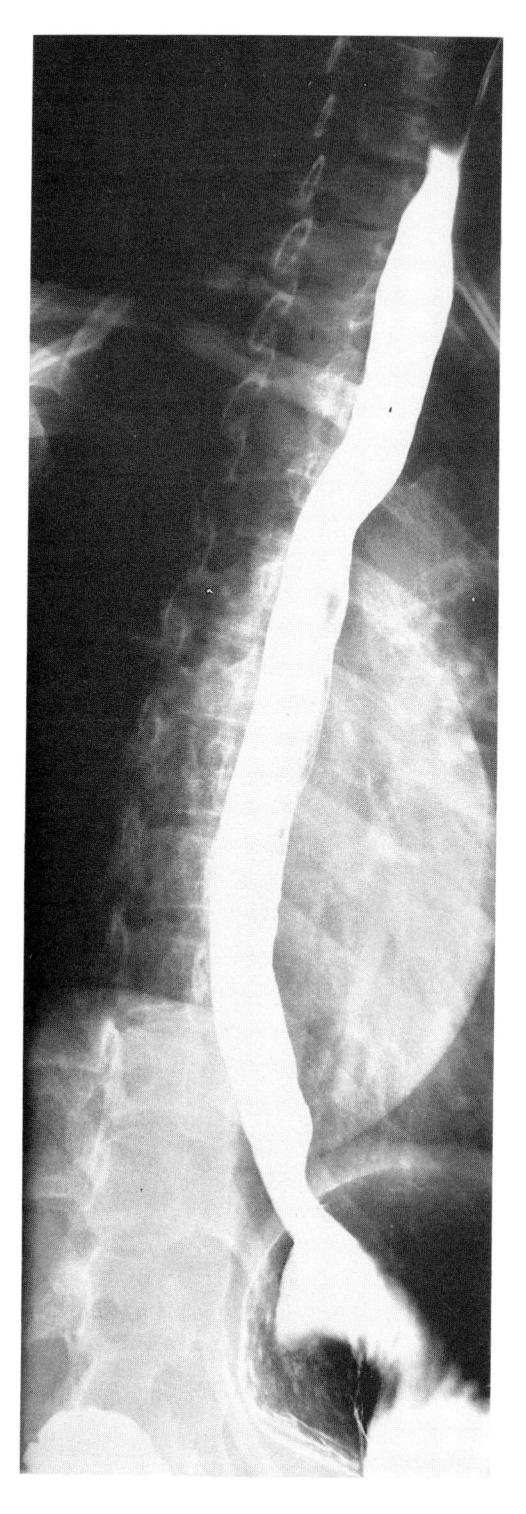

A

(*A*) Oblique chest film, (*B*) AP supine abdominal film, and (*C*) PA prone abdominal film of a double-contrast study of the upper gastrointestinal tract of a 28-year-old woman. The patient's upper gastrointestinal tract appears normal. Identify the segments of the upper gastrointestinal tract filled with contrast material in each radiograph.

continued on next page

Case 29 *continued*

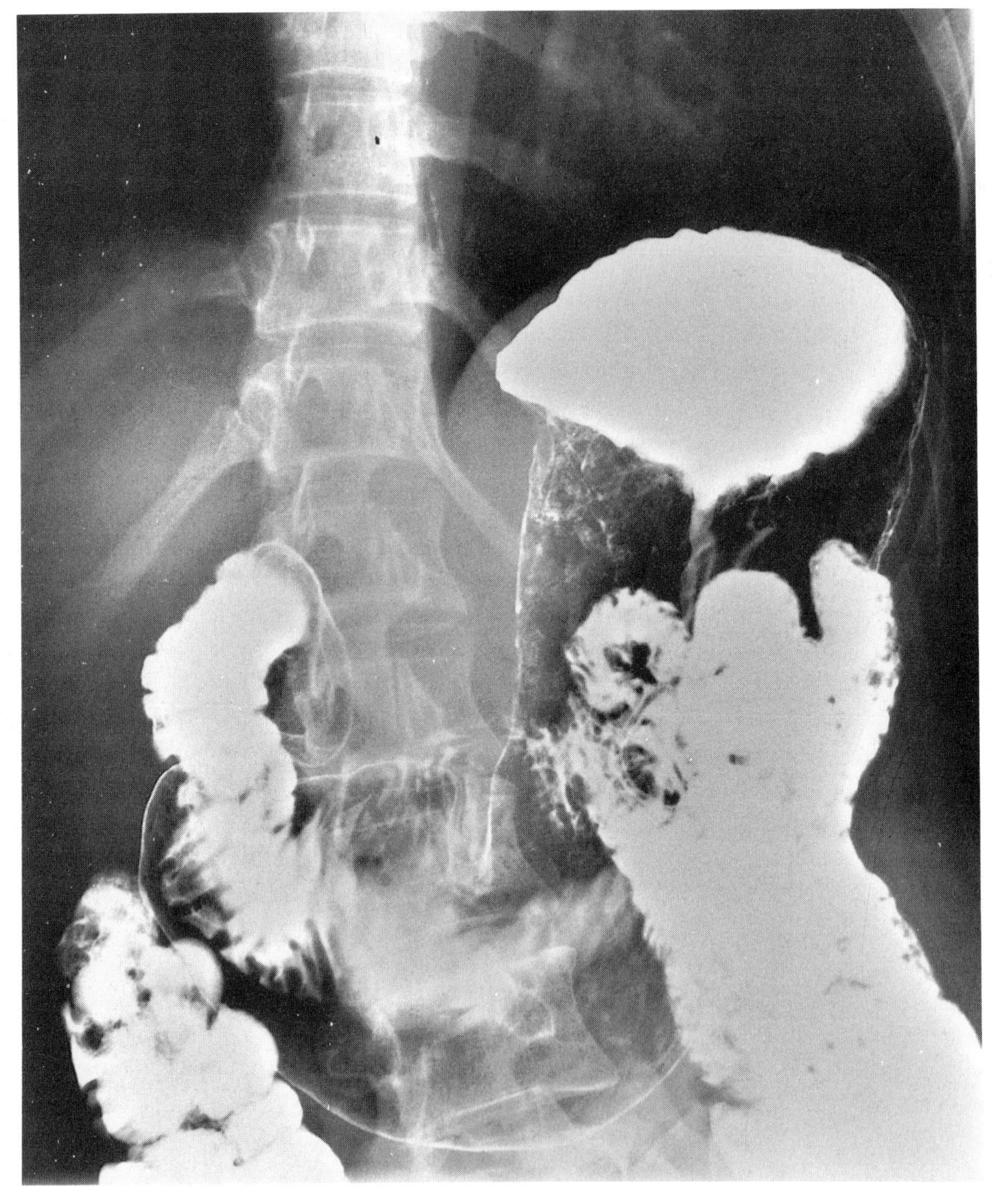

B

Case 29 *continued*

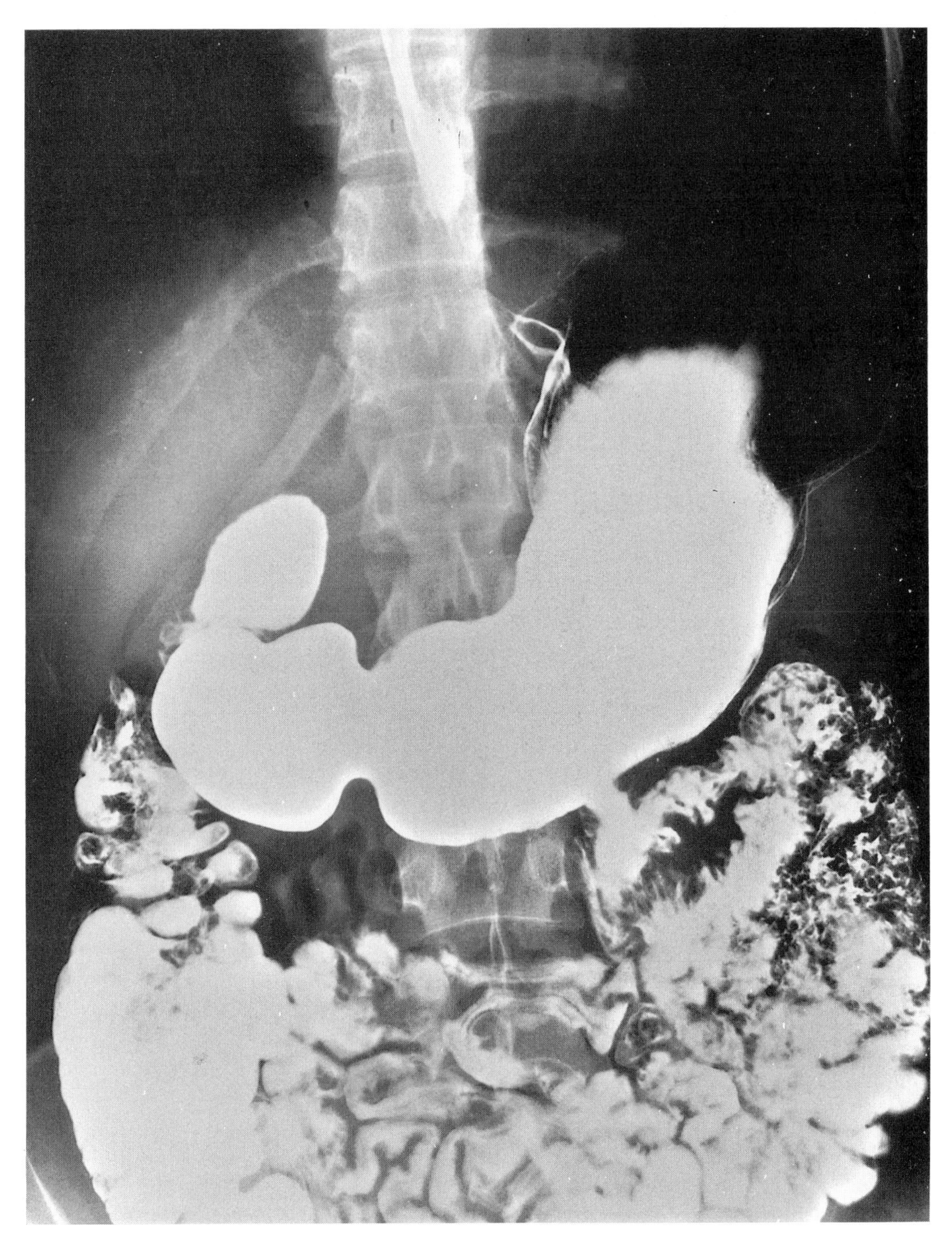

C

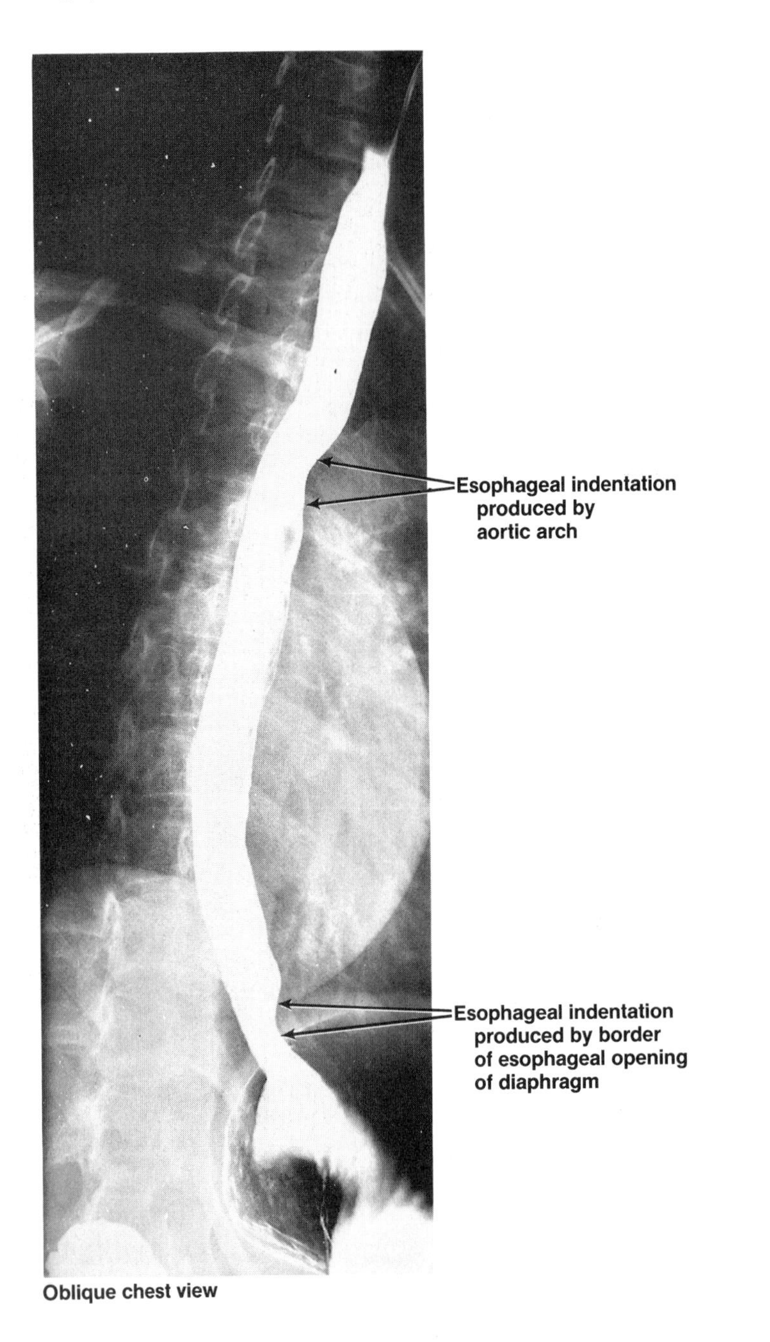

Oblique chest view

Case 29 discussion. [*Chapter 4 I C 2 c*] The radiologic procedure most commonly employed to study the mucosal lining of any segment of the gastrointestinal tract from the stomach to the rectum is to take radiographs of the segment under conditions in which its lumen is distended with gas or air and its mucosa is thinly coated with a barium sulfate suspension. The thin barium coating accurately portrays the topography of the mucosal lining, and this topography can be finely examined radiographically because of the marked contrast between the radiodensity of the barium coating and the gas- or air-filled lumen.

Barium sulfate's chemical inertness and virtual insolubility render it the contrast medium of choice for radiologic studies of the gastrointestinal tract. However, barium sulfate is not used if surgery is planned immediately following the examination or if a segment of the tract may have been perforated; this is because, in either situation, the barium sulfate would ultimately extravasate from the gastrointestinal tract into either the mediastinum or the peritoneal cavity.

The double-contrast procedure used to study the mucosal lining of the stomach and duodenum is

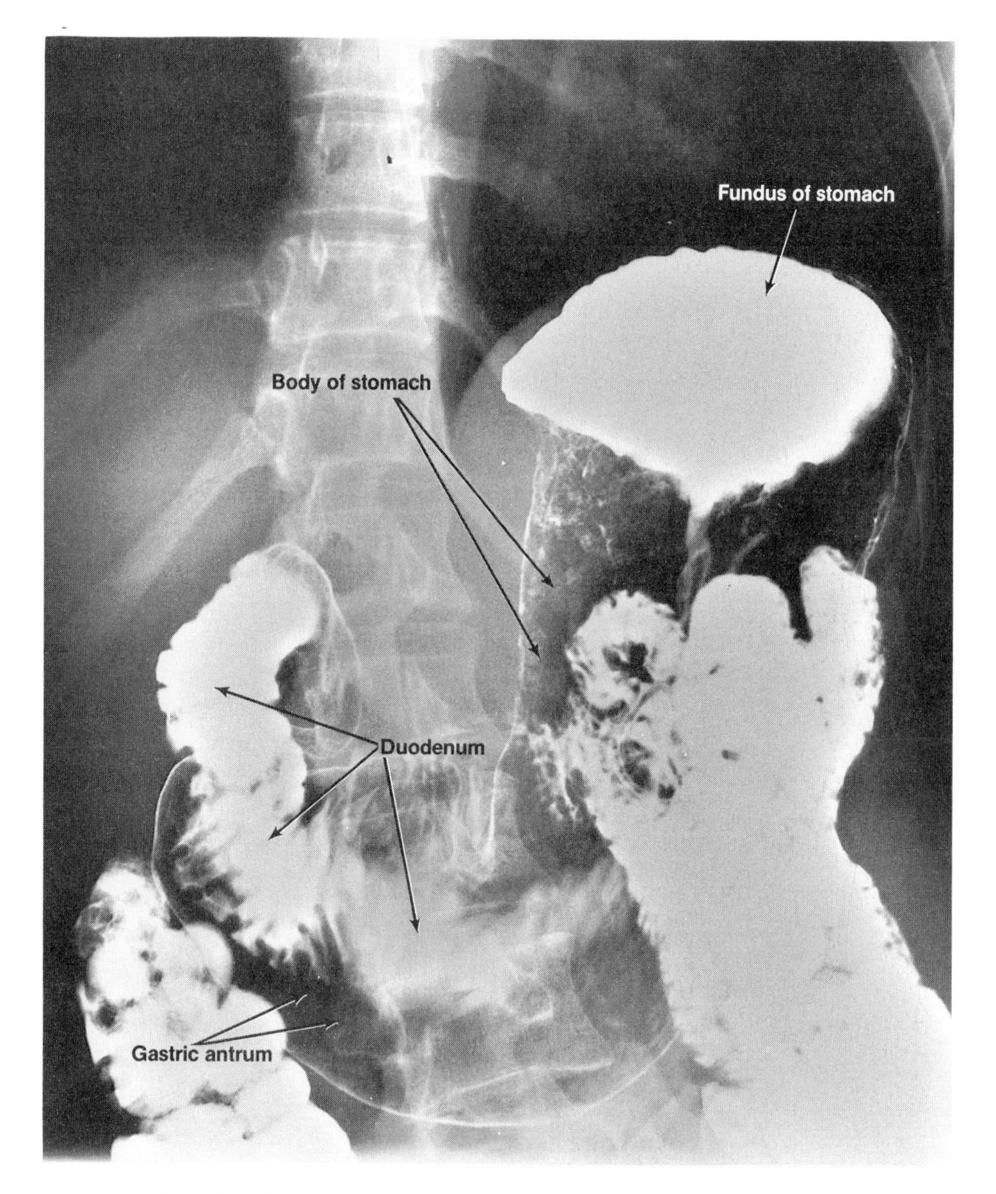

AP supine abdominal film

called a "double-contrast barium meal." The patient frequently fasts overnight prior to the examination in order to rid the stomach and duodenum of food contents. The procedure begins with the patient swallowing a barium sulfate suspension. Transport of the contrast material down the esophagus and through the stomach and duodenum can be monitored by fluoroscopy and documented with spot radiographs; the fluoroscopic monitoring distinguishes permanent strictures in the caliber of segments from those temporarily produced by peristalsis. A gas-producing agent is then administered to achieve gastric distension and double contrast. Multiple radiographs, taken with the patient in different positions, provide images of gastric regions both in dependent positions, in which the lumen is filled with contrast material, and in nondependent positions, in which the mucosa is lined by a thin coating of the contrast material and overlies a gas bubble.

The oblique chest film (radiograph A) shows the esophageal lumen uniformly expanded and filled with the barium sulfate suspension. The radiograph shows the origin of the esophagus at the lower border of the laryngopharynx, the course of the esophagus as it descends through the superior and then posterior mediastinum, and finally its passage through the diaphragm and termination at the cardiac opening of the stomach. The upper and lower indentations in the esophagus represent the physical restrictions to the expansion of the esophagus normally imposed by the aortic arch and the border of the

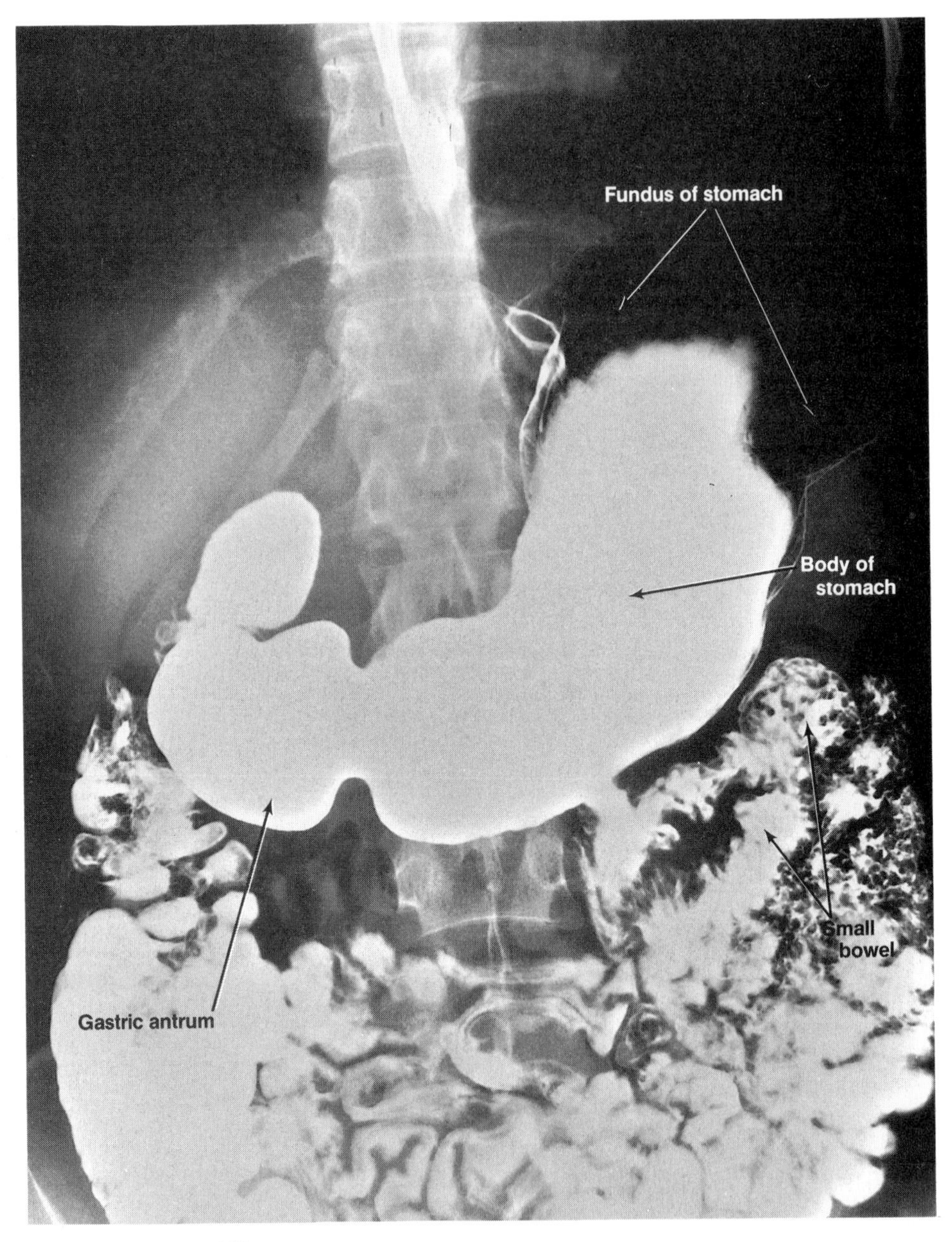

PA prone abdominal film

esophageal opening of the diaphragm, respectively. Note that these physical restrictions appear as filling defects; in descriptions of radiographs of the gastrointestinal tract, the expression "filling defect" is used to refer to any defect which prevents the normal filling of the lumen with barium sulfate suspension. Filling defects that are produced via compression from external structures (be these normal or pathologic) exhibit a characteristic feature: the outline of the defect makes a shallow angle (generally between 130° and 180°) with the outline of the unrestricted, radiopaque lumen.

Radiograph B was taken with the patient lying supine, a position which tends to pool the contrast suspension in the most posterior parts of the stomach. Accordingly, the radiograph shows the fundus filled with contrast material and the body of the stomach outlined by only a thin coating. (Some of the contrast material has already passed into the small bowel.) Radiograph C was taken with the patient lying prone, a position which tends to pool the contrast suspension in the most anterior parts of the stomach. Accordingly, the body of the stomach is filled with contrast material and the fundus is outlined by only a thin coating. Radiograph C has also captured a peristaltic wave transporting contrast material into the gastric antrum and proximal end of the duodenum.

Case 30

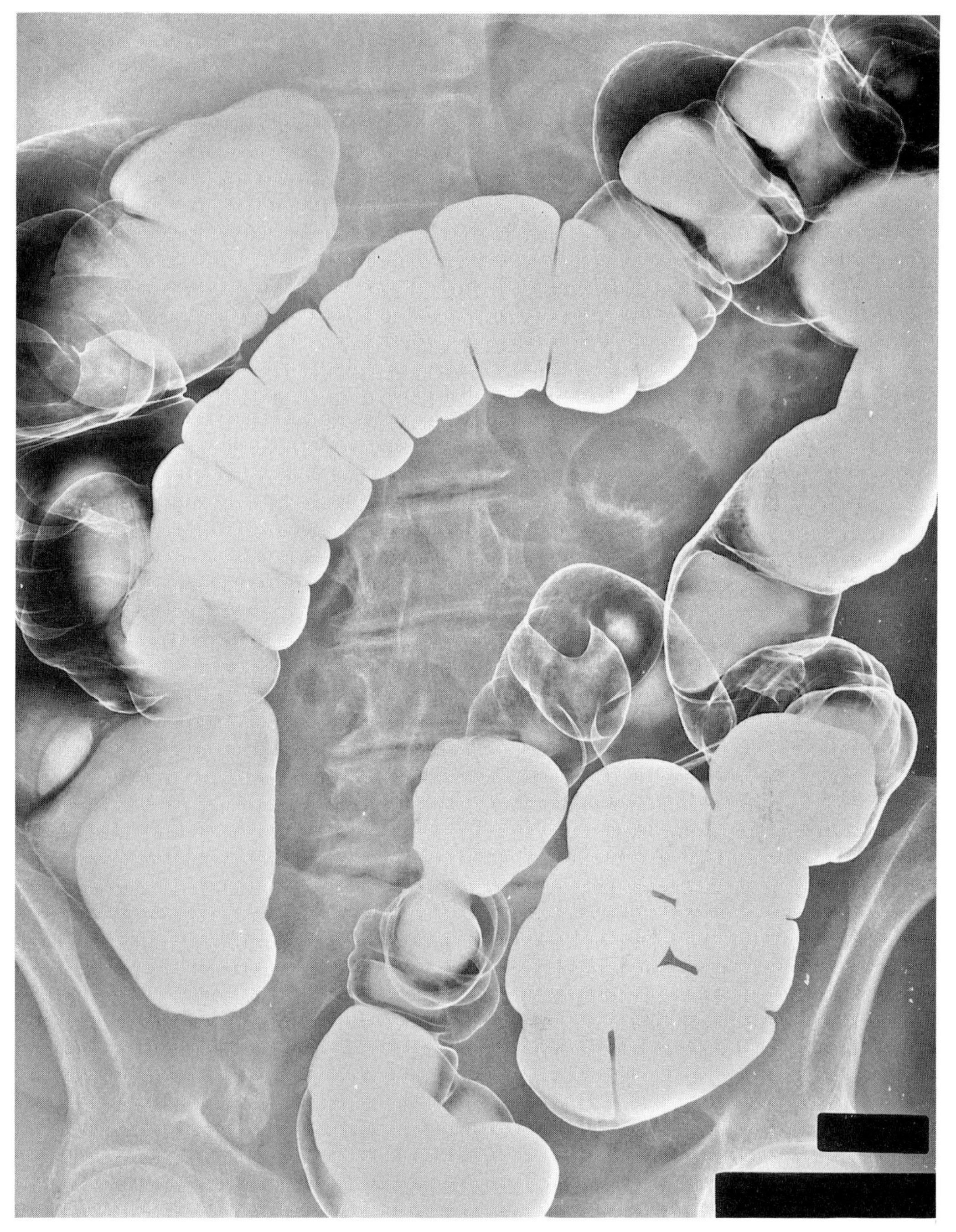

A

Four abdominal films of a double-contrast barium enema study of the large bowel of a 73-year-old woman. The radiographs are (*A*) a PA prone film, (*B*) an AP supine film, (*C*) a right lateral decubitus film, and (*D*) a left lateral decubitus film. The patient's large bowel appears normal. Identify the major segments of the patient's large bowel for each of the radiographs.

continued on next page

Case 30 *continued*

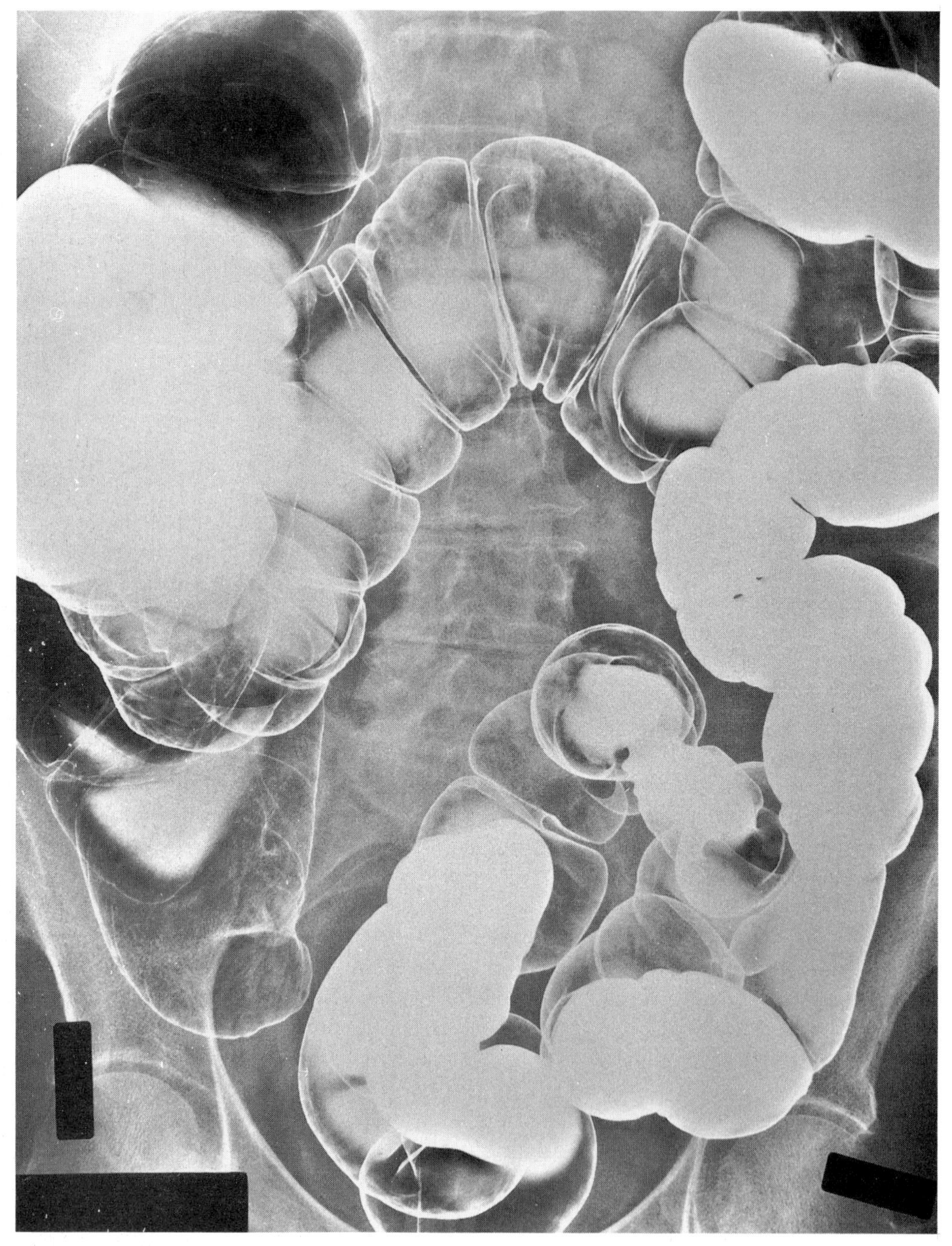

B

Case 30 *continued*

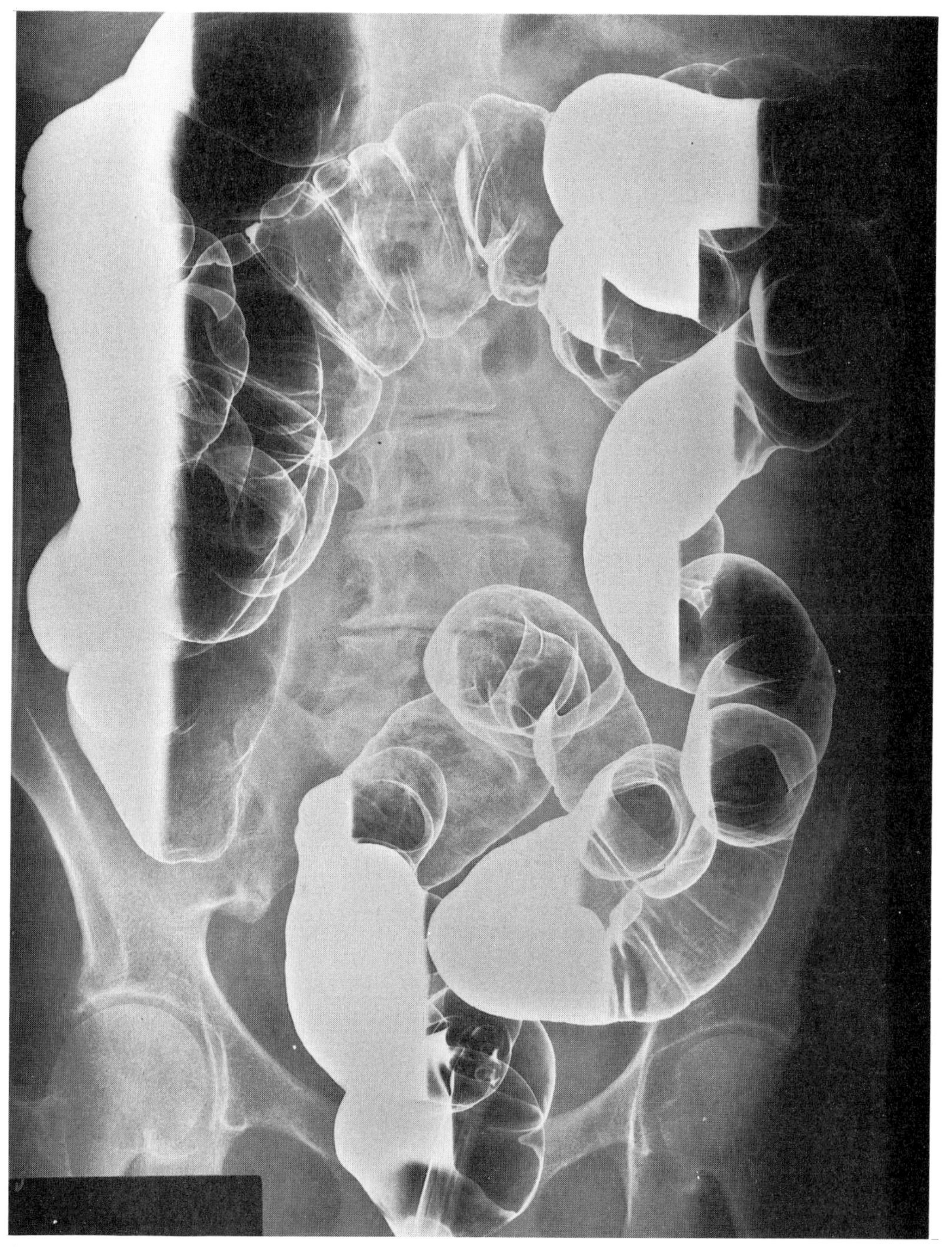

C

continued on next page

Case 30 *continued*

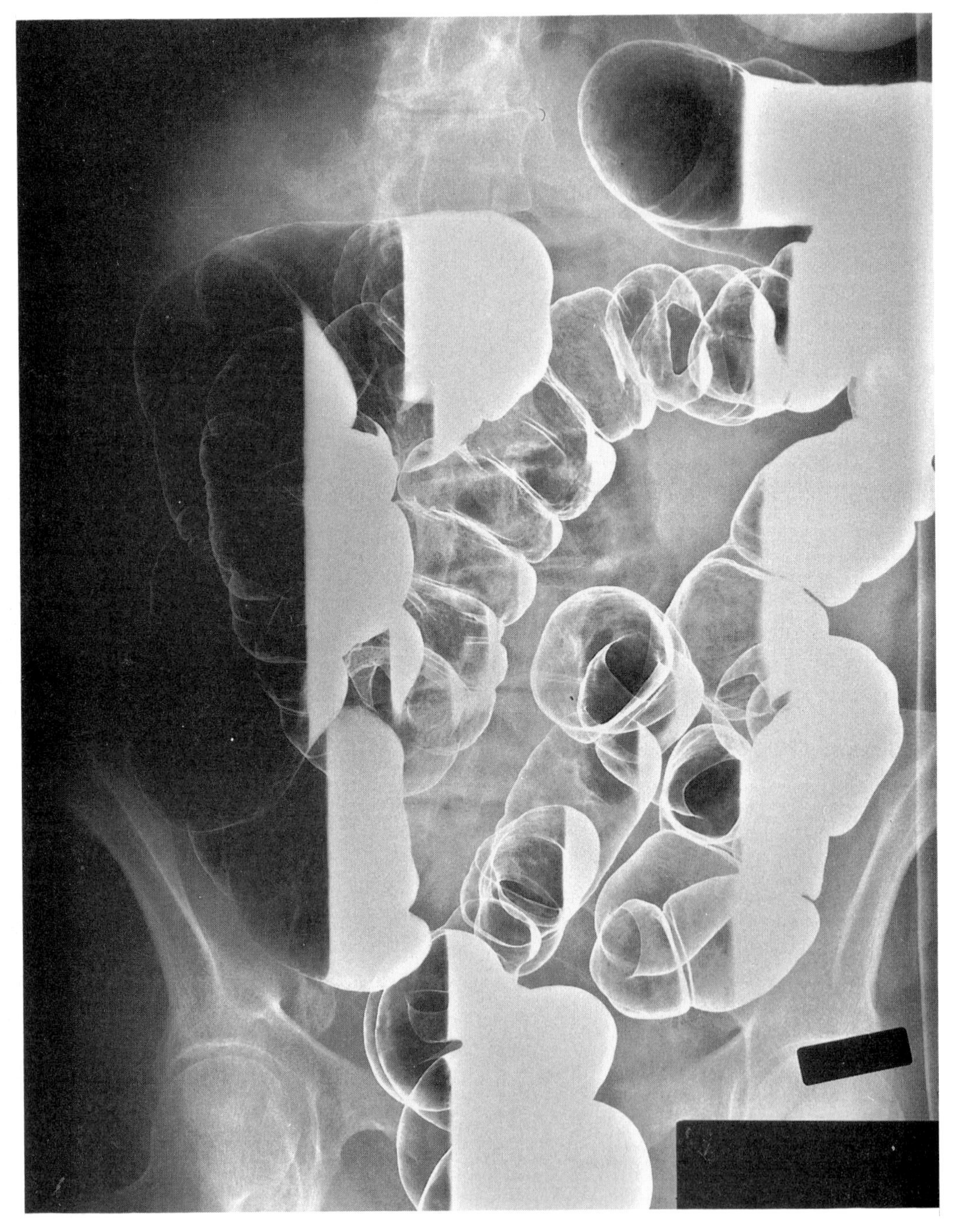

D

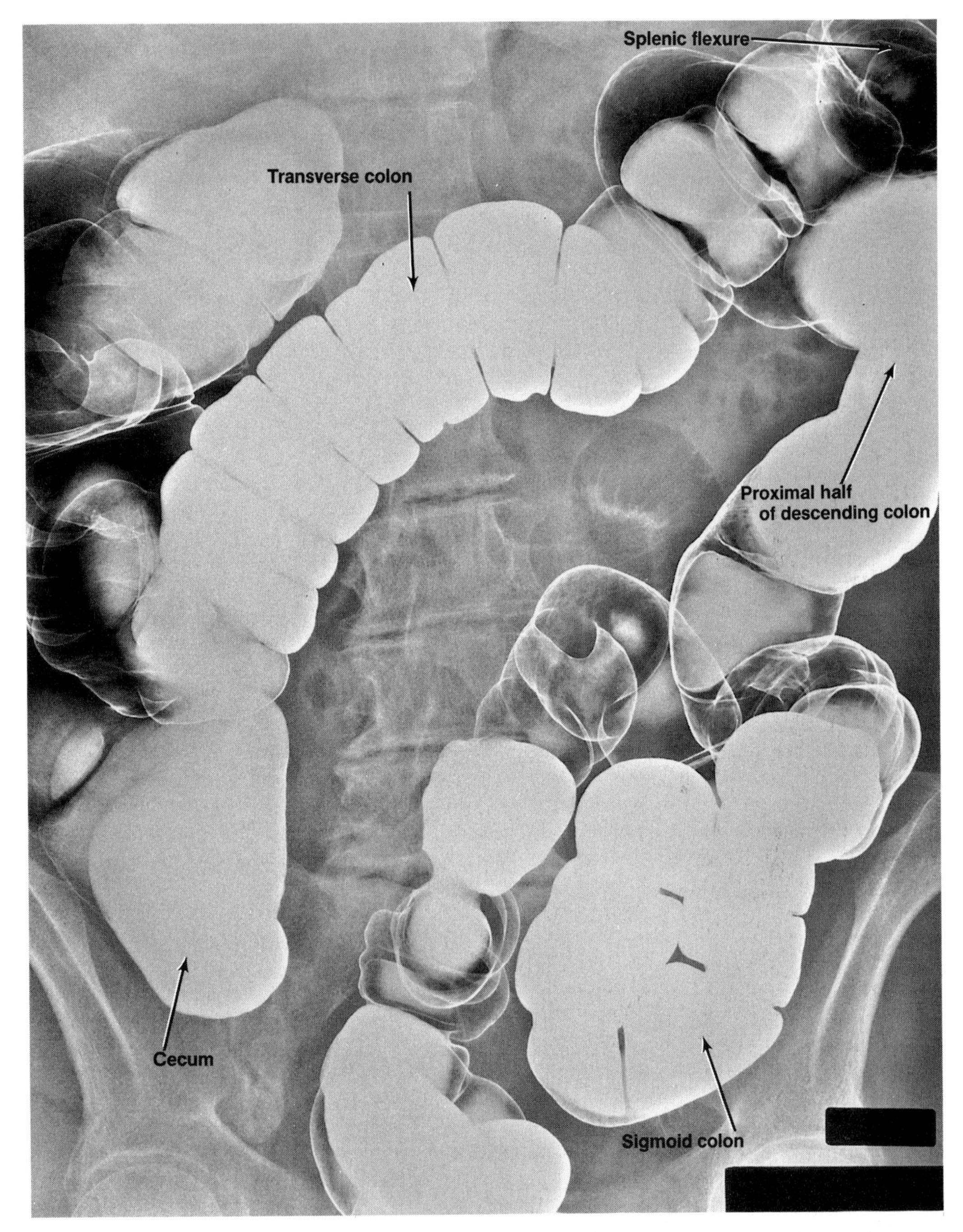

A. PA prone film

Case 30 discussion. [*Chapter 4 I D 5–7, E; II D 6*] A double-contrast barium enema study is the radiologic method most commonly used to study the mucosal lining of the large bowel. The patient is frequently prepared for the study by cleansing the large bowel of fecal material through the administration of a low-residue diet and oral laxatives over a 24- to 48-hour period, followed by tap-water enemas until returns are clear. A rectal catheter is first used to introduce a thick suspension of barium sulfate into the large bowel as far back as the splenic flexure or midregion of the transverse colon. Air is then injected through the catheter to spread the barium suspension retrogradely and to distend the large

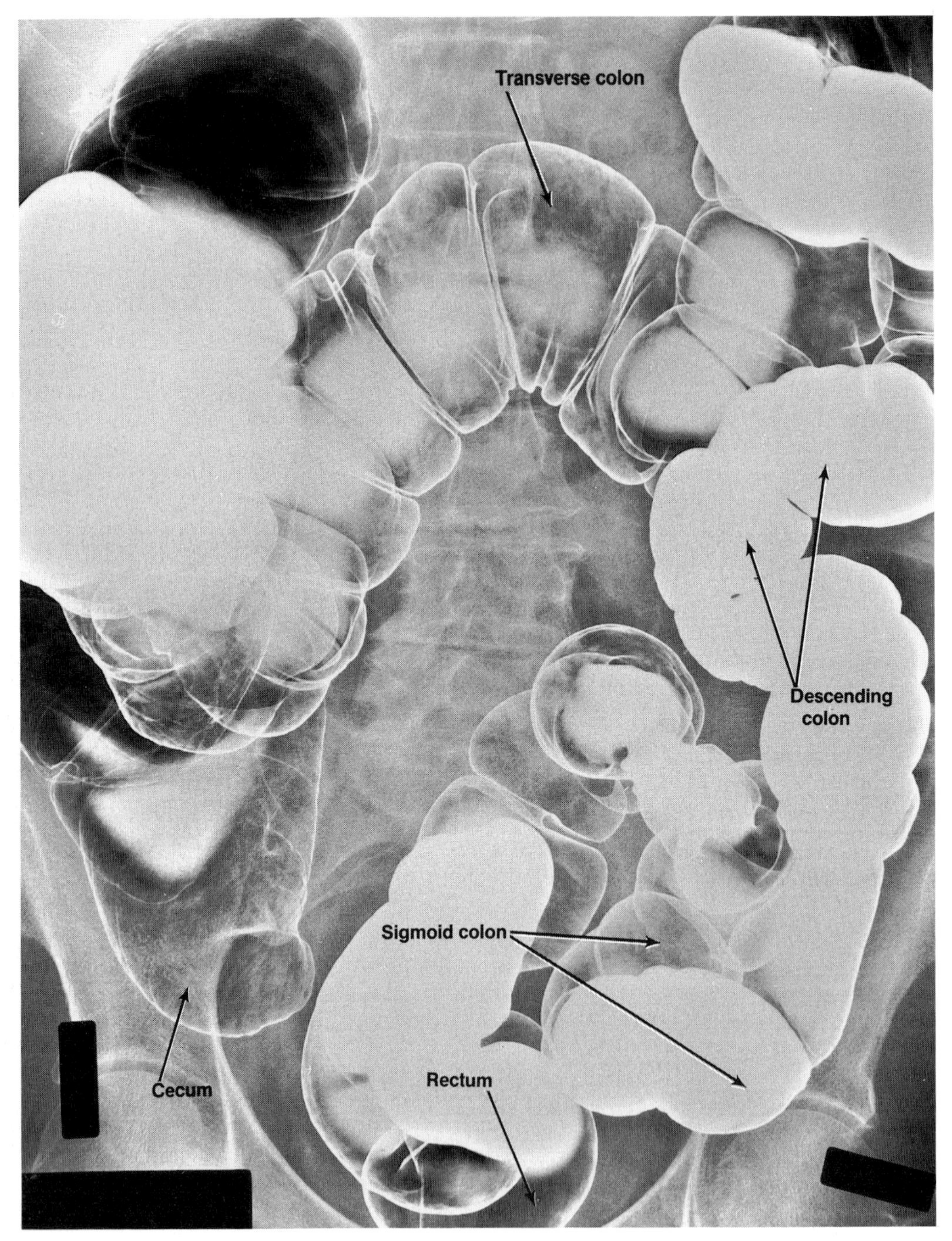

B. AP supine film

bowel. Multiple radiographs, taken with the patient in different positions, provide images of bowel segments both in dependent positions, in which the lumen is filled with contrast material, and in nondependent positions, in which the mucosa is lined by a thin coating of contrast material and distended by air.

Radiograph A was taken with the patient lying prone, a position which tends to pool the contrast suspension in the most mobile and anterior segments of the large bowel. Accordingly, radiograph A shows the cecum, most of the transverse colon, the proximal half of the descending colon, and the

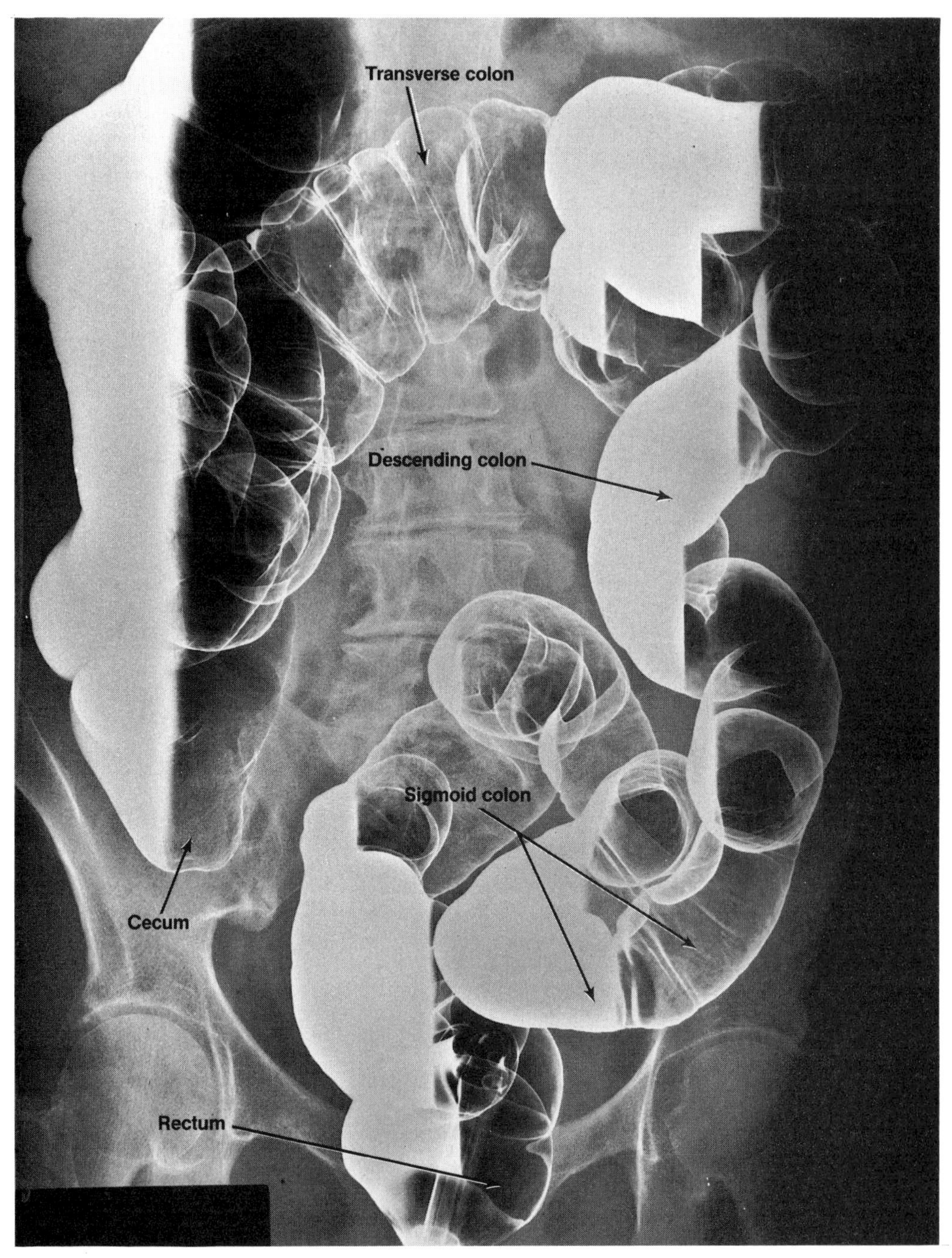

C. Right lateral decubitus film

midregion of the sigmoid colon filled with contrast material; the mucosal lining of much of the ascending colon, the splenic flexure, and the distal half of the descending colon are shown in relief. Radiograph B was taken with the patient lying in the supine position and, accordingly, shows a distribution of contrast material that is largely reversed from that in radiograph A. Radiographs C and D were taken with the patient lying, respectively, in the right and left lateral decubitus positions.

continued on next page

Case 30 discussion *continued*

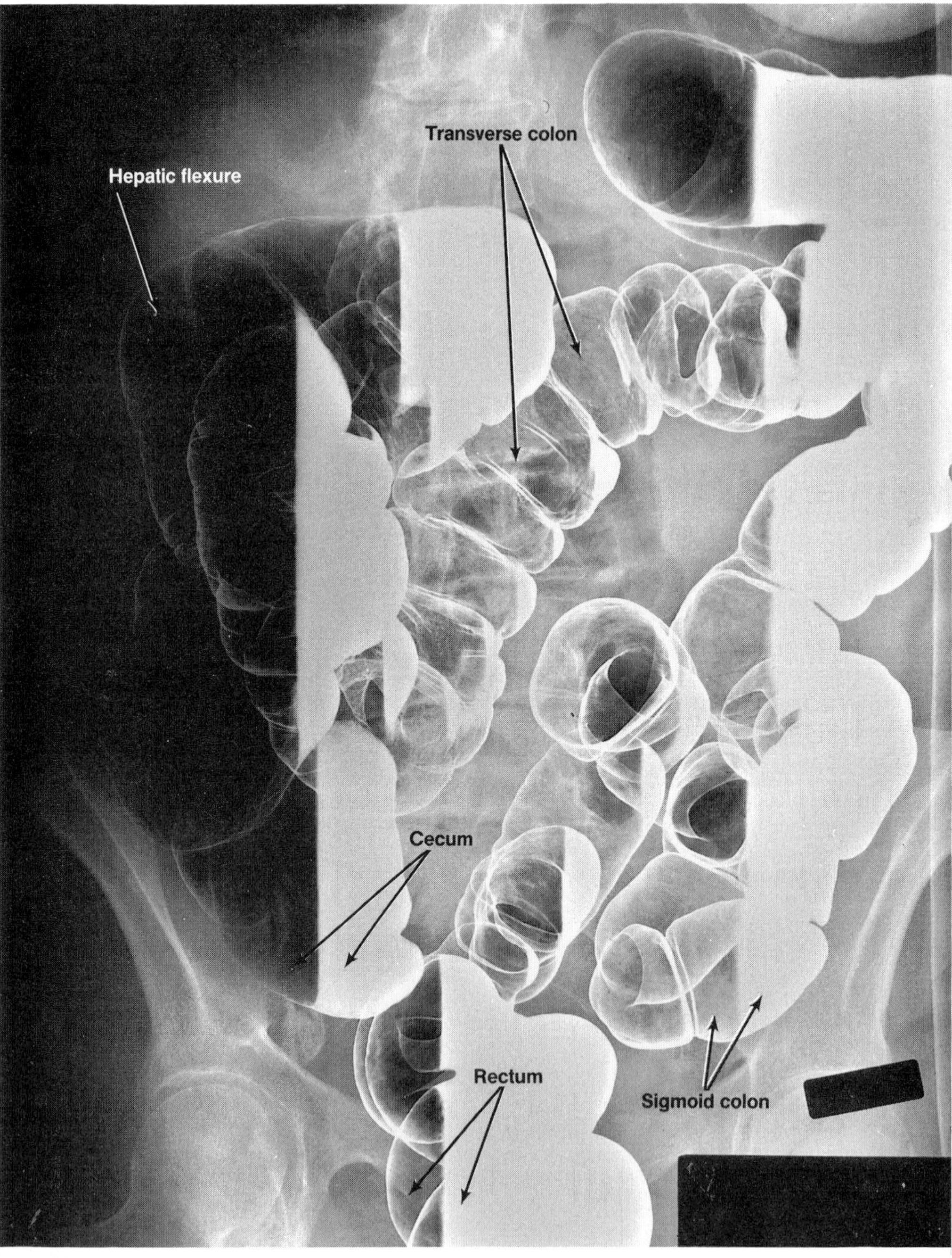

D. Left lateral decubitus film

Case 31

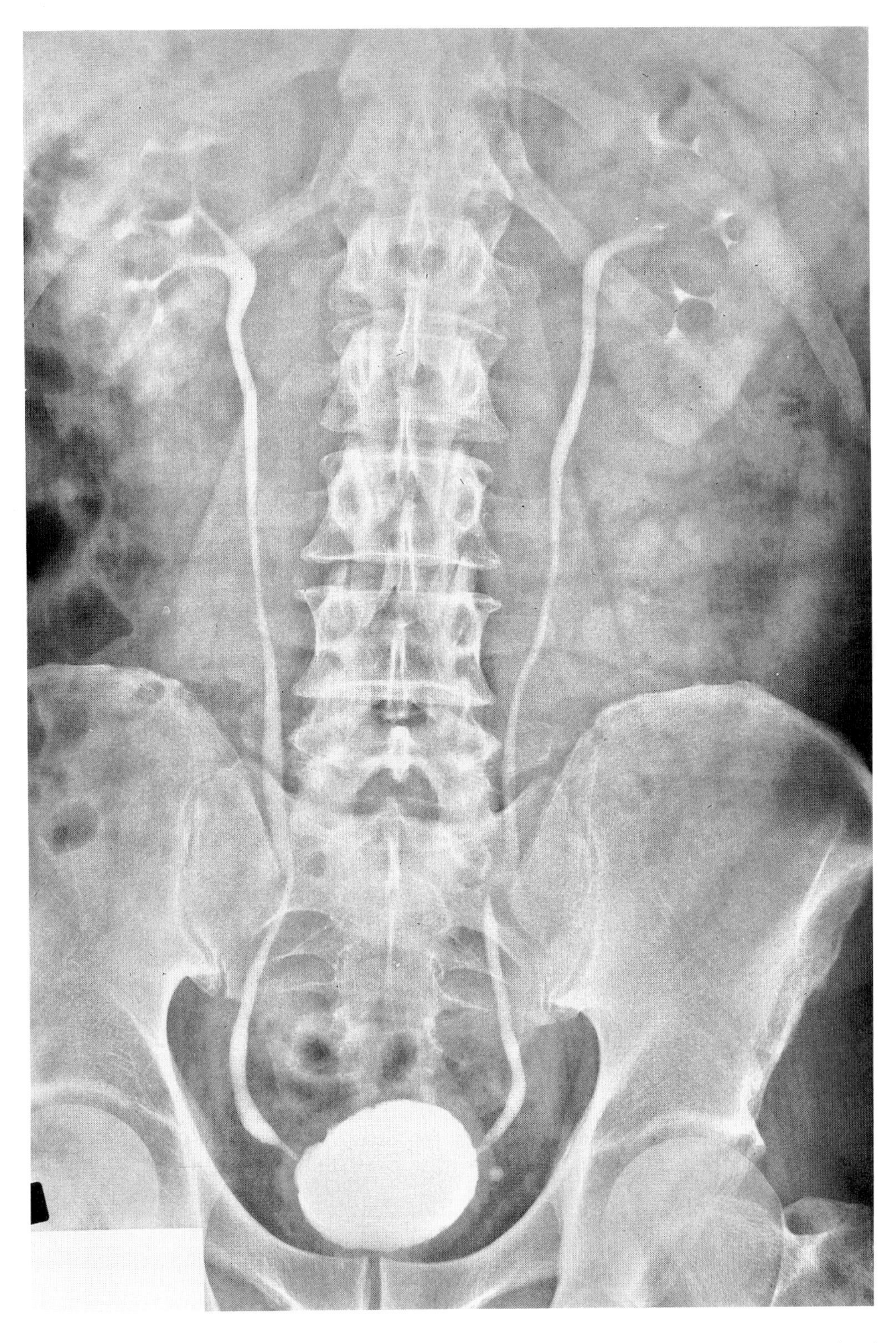

Normal intravenous urogram of a 62-year-old man. Identify the parts of the urinary system visualized with contrast material.

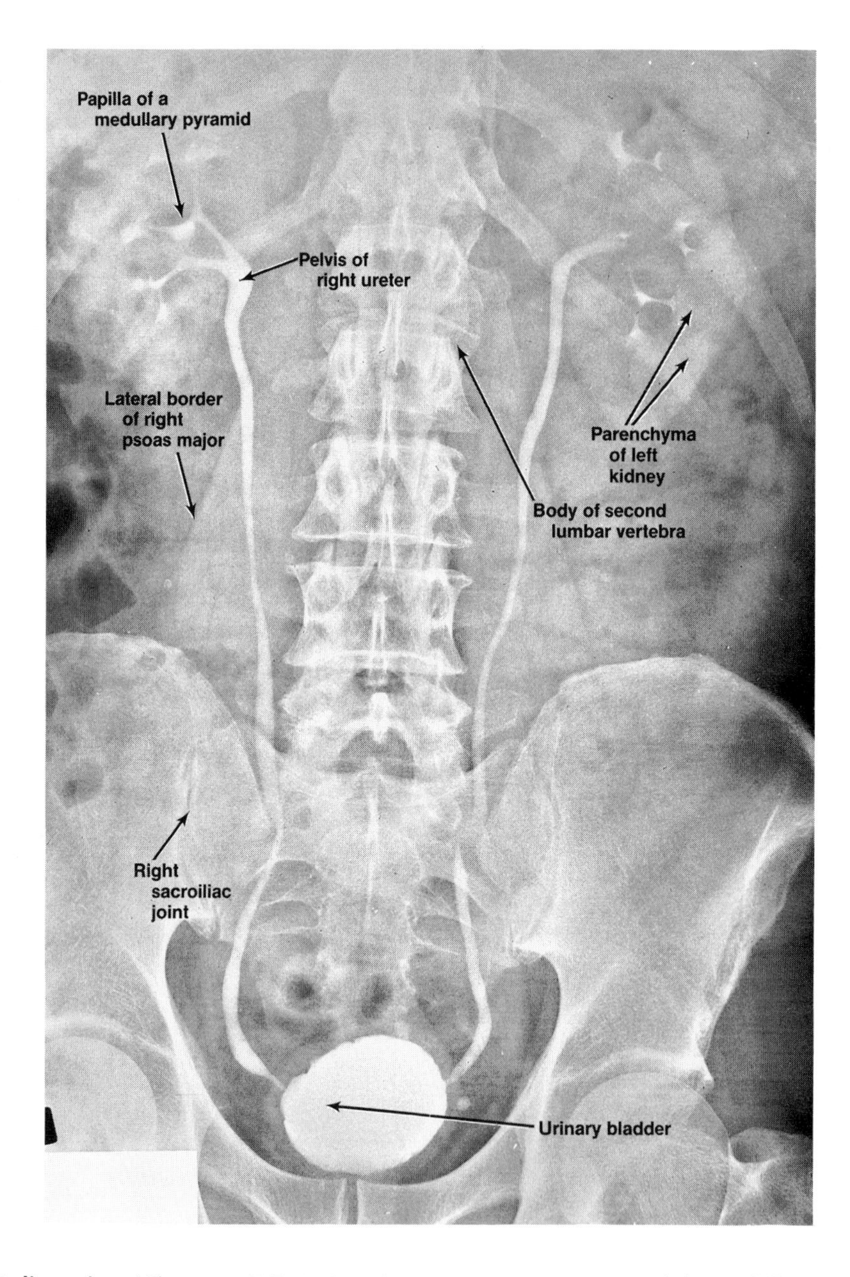

Case 31 discussion. [*Chapter 4 II D 2, 7*] An intravenous urogram is an abdominal film which shows the distribution of contrast material within the urinary system following intravenous injection of a radiopaque substance that is excreted by the kidneys. The urogram depicted was taken after most of the contrast material had already been excreted into the calyces and transported by peristalsis down the ureters into the urinary bladder. Each kidney's parenchyma is still slightly radiodense from residual contrast material; the kidneys can be seen to extend from the level of the eleventh thoracic vertebra to that of the second lumbar vertebra, with the left kidney uncharacteristically lying slightly lower than the right kidney. The thickness of the left kidney's parenchyma and the conical shape of the papilla of some of the right kidney's medullary pyramids are well defined. Each ureter can be seen to descend vertically through the abdominal cavity on the anterior surface of the psoas major muscle, cross the boundary of the pelvic inlet just medial to the sacroiliac joint, and finally descend through the pelvic cavity to the urinary bladder.

Case 32

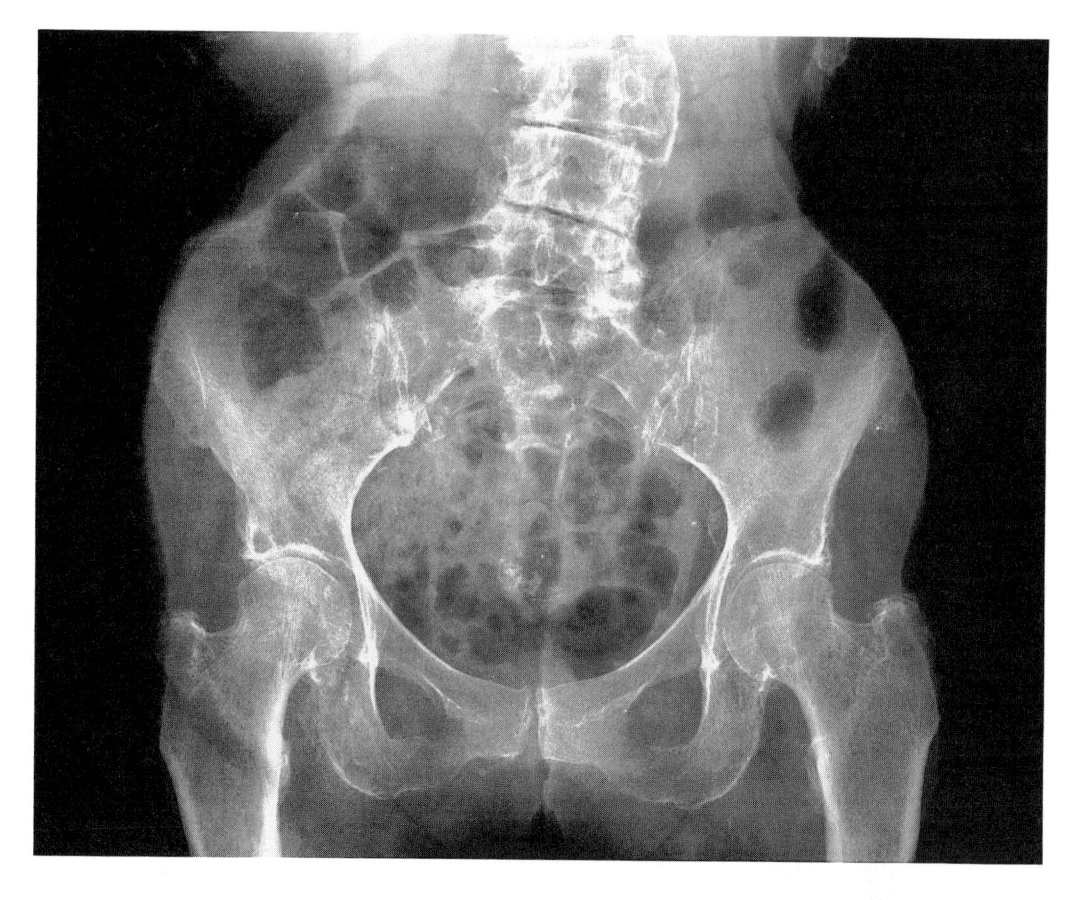

AP radiograph of the pelvis of an 86-year-old woman with low back pain.

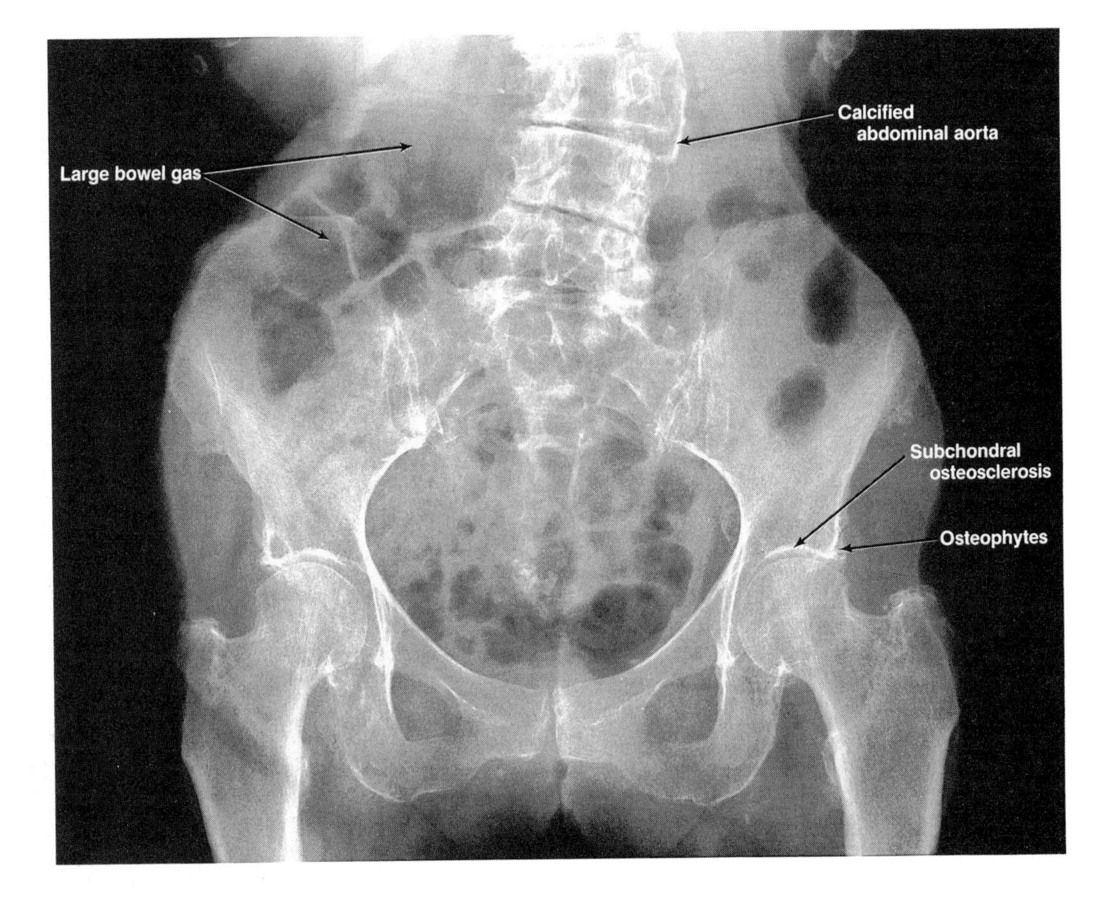

Case 32 discussion. The radiograph shows scoliosis of the lumbar portion of the vertebral column (deviation to the left) and a tortuous calcified abdominal aorta deviated to the left at the level of the third lumbar vertebra. The gas pattern is nonspecific; the large gas bubbles superimposed upon the ileal wing of the right innominate bone are outlined by the distinctive sacculated intraluminal border of the walls of a large bowel segment. As expected from the age of the patient, both hip joints exhibit signs of osteoarthritis; namely, narrowing of the superior joint space, subchondral osteosclerosis in the roof of the acetabular cavity, and osteophytes along the rim of the acetabular cavity.

Case 33

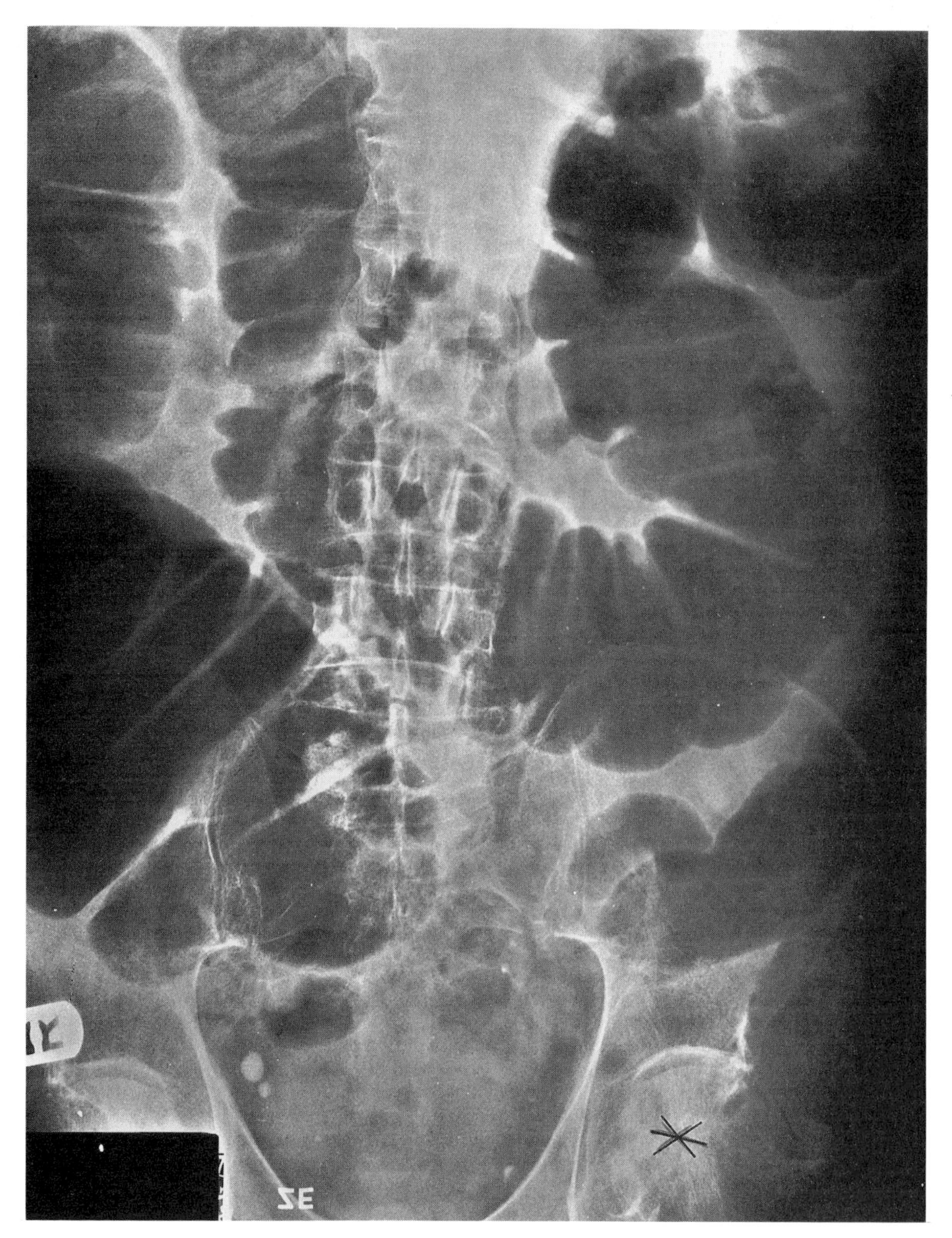

AP supine abdominal radiograph of an 88-year-old man with acute abdominal pain.

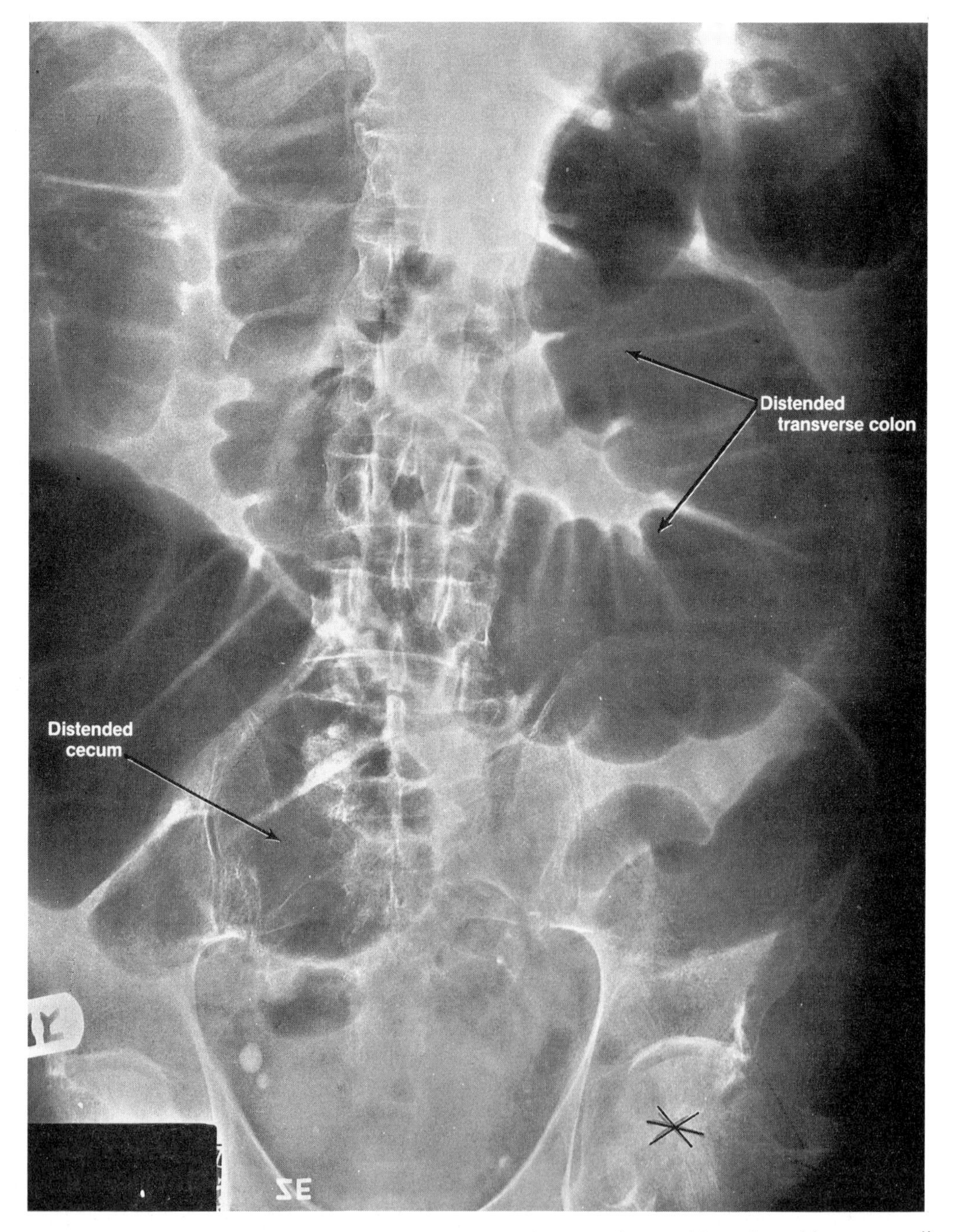

Case 33 discussion. [*Chapter 4 IV B 3*] The radiograph shows evidence of large bowel but not small bowel distension, as all of the distended, gas-filled loops are traversed by the thick, incomplete, water-density bands that represent the semilunar submucosal folds of the large intestine. The large, circularly outlined gas collection in the lower left quadrant of the abdomen marks the distal end of the large bowel distension. The S-shaped distended loop extending across the upper abdomen represents the distended transverse colon. The large gas collection in the lower right quadrant represents the distended cecum. The absence of small bowel distension suggests that the ileocecal valve is competent and functional. In this case, the large bowel distension is due to an incarcerated, indirect inguinal hernia of the sigmoid colon (the asterisk marked on the radiograph indicates the location of the left deep inguinal ring and the neck of the hernia).

Case 34

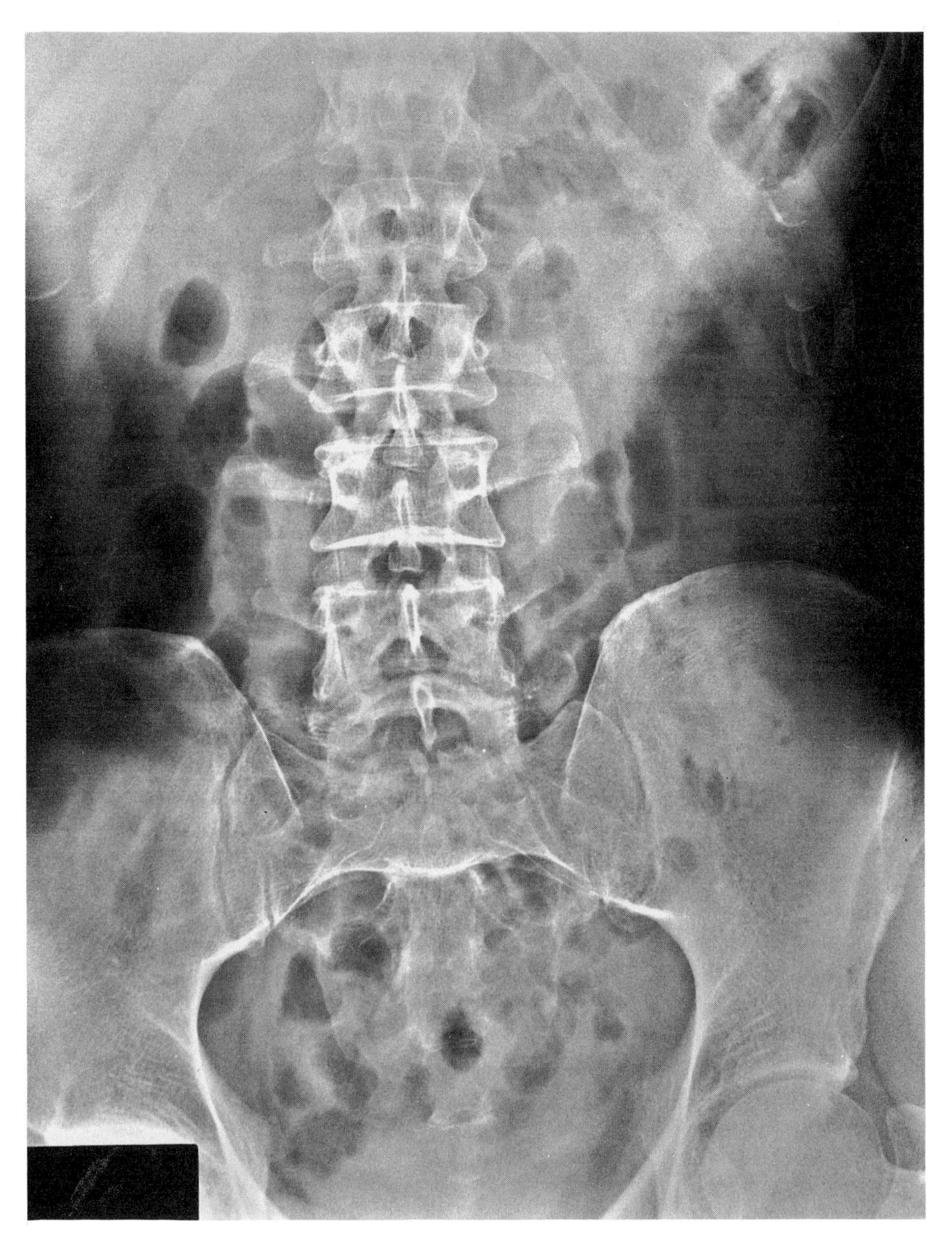

AP supine abdominal radiograph of a 47-year-old man.

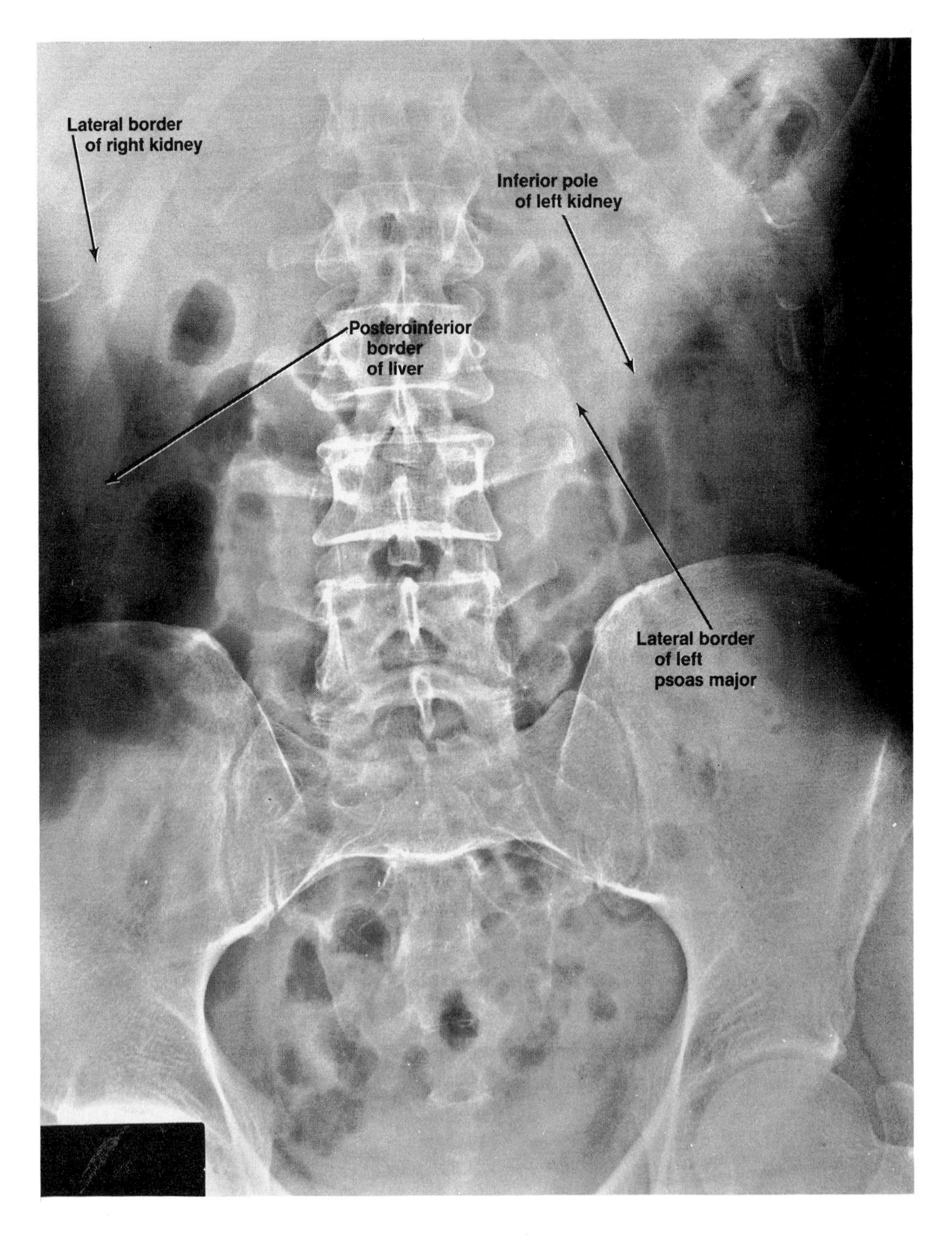

Case 34 discussion. [*Chapter 4 II A, C 2, D*] The radiograph shows a nonspecific gas pattern and no abnormalities. Part of the lateral border of the left psoas major is discernible. The liver's posteroinferior border, the lateral border of the right kidney, and the inferior pole of the left kidney are also discernible.

Index

Note: Page numbers in *italics* denote illustrations; those followed by (t) denote tables; those followed by Q denote questions; and those followed by E denote explanations.

N

O

T

U

V

W

Z